A. Shai

H. I. Maibach

Wound Healing and Ulcers of the Skin

Diagnosis and Therapy –

The Practical Approach

A. Shai

H. I. Maibach

Wound Healing and Ulcers of the Skin

Diagnosis and Therapy –
The Practical Approach

With 115 Figures and 25 Tables

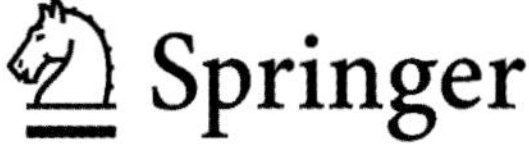 Springer

Dr. Avi Shai
Department of Dermatology
Soroka University Medical Center
Faculty of Health Sciences
Ben-Gurion University of the Negev
Beer-Sheva 84105
Israel

Professor Howard I. Maibach
Department of Dermatology
University of California
San Francisco School of Medicine
Box 0989
San Francisco, CA 94143-0989
USA

Library of Congress Control Number: 2004104389

ISBN 3-540-21275-2 Springer Berlin Heidelberg New York

Springer is a part of Springer Science+Business Media
springeronline.com
© Springer-Verlag Berlin Heidelberg 2005
Printed in Germany

Editor: Marion Philipp
Desk Editor: Irmela Bohn
Production: ProEdit GmbH, 69126 Heidelberg, Germany
Cover: Frido Steinen-Broo, EStudio Calamar, Spain
Typesetting: K. Detzner, 67346 Speyer, Germany

Printed on acid-free paper   21/3150 ML   5 4 3 2 1 0

Preface

In recent years, the amount of knowledge surrounding the processes of wound healing has significantly increased, resulting in a vast array of therapeutic options. The assortment of preparations currently available may become somewhat perplexing to physicians and medical personnel.

We have become aware of the difficulty involved in selecting the most appropriate therapy for a specific type of wound. Our main purpose in writing this book, therefore, is to present a step-by-step algorithmic approach to the treatment of chronic wounds.

The caring of wounds has always been the realm of the various branches of surgery. Dermatology, on the other hand, being the medical science that specializes in skin and cutaneous physiology, deals with the essential and fundamental aspects of wound healing. Due to its very nature, wound healing overlaps into the many disciplines of medicine in general. Internists, diabetologists, and geriatricians are becoming increasingly involved in the field of wound care. General practitioners and family physicians are frequently required to treat acute and chronic wounds.

In this book, we introduce the dermatologic perspective of wound healing which applies to the diagnosis of cutaneous ulcers, based on history, physical examination, biopsy, and laboratory tests. We also present a therapeutic approach to ulcers according to their appearance.

We believe that this guidebook will assist physicians in the treatment of chronic wounds, and that it will ultimately serve to reduce the immense suffering of those afflicted.

■ **Note to the Reader.** Neither the authors nor the publishers are liable for any consequences arising from the use of information presented in this book. The readers are advised to check for up-dated information provided by the manufacturers, including dosage and safety regulations, for each of the products described in this book. Ultimate responsibility rests with the treating physician.

Some of the chapters include lists of commercial names of preparations used in the healing of chronic ulcers. This is by no means intended as a commercial recommendation. It is simply intended to provide the readers with a guide to the range of brand names in use for a certain biologic substance. We have done our best to provide up-dated and accurate lists. However, this area is subject to frequent changes, and the readers are advised to gather information from other currently available sources.

Acknowledgements

The authors wish to thank the following for providing this book with illustrations and pictures: Dr. Emanuela Cagnano for Figs. 12.1 (modified by Inanit Ashtamker as Fig. 1.1), 2.2, 6.1, 6.3, and 6.6; Dr. Oren Lapid for Figs. 12.3 and 12.4; Dr. David Vigoda for Fig. 12.5; Dr. Tidhar Steiner and the Semmelweis Museum of the History of Medicine for Figs. 3.5 and 3.6; Dr. Alex Zvulunov for Fig. 4.2; Dr. Kosta Mumcuoglu for Figs. 9.6–9.8; Professor Sima Halevy for Figs. 14.1–14.7; Audra J. Gera and Novartis for Figs. 2.6 and 3.9, from *Dermatology: A Medical Artist's Interpretation*, copyright 1990 by Sandoz Pharma LTD; The Wellcome Library, London, for Figs. 3.1–3.4, 3.7, and 8.8; Taylor & Francis Publishing House for Fig. 8.6, reprinted from Jacobsson et al: A new principle for the cleansing of infected wounds. *Scandinavian Journal of Plastic & Reconsructive Surgery*, 10:65–72, 1976; Taylor & Francis Publishing House for Fig. 20.2, reproduced from *Handbook of Cosmetic Skin Care*, published by Martin Dunitz, 2001. Figure 18.1 is reprinted from T.J. Ryan: Wound healing and current dermatologic dressings. *Clinics in Dermatology* 8:21–29, copyright 1990, with permission from Elsevier Science; Fig. 2.5 is reprinted from Germain et al: Human wound healing fibroblasts have greater contractile properties than dermal fibroblasts. *Journal of Surgical Research* 57:268–273, copyright 1994, with permission from Elsevier Science; Fig. 18.2 is reprinted from *Dermatologic Therapy in General Practice*, by M. Sulzberger and J. Wolf, (p 116), published by The Year-Book Publishers, copyright 1943, with permission from Elsevier Science; Fig. 6.2 is reprinted from Falanga et al: The cutaneous manifestations of cholesterol crystal embolization, *Archives of Dermatology* 122:1194–1198, copyright 1986, with permission from the American Medical Association; Fig. 4.4 is reprinted from S.W. Graeca et al: A painful precursor for necrosis. *Postgraduate Medicine* 106:249–250, copyright 1999, with permission from Postgraduate Medicine (photographed by Scott Dornbaser). Fig. 6.4 is reprinted from J. Lima-Maribona et al: Self-assessment examination. *The American Academy of Dermatology Journal* 29:803, 1993, with permission from Mosby-Year Book, Inc.; part of Fig. 2.1 is reprinted from CIBA Clinical Symposia on common bleeding disorders, vol 35, no 3, p 8, copyright 1983, with permission from Novartis; part of Fig. 2.1 is taken from *Dermatology: A Medical Artist's Interpretation*, copyright 1990 by Sandoz Pharma LTD.

Many thanks are due to the following for their assistance in the preparation of the text and for their valuable comments: Dr. Gary Zentner; Professor Ilana Harman-Bohem; Professor Pablo Yagupsky; Dr. Batya Davidovici; Dr. Marcelo H. Grunwald; Dr. Dafna Hallel-Halevy; and Dr. Emmilia Hodak. Our particular thanks go to all the reviewers of the chapters in this book for their efforts and assistance (see below); to Professor Sima Halevy, for advancing the field of wound healing in Soroka University Medical Center and for actively supporting the production of this book; to Mrs. Rina Ben-Zeev for her assistance in the preparation of the Appendix section of the book and for constructive collaboration at the Chronic Wound Clinic; to Dr. Alex

Zvulunov and Mr. Naftali Oron for their most valuable ongoing advice stemming from sheer wisdom and clear reason. We would like to especially thank Miss Kristina Hawthorne for contributing her vast experience in the production of books, for her creative ideas, and for her indispensable support and assistance throughout the whole course of this project.

Contents

List of Reviewers

Natural Course of Wound Repair versus Impaired Healing in Chronic Cutaneous Ulcers

Theodora Mauro, MD
Associate Professor in Residence and Vice-Chairman
Department of Dermatology
University of California, San Francisco
Service Chief, Dermatology
San Francisco Veteran's Hospital
San Francisco, California
USA

Milestones in the History of Wound Healing

David T. Rovee, PhD
Cambridge, MA
USA

Etiology and Mechanisms of Cutaneous Ulcer Formation

Jürg Hafner, MD, PD
Dermatology, Vascular Medicine, Phlebology, Dermatologic Surgery
Senior Staff Member
Department of Dermatology
University Hospital of Zürich
Zürich
Switzerland

Determining Etiology: History and Physical Examination

Irwin M. Braverman, MD
Professor of Dermatology
Department of Dermatology
Yale Medical School
New Haven, CT
USA

Determining Etiology: Biopsy and Laboratory Investigation

Robert S. Kirsner, MD
Department of Dermatology and Cutaneous Surgery
Department of Epidemiology and Public Health
University of Miami School of Medicine
Veterans Administration Medical Center
Miami, Florida
USA

Ulcer Measurement and Patient Assessment
Marco Romanelli, MD, PhD
Consultant Dermatologist
Department of Dermatology
University of Pisa
Pisa
Italy

Dressing Materials
Marketa Limova, MD
Associate Clinical Professor
Wound and Ulcer Clinic
University of California, San Francisco
San Francisco, CA
USA

Debridement
William H. Eaglstein, MD
Harvey Blank Professor
Department of Dermatology and Cutaneous Surgery
University of Miami School of Medicine
Miami, FL
USA

Antibiotics, Antiseptics and Cutaneous Ulcers
Keith G. Harding, MD MB ChB MRCGP FRCS
Professor of Rehabilitation Medicine (Wound Healing)
Head of Department of Surgery
Wound Healing Research Unit
University of Wales College of Medicine
Cardiff
UK

Topical Antibacterial Agents
Raza Aly, PhD
Professor of Dermatology and Microbiology
Department of Dermatology
University of California
San Francisco, CA
USA

Skin Grafting
I. Kelman Cohen, MD
Emeritus Professor
Plastic and Reconstructive Surgery
Virginia Commonwealth University
Health Science Center
Richmond, Virginia
USA

Skin Substitutes and Tissue-Engineered Skin Equivalents

Tania J. Phillips, MD FRCPC
Professor of Dermatology
Boston University School of Medicine
Department of Dermatology
Boston, MA
USA

Growth Factors

Martin C. Robson, MD
Emeritus Professor of Surgery
Department of Surgery
University of South Florida, Tampa
Florida
USA

Drugs, Wound Healing and Cutaneous Ulcers

Sima Halevy, MD
Professor of Dermatology
Ben-Gurion University
Chairman, Department of Dermatology
Soroka University Medical Center
Beer Sheva
Israel

Nutrition and Cutaneous Ulcers

Nancy Collins, PhD, RD, LD/N
Nutrition Guidance Center
Pembroke Pines
Florida
USA

Basic Definitions and Introduction

> The treatment of leg ulcers is generally looked upon as an inferior branch of practice, an unpleasant and unglorious task where much labor must be bestowed, and little honor gained.
>
> *(Edinb Med Surg*, 1805)

Contents

1.1 Definitions

Dorland's Medical Dictionary defines 'wound' as "a disruption in the normal continuity of a body structure". The term 'wound', as found in dictionaries and in the commonly accepted terminology, usually relates to an acute injury or an acute mechanical trauma, such as a gunshot wound, a stab wound, etc.

The accepted definition of 'chronic wound' relates to any wound that fails to heal within a reasonable period. There is no clear-cut definition that points to the chronicity of a wound. However, most physicians would agree that a wound that fails to heal within 3–4 months may be regarded as chronic. The estimated time for healing is not arbitrary but depends on factors such as the size of the wound, its cause, and the patient's general clinical status.

In dermatology, the preferred term for 'chronic wound' is 'chronic cutaneous ulcer'. An ulcer, in turn, is defined as a depressed lesion in which the epidermis and at least the upper dermis have been destroyed [1] (Figs. 1.1, 1.2). An 'erosion', on the other hand, is a focal loss of the epidermis without involvement of the dermis (Fig. 1.3).

Note that a cutaneous ulcer is not a primary lesion. An ulcer does not develop *de novo*, from

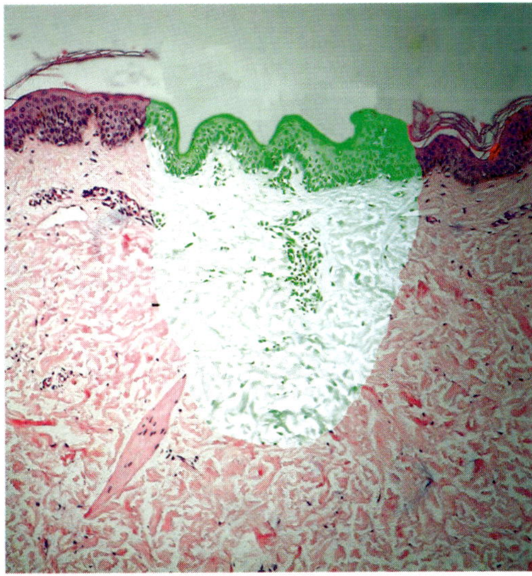

Fig. 1.1. Schematic illustration of an ulcer. There is involvement of the epidermis and at least part of the dermis

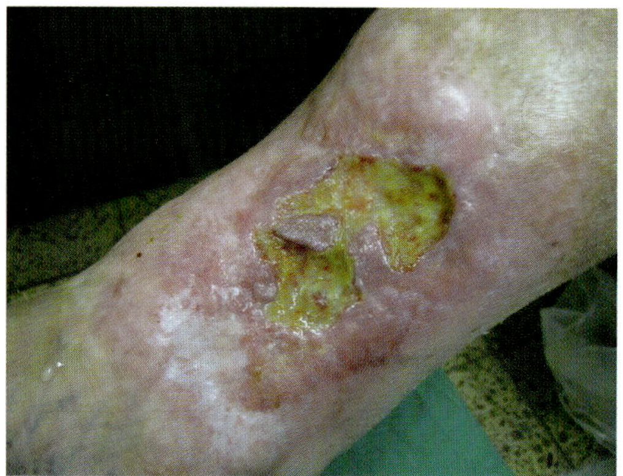

Fig. 1.2. A cutaneous ulcer. Note that the destruction extends deeper into the epidermis

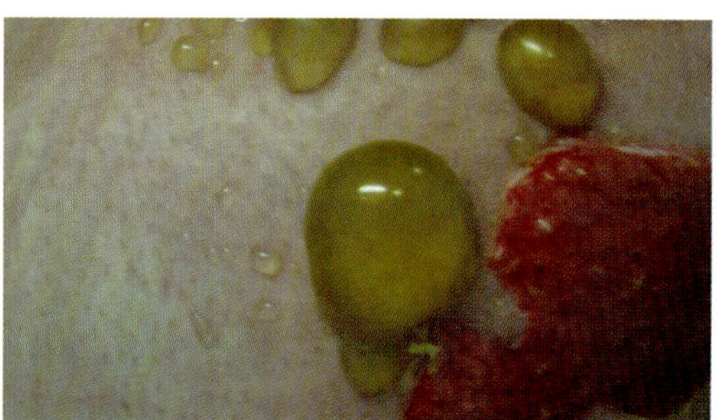

Fig. 1.3. An erosion that developed following blister rupture

intact normal skin. It is preceded by another initial pathologic lesion, such as a papule or a pustule, from which the ulcer evolves.

1.2 Three Aspects of Treatment in Wounds and Ulcers

In recent years, accumulating knowledge regarding wound healing processes has led to the development of numerous therapies. A bewildering plethora of novel topical preparations, dressing materials, and advanced methods of debridement are now at the hands of physicians and medical personnel. In many cases, even those who specialize in the field of wound healing, such as dermatologists or plastic surgeons, may find it difficult to choose the most appropriate treatment.

This book places this flood of information and the many modes of therapy currently suggested into some order and offers a reasonable approach to the treatment of cutaneous ulcers. The following chapters put forward a practical and algorithmic therapeutic approach, according to specific features of the ulcer.

As a rule, the treatment of a cutaneous ulcer is determined by three aspects:
- Etiology
- Clinical appearance of the ulcer
- Adjuvant therapy

1.2.1 Etiology

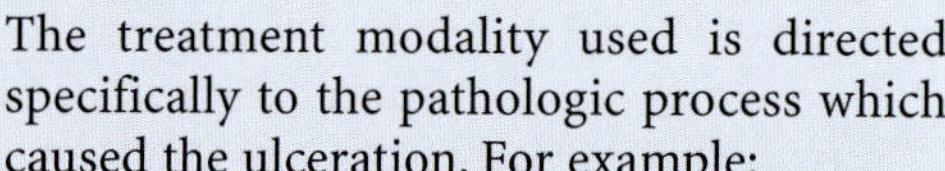

The treatment modality used is directed specifically to the pathologic process which caused the ulceration. For example:
- Glucocorticoid therapy should be considered when the ulcer is attributed to a vasculitic process or to a certain connective tissue disease. It is often advisable for pyoderma gangrenosum. However, since glucocorticoids have an inhibitory effect on wound-healing processes, their use is not desirable for other kinds of cutaneous ulcers.
- In an ulceration diagnosed as caused by leishmaniasis, one may consider applying a topical preparation containing parmomycin. In cases of unresponsive or destructive ulceration, intravenous pentostam may be considered.
- Splenectomy may be considered for recalcitrant ulcerations due to hereditary spherocytosis.

Due to the vast array of diseases and pathologic processes characterized by the appearance of cutaneous ulcers, a comprehensive dermatology textbook would be needed to fully cover each issue. In this book we limit the discussion to the appropriate identification of an ulcer's cause based on clinical features, histology, and laboratory tests (see Chaps. 5 and 6). A structured diagnostic process is suggested as an algorithmic approach.

1.2.2 Clinical Appearance of the Ulcer

The currently accepted classification of cutaneous ulcers is based on their clinical appearance [2–9]. A practical distinction is made between 'yellow', 'black', and 'red' ulcers. In most cases, the topical therapeutic method to be used depends on the ulcer's clinical appearance.

In Chap. 20, a flow chart is presented for the treatment of cutaneous ulcers, when the ulcer's clinical appearance is the major determinant regarding choice of topical treatment.

For the time being, there is no evidence that a certain dressing type or a certain method of debridement is more beneficial for a cutaneous ulcer of specific etiology (e.g., venous ulcers or diabetic ulcers).

1.2.3 Adjuvant Therapy

Modalities of adjuvant therapy are those intended to improve a patient's general condition, thereby providing wounds with better healing conditions.

Improvement of a patient's nutritional status and supplementation of certain nutritional ingredients, as described in Chap. 19, is applicable here. The treatment of a patient's other medical problems that can increase the severity of the ulcer can be included in this category. For example, treatment of congestive heart failure can reduce edema in the lower limbs, allowing enhanced healing of leg ulcers.

Similarly, hyperbaric-oxygen therapy can be regarded as another mode of adjuvant therapy that may have a beneficial effect on the healing of a large spectrum of cutaneous ulcers. It should always be considered in cases of difficult-to-heal cutaneous ulcers, in which ischemia is involved in the pathogenesis.

1.3 Ulcer Depth

A further classification of ulcers refers to their depth. Definitions of ulcer staging, based on depth and severity, were originally used for pressure ulcers (Figs. 1.4–1.7). The staging

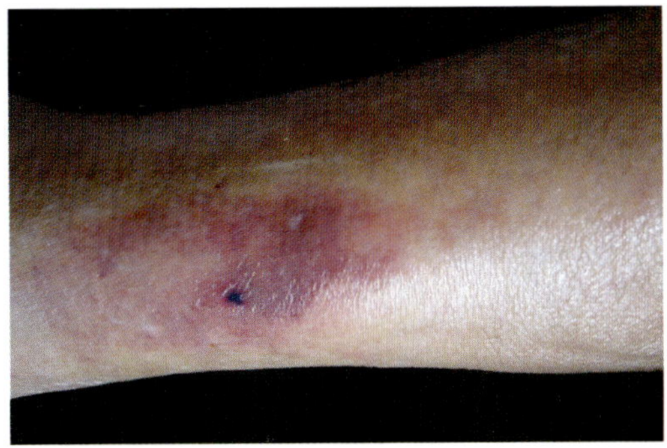

Fig. 1.4. A stage-I pressure ulcer

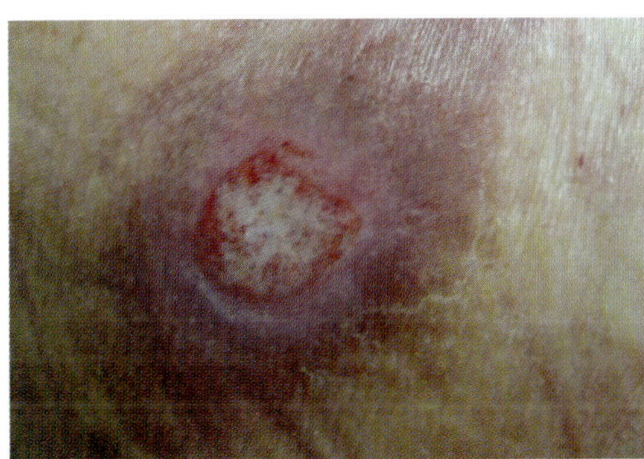

Fig. 1.5. A stage-II pressure ulcer

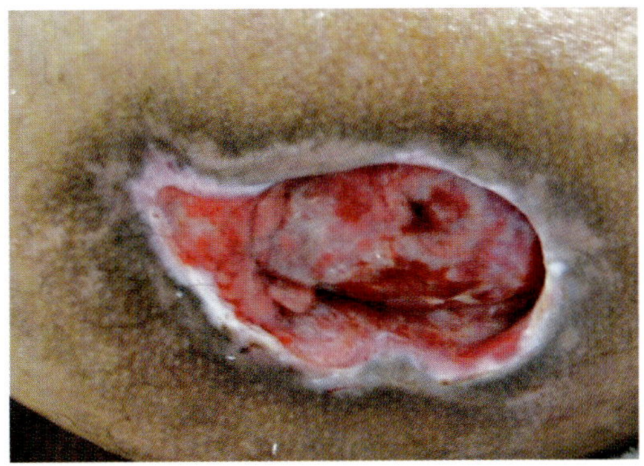

Fig. 1.6. A stage-III pressure ulcer

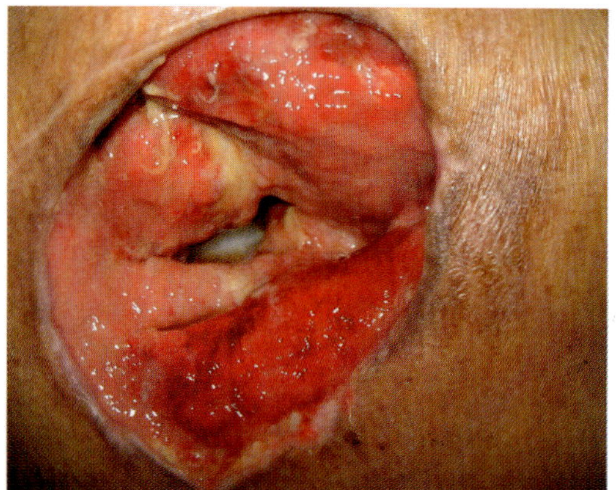

Fig. 1.7. A stage-IV pressure ulcer. Note that the bone is exposed

system was developed with the objective of creating better communication between medical personnel. Obviously, these definitions can be implemented for any other sorts of cutaneous ulcers as well.

A commonly accepted system was developed in 1987 in the USA by The National Pressure Ulcer Advisory Panel (NPUAP) [10], as follows:

- Stage I: Blanchable erythema of intact skin
- Stage II: Partial-thickness skin loss involving the epidermis and dermis, presenting clinically as an abrasion
- Stage III: Full-thickness skin loss, including the subcutaneous layer with extension down to (but not through) the underlying fascia
- Stage IV: Full-thickness skin loss with involvement of muscle, bone, or other deep structures such as tendons or joint capsules

1.4 Comments on Current Treatments

Accepted modes of treatment are discussed in various chapters of this book, including dressing materials, methods of debridement, biological dressings and skin substitutes, and growth factors. Other therapeutic measures have not been sufficiently established, thus they cannot be recommended as evidence-based methods in the treatment of cutaneous ulcers for the time being. These are mainly physical therapeutic modalities such as infrared light, low-energy laser irradiation, ultrasonography, and electrical stimulation. These modalities are not discussed in this book.

As a rule, it is difficult to accurately determine the efficacy of various treatments for cutaneous ulcers on the basis of current data. Researchers have indicated that in some studies, basic information such as history of previous ulceration, ulcer duration, or its appearance, has not been provided [11, 12]. Similarly, other studies have included too small a sample of patients or have not been controlled. Nevertheless, some idea of the efficacy of current treatments may be obtained, allowing a treatment approach to be suggested, as presented in subsequent chapters.

References

1. Stewart MI, Bernhard JD, Cropley, Fitzpatrick TB: The structure of skin lesions and fundamentals of diagnosis. In: Freedberg IM, Eisen AZ, Wolff K, Austen KF, Goldsmith LA, Katz SI (eds) Fitzpatrick's Dermatology in General Medicine, 6th edn. New York: McGraw-Hill. 2003; pp 11–30
2. Hellgren L, Vincent J: Debridement: an essential step in wound healing. In: Westerhof W (ed) Leg Ulcers: Diagnosis and Treatment. Amsterdam: Elsevier. 1993; pp 305–312
3. Hellgren L, Vincent J: A classification of dressings and preparations for the treatment of wounds by second intention based on stages in the healing process. Care Sci Pract 1986; 4:13–17
4. Stotts NA: Seeing red and yellow and black. The three-color concept of wound care. Nursing 1990; 20:59–61
5. Eriksson G: Local treatment of venous leg ulcers. Acta Chir Scand [Suppl] 1988; 544:47–52
6. Lorentzen HF, Holstein P, Gottrup F: Interobserver variation in the red-yellow-black wound classification system. Ugeskr Laeger 1999; 161:6045–6048.
7. Goldman RJ, Salcido R: More than one way to measure a wound: An overview of tools and techniques. Adv Skin Wound Care 2002; 15:236–243
8. Findlay D: Modern dressings: what to use. Aust Fam Phys 1994; 23:824–839
9. Romanelli M, Gaggio G, Piaggesi A, et al: Technological advances in wound bed measurements. Wounds 2002; 14:58–66

10. Pressure ulcer prevalence, cost and risk assessment: consensus development conference statement. The National Pressure Ulcer Advisory Panel. Decubitus 1989; 2:24–28

11. Nelson EA, Bradley MD: Dressing and topical agents for arterial leg ulcers (Cochrane Review). In: The Cochrane Library, issue 1, 2003. Oxford: Update Software

12. Stephens P, Wall IB, Wilson MJ, et al: Anaerobic cocci populating the deep tissues of chronic wounds impair cellular wound healing responses *in vitro*. Br J Dermatol 2003; 148:456–466

Natural Course of Wound Repair
Versus Impaired Healing
in Chronic Skin Ulcers

2

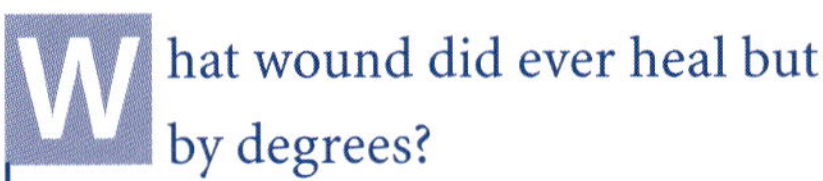

What wound did ever heal but by degrees?

(William Shakespeare, Othello II: iii, 379)

Contents

2.1 Overview

Wound healing is a complex alignment of various dynamic processes which are not yet fully understood. The natural processes that occur during normal wound healing, including the various aspects of molecular and cellular events, will be briefly discussed in this chapter, the aim of which is to describe the practical basis for treating acute and chronic cutaneous ulcers.

It is recommended that whoever is interested in a wider view of the basic scientific aspects of this matter consult *Cutaneous Wound Healing*, edited by Vincent Falanga (Martin Dunitz); *The Molecular and Cellular Biology of Wound Repair*, edited by R.A.F. Clark (Plenum Press); and *The Epidermis in Wound Healing* by David T. Rovee and Howard I. Maibach (CRC Press).

In its usual schematic presentation, the course of normal wound healing is divided into three phases (Fig. 2.1):
- Inflammation phase
  (also called 'lag phase')
- Tissue formation phase
  ('proliferative phase')
- Tissue remodeling phase

Note that this traditional division is somewhat arbitrary and these phases partially overlap. For example, processes of tissue formation begin while active events of the inflammation phase are still occurring.

Wound healing is regulated and synchronized by a unique group of cytokines, known as growth factors, secreted from thrombocytes,

Fig. 2.1.
The three phases
of wound healing

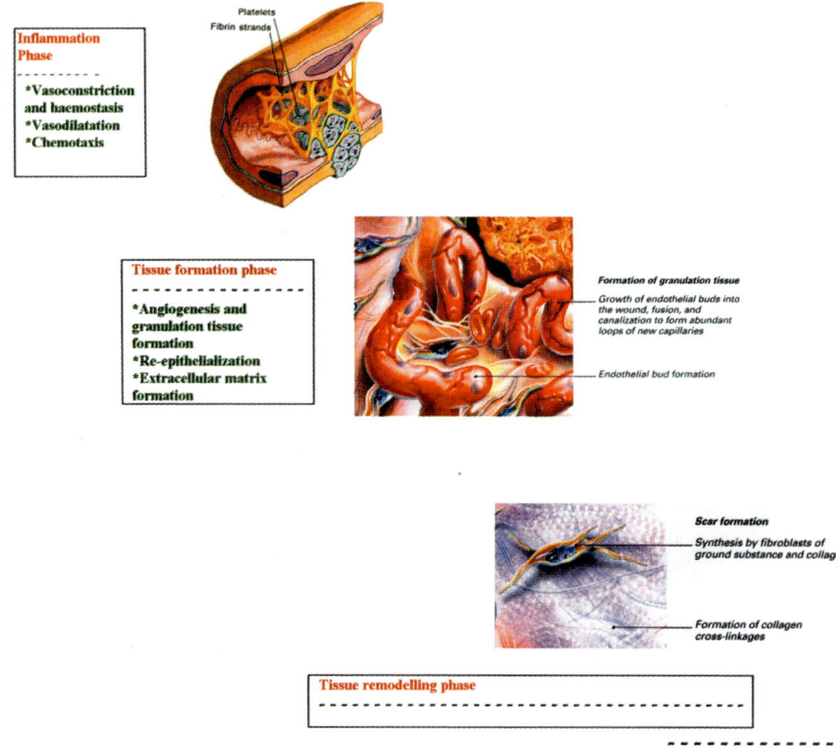

macrophages, neutrophils, lymphocytes, endothelial cells, and fibroblasts [1–7]. Many cytokines have been identified as having a certain role in the processes of wound healing, such as platelet-derived growth factor (PDGF), fibroblast-derived growth factor (FGF), epidermal growth factor (EGF), tumor necrosis factor (TNF), granulocyte-macrophage colony-stimulating factor (GM-CSF), insulin-like growth factor (IGF), and transforming growth factors (TGF) α and β.

Growth factors induce proliferation of certain cell lines, including fibroblasts, endothelial cells, and epithelial cells with subsequent tissue formation. Growth factors also induce processes such as chemotaxis of white cells, wound contraction, and extracellular matrix deposition.

The three phases mentioned above will be briefly summarized here. The practical approach to the management of a chronic cutaneous ulcer, or of a surgical wound, requires a broad understanding of the physiological events described below.

2.2 Inflammation Phase

In the normal course of wound repair, the inflammation phase usually lasts about 4–6 days. The main processes that take place during this phase are described below.

2.2.1 Vasoconstriction and Hemostasis

The initial events of the inflammation phase begin immediately after the wounding: The injured blood and lymphatic vessels undergo rapid vasoconstriction that lasts a few minutes [8]. Thrombocytes aggregate along the endothelium of injured vessels. The wounding process also activates a cascade of coagulation. Eventually, fibrinogen is cleaved to fibrin monomers with the subsequent formation of a hemostatic clot. Thrombocyte aggregation and clot formation prevent leakage of blood from the injured vessels.

The forming clot is composed of a matrix of fibrin, together with small amounts of fibronectin, vitronectin, and thrombospondin [1], in which platelets and various blood cells are embedded.

Later on, a process of fibrinolysis takes place, in which plasmin dissolves the fibrin clot. As discussed below, in more advanced phases of wound repair, newly forming granulation tissue gradually replaces the fibrin clot within the wound defect. In the final stages, healing is completed by the formation of scar tissue.

2.2.2 Vasodilatation and Increased Permeability

Certain chemicals such as prostaglandins released from injured tissue and histamine secreted by mast cells induce vascular dilatation with increased capillary permeability [8,9]. Leaking of plasma through the permeable vessels into surrounding tissue causes the site of the injury to become swollen. Due to the secretion of various chemical substances, the area may show other typical signs of inflammation such as redness, local warmth, and pain. Vasodilatation lasts approximately one hour.

2.2.3 Chemotactic Growth Factors and Phagocytosis

During the initial stages of the inflammation phase, thrombocytes initiate a complex chain of events by secreting growth factors, leading to an influx of white blood cells through the capillary pores to the wound site. This commences just minutes after wounding. A few hours after wounding, neutrophils are seen within the site of injury; their number reaching a peak 1 or 2 days thereafter. If there is no infection, they gradually start to drop in number from the sec-

ond day after wounding. Within the following 3–4 days their number is significantly reduced [10, 11]. Together with the appearance of neutrophils, macrophages transformed from circulating monocytes accumulate. The increase is relatively slower; they reach a maximum number after 4–5 days and become the most significant cells in the phagocytic processes. Lymphocytes reach their maximal number approximately six days after the wound occurs. White blood cells and tissue macrophages act against pathogenic organisms, debride necrotic tissue, and secrete various other growth factors that further activate the wound-healing processes [12–14].

2.3 Tissue Formation Phase

The tissue formation phase includes the most prominent events of wound healing. It begins about 4–5 days after wounding and lasts for a few weeks thereafter in the case of a normal, 'healthy' healing process.

The main processes that take place during this phase are angiogenesis and granulation tissue formation, re-epithelialization, and extracellular matrix formation. All these processes are detailed below (see also Fig. 3.9).

2.3.1 Angiogenesis and Granulation Tissue Formation

Release of growth factors induces migration and proliferation of endothelial cells [12, 13]. Endothelial proliferation results in **angiogenesis**, i.e., the formation of new blood vessels. The new capillaries that are formed branch out and invade the fibrin matrix within the wound site, thereby forming a complex and branched vascular network. This vascular alignment is clinically manifested as the new **granulation tissue** covering the ulcer surface area during the normal healing process.

Granulation tissue consists of immature collagen (type III) and ground substance, in which white blood cells, fibroblasts, and young endothelial cells are embedded [12]. The term 'granulation' is derived from the general appearance of the tissue – upon close inspection, the tissue seems to contain numerous tiny granules, which are actually young blood vessels (Figs. 2.2, 2.3).

The transforming growth factor-β (TGF-β) superfamily encompasses a large number of different cytokines which mediate various physiologic processes. Cytokines of the TGF-β superfamily seem to play a significant role in wound healing, and especially in the process of granulation tissue formation. TGF-β enhances angiogenesis, proliferation of fibroblasts, and differentiation of myofibroblasts, and induces extracellular matrix deposition [15, 16]. The angiogenetic activity of TGF-β is influenced by its concentration and the presence (and amount) of other growth factors in the wound area.

Leptin, a protein produced primarily in the adipose tissue, is involved in processes of wound healing. Leptin regulates various metabolic and endocrine functions. In addition, it acts as an angiogenic factor and induces proliferation of endothelial cells. Its activity seems to be regulated by hypoxia [15, 17, 18]. These findings may support earlier observations indicating that the hypoxic environment induced by hydrocolloid dressing may stimulate angiogenesis [19, 20].

2.3.2 Extracellular Matrix Formation

Two or three days after wounding, fibroblasts migrate and appear in the wound bed. They proliferate, and after a few days, an active synthesis of collagen takes place [1, 21]. Initially, the collagen produced is type III collagen. Deposition of collagen is the initial process that creates some sort of structural alignment that gradually enables skin integrity to be restored.

The proliferation of fibroblasts results in the formation of an extracellular matrix of the granulation tissue (Figs. 2.4). Apart from collagen, fibroblasts also produce substances such as proteoglycans and glycosaminoglycans.

The migration of fibroblasts is dependent on the normal functioning of peripheral innervation in the wounded area with adequate secretion of nerve growth factor [22–24].

Note that the synthesis of collagen requires hydroxylation of proline and lysine residues. Certain cofactors such as oxygen, iron, or vitamin C are needed for collagen synthesis. A defi-

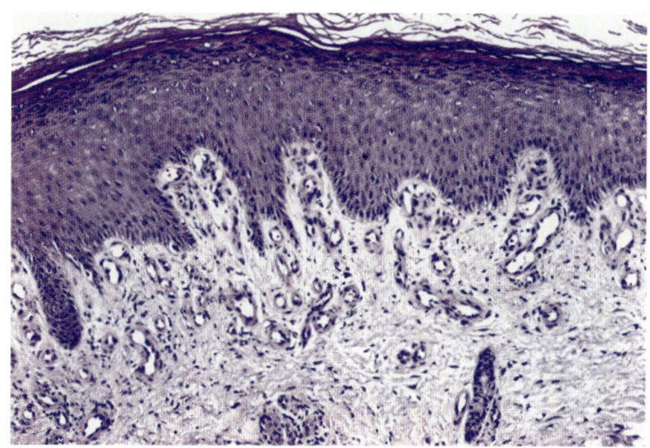

Fig. 2.2. Granulation tissue; histologic view. Note numerous vertical blood vessels in the upper dermis and proliferation of fibroblasts

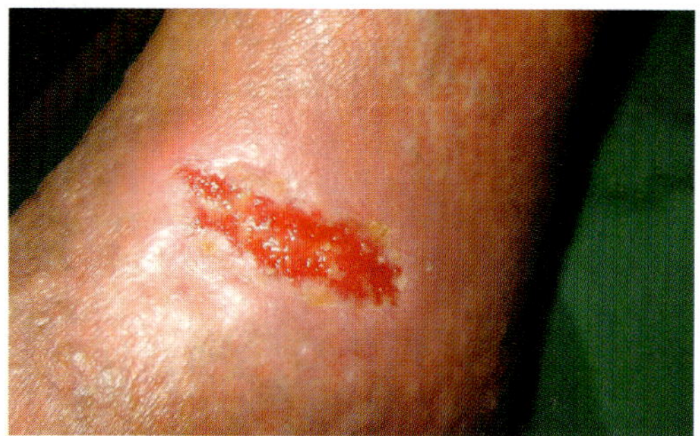

Fig. 2.3. A clean red wound covered by healthy granulation tissue

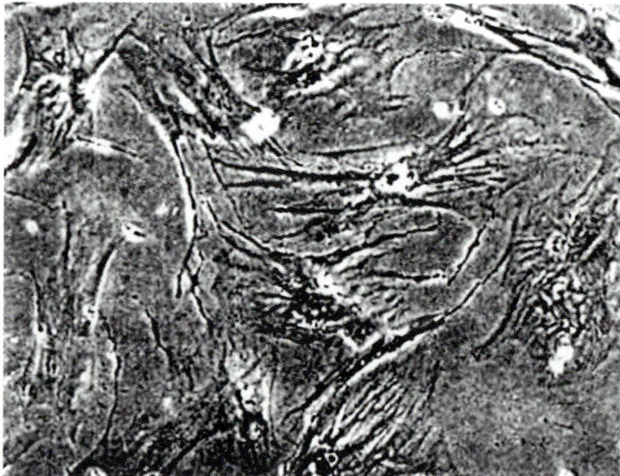

Fig. 2.4. Phase-contrast micrographs of human fibroblasts cultured from wound healing tissue

ciency of one of these cofactors may result in impaired healing [8].

As previously mentioned, TGF-β induces extracellular matrix deposition. In addition, recent studies have indicated the main role of activins, i.e., members of the TGF-β superfamily, in various processes of wound healing. Animal studies suggest that activins may affect dermal components with the induction of matrix formation and dermal fibrosis [15, 25].

2.3.3 Re-epithelialization

Re-epithelialization is achieved by migration, proliferation, and differentiation of epidermal keratinocytes. The overall purpose is complete ulcer healing, when the whole ulcer surface area is covered by a layer of epithelium.

Note that in most cases, epithelial cells tend to behave as stationary cells. Yet, they may become migratory cells under certain unique conditions: embryonic development, the normal course of wound healing, and malignancy [26, 27].

■ **Migration.** Initial re-epithelialization of a cutaneous wound is discerned several hours after wounding, when a gradual flattening and pseudopodium-like projections are seen in epidermal cells adjacent to the wound margin. Within 24 h, epidermal cells detach themselves from the basal lamina to which they are attached. The movement, or migration, of epidermal cells is seen from the margins of the wound towards the wound matrix [13]. This type of movement is obtained by contraction and reinsertion of intracellular filaments of actinomyosin [28]. The ameboid motion of each cell is in the form of a unique pattern called **lamellopodial crawling.** The advancing epithelialization also combines movement of cells in groups or sheets, with sliding over other epidermal cells [29,30]. Under optimal conditions, a single cell does not advance more than two or three cell diameters from its original, initial location [31]. Therefore, appropriate epidermal coverage has to be accomplished by proliferation.

■ **Proliferation.** A few hours following initial migration, epithelial cells in this area undergo a phenomenon called **proliferative burst** [1, 32, 33]. In the following days, due mainly to the stimulus of growth factors, epidermal cells proliferate, forming and producing new epidermal cells and enabling the process of epithelialization to be completed [12, 13].

In a simple incisional/surgical wound, re-epithelialization is expected to be completed within 24 h, when cells from both sides of the wound margin touch one another and seal the area.

2.3.4 Wound Contraction

Wound contraction is a major process that further contributes to wound closure (Fig. 2.5). This process does not involve the formation of

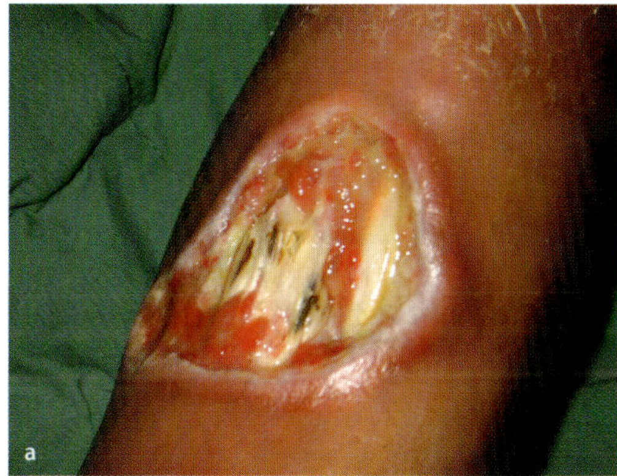
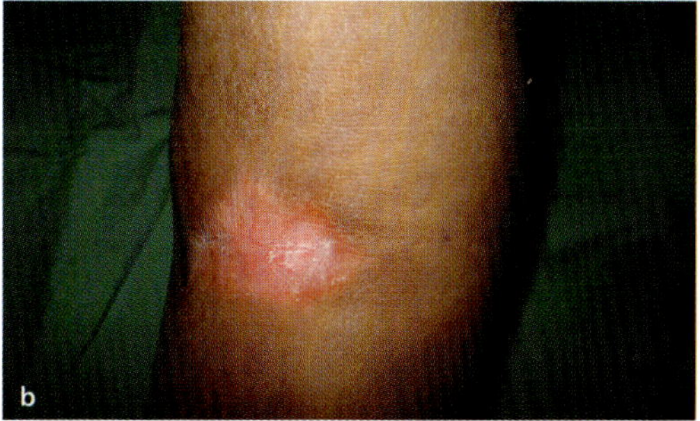

Fig. 2.5 a, b. **a.** A cutaneous ulcer. **b.** A scar following complete healing of the same ulcer. From the size of the scar, it is clear that a significant part of the healing process is achieved by contraction

new tissues, as discussed above. It is based on the centripetal movement of healthy tissues peripheral to the site of injury, so that when the wound is eventually closed, the scar in its center will be of the minimal possible size. Wound contraction begins a few days after injury, simultaneous to the tissue remodeling phase. This process is conducted via modified fibroblasts, called myofibroblasts. Certain growth factors, such as TGF-β1, regulate the conversion of fibroblasts to contractile myofibroblasts [1, 34]. Myofibroblasts resemble smooth muscle cells; having actin-containing contractile filaments, they can induce contractile forces on the edges of a wound towards its center [35–38].

The rate of contraction is dependent on all factors that dictate the ability to heal in general, such as the patient's general and nutritional condition, the etiology of the wound, and the presence of local infection. It is also determined by the geometric shape of the healing wound. In round wounds, for example, the process of contraction tends to be slower.

2.3.5 Role of Nitric Oxide in Wound Healing

Nitric oxide (NO) is a free radical synthesized from L-arginine. In recent years, data have been accumulating on the significant role of NO in the processes of wound healing. NO is a vasodilator and apparently regulates proliferation and differentiation of several cell types such as macrophages, keratinocytes, fibroblasts, and endothelial cells during the inflammatory and proliferative phases of wound healing. Hence, it affects angiogenesis, collagen deposition, and wound contraction [39–41]. Most evidence suggests that a certain increase in NO production may be beneficial to normal healing [42].

Further research is required to identify the exact mechanisms by which NO affects healing. The clinical implications of the above have not yet been determined.

2.4 Tissue Remodeling Phase

The tissue remodeling phase represents the late processes of healing, taking place up to two years following injury in normal healing conditions. A continuous process of dynamic equilibrium between the synthesis of new stable collagen and the lysis of old collagen is the hallmark of this phase. Collagen type III, synthesized in the first few weeks, is replaced by the more stable collagen type I. The fibers of collagen are arranged in a desired alignment. These processes lead, eventually, to the formation of scar tissue (Fig. 2.6).

The increasing amount of stable collagen and the alignment of its fibers gradually increase the strength of the healing wound [13, 43]. Two weeks after injury, an average wound has about 5% of its original strength; after one month, it reaches about 40% of its original strength. A healed wound will never regain more than 80% of its original strength. It always has a higher risk of breakdown compared with intact skin.

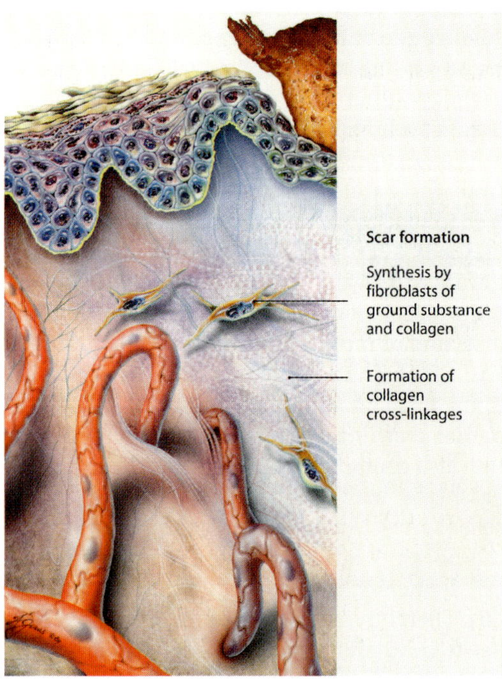

Fig. 2.6. Formation of scar tissue. (From [76])

2.5 Types of Repair

From the surgical point of view, one may distinguish between three different modes of wound management, relating mainly to approximation of the wound's edges:

- **Repair by Primary Intention.** Repair by primary intention is intended for acute, clean surgical wounds. The skin edges are approximated to each other, either by suturing, by staples, or by adhesive plasters. This procedure facilitates a relatively rapid process of wound healing [44].

- **Repair by Secondary Intention.** In the case of chronic ulcers, or in wounds that have a higher probability of developing infection, repair should be achieved by secondary intention. The edges of such wounds should not be approximated. Closure and complete healing is achieved gradually by granulation tissue formation and re-epithelialization [44].

- **Repair by Tertiary Intention.** Tertiary intention, also called delayed primary closure, is intended for wounds where the surgeon approximates the wound edges only after a few days. The delay allows natural physiological processes to take place, such as drainage of exudates or reduction in the extent of edema [44, 45].

2.6 Chronic Ulcers and Protracted Inflammation

In contrast to the normal, natural course of wound repair described above, chronic cutaneous ulcers are considered to be arrested and 'trapped' in an ongoing inflammatory phase [46–48]. A protracted inflammatory process develops in ulcers where normal mechanisms of wound healing are not sufficient to enable the wound to heal completely. This may occur due to bacterial infection or to the presence of foreign material that cannot be removed, solubilized or phagocytized.

Clinically, the bed of a chronic cutaneous ulcer tends to appear fibrotic and to contain a variable amount of necrotic debris. It cannot be regarded as an appropriate matrix for the processes of normal wound healing, such as migration of keratinocytes or epithelialization of the wound surface.

> The main features that characterize chronic ulcers are as follows:
> - Increased enzymatic activity of matrix proteases
> - Reduced response to growth factors
> - Cell senescence

2.6.1 Increased Enzymatic Activity of Matrix Proteases

Chronic ulcers have been shown to have high enzymatic activity of matrix metalloproteases (MMP), which act to degrade growth factors and extracellular matrix components such as collagen, fibronectin, and vitronectin [47, 49–53].

At the same time, the activity of MMP inhibitors, which could neutralize those unwanted effects, is reduced [54, 55]. The ongoing degradation of a newly formed matrix by MMP impairs and prevents normal wound healing, perpetuating the continuous inflammatory processes that characterize chronic ulcers.

2.6.2 Reduced Responsiveness to Growth Factors

The level of growth factors is not necessarily lower in chronic ulcers than in acute lesions. Numerous studies of growth factor levels in chronic ulcers have reported a wide range of results [47, 54–58]. Nevertheless, the general impression is that the growth factors of chronic ulcers are subjected to ongoing degradation due to increased protease activity, as described above. Accumulating evidence suggests that in chronic ulcers there may be reduced expression of growth factor receptors [59, 60]. It seems that these pathophysiologic changes are, at least in part, an expression of cell senescence that occurs in the chronic ulcer bed.

2.6.3 Cell Senescence

Recently, research studies have focused on the issue of **cellular senescence**. The term 'senescence' is derived from the Latin word *senescere,* meaning to grow old. According to *Dorland's Medical Dictionary*, 'senescence' indicates the process of growing old, especially the condition resulting from the transitions and accumulations of the deleterious aging process.

Old cells, in general, are characterized by reduced proliferative capacity [61–64]. The current concept suggests that each human cell is programmed to have a limited number of cellular divisions, determined by its specific origin and nature. Following a finite number of divisions, the cells reach a state of senescence, with subsequent reduced proliferative capacity. An in-vivo model of neonatal fibroblasts demonstrated that these cells reached growth arrest after 40–60 population doublings [65].

Senescent cells have characteristic morphological features; i.e., they tend to be larger than cells that have not undergone such changes [66, 67]. In addition, they have specific biochemical changes, such as an over-expression of matrix proteins (e.g., cellular fibronectin). Senescent cells have a decreased response to growth factors [66].

Mendez et al. [66] and Vande-Berg et al. [67] demonstrated that fibroblasts derived from the margins and beds of chronic cutaneous ulcers become prematurely senescent. It is logical to assume that the presence of senescent cells on the surface and edges of a cutaneous ulcer results in impaired healing.

Agren et al. [68] demonstrated that fibroblasts obtained from chronic cutaneous ulcers showed characteristics of senescence; their in-vitro growth was significantly slower compared with that of fibroblasts isolated from acute wounds or normal skin.

Possible explanations for the presence of senescent cells in cutaneous ulcers are as follows:

1. Cells within the surface or margin of a cutaneous ulcer are continuously stimulated to proliferate (since the ulcer is not closed). On the other hand, the basic pathologic processes leading to ulceration (e.g., infection, poor vascularization, external pressure) still exist and prevent healing. Mendez [66] suggests that in these cases, cells undergo many unnecessary futile divisions and gradually lose their proliferative capacity.

2. It is suggested that chronic wound fluid and the ulcer microenvironment contain certain components that lead to cellular senescence. Certain cytokines [69] or bacterial toxins [70] may be involved in this process. Research studies have shown that chronic wound fluid suppresses in-vitro proliferation of fibroblasts, keratinocytes and endothelial cells [70].

There are several clinical implications arising from the fact that cell senescence could be an important factor in the failure of ulcers to heal.

- Meticulous debridement has an important part in the optimal treatment of a chronic ulcer. Debridement helps to remove senescent cells from the ulcer's surface and margin. The value of debridement procedures prior to applications of growth factors, keratinocyte transplantation, and the use of composite grafts has been documented [71–75].

- Autologous skin grafting should be considered for chronic ulcers that are relatively large. As described in Chap. 13, the main mechanism by which allogeneic grafting is considered to exert its beneficial effect is via the production of growth factors, which, in turn, enhance proliferation of epithelial cells, fibroblasts, and endothelial cells of the ulcer bed. However, it is reasonable to assume that in large, long-standing ulcers cell senescence has occurred. Consequently, the patient's own cells would not be able to heal and close a relatively large ulcer. Moreover, in such cases, growth factors do not actually have an appropriate and functional target tissue to affect. Therefore, under appropriate conditions, it may be preferable to consider using autologous skin grafting, which may 'take' and cover the ulcer bed, rather than allogeneic grafting. Future research studies may identify specific components that lead to senescence, which would then enable the development of new treatment modalities specifically aimed at preventing senescence and thereby improving the healing of cutaneous ulcers.

2.7 Concluding Remarks

In contrast to the normal healing of an acute wound, chronic ulcers tend to be 'stuck' in an ongoing inflammatory process. Today, chronic ulcers are considered to represent a unique pathophysiologic entity, in which the precise process remains an enigma.

The optimal treatment of a chronic ulcer requires appropriate ulcer bed preparation, followed by advanced therapeutic measures such as cultured keratinocyte grafts, composite grafts, or preparations containing growth factors. These steps are aimed at breaking the cycle of futile events that occur in a chronic ulcer and to divert its course to a pathway of normal wound healing.

References

1. Mehendale F, Martin P: The cellular and molecular events of wound healing. In: Falanga V (ed) Cutaneous Wound Healing, 1st edn. London: Martin Dunitz. 2001; pp 15–37

2. Clark RAF: Wound repair: overview and general considerations. In: Clark RAF (ed) The Molecular and Cellular Biology of Wound Repair, 2nd edn. New York: Plenum Press. 1996; pp 3–50

3. Harding K: Introduction to growth factors. In: Meeting the challenge of managing the diabetic foot: use of growth factor therapy. Proceedings from a symposium preceding the 35th Annual Meeting of the European Association for the Study of Diabetes. Antwerp, Belgium. 1999; pp 31–40

4. Cohen K: An overview of wound healing biology. In: Ziegler TR, Pierce GF, Herndon DN (eds) Growth Factors and Wound Healing: Basic Science and Potential Clinical Applications. Berlin Heidelberg New York: Springer. 1997; pp 3–7

5. Kiritsy CP, Lynch AB, Lynch SE: Role of growth factors in cutaneous wound healing: a review. Crit Rev Oral Biol Med 1993; 4:729–760

6. Schaffer CJ, Nanney LB: Cell biology of wound healing. Int Rev Cytol 1996; 169:151–181

7. Bennett NT, Schultz GS: Growth factors and wound healing. Role in normal and chronic wound healing, part II. Am J Surg 1993; 166:74–81

8. Iocono JA, Ehrlich HP, Gottrup F, et al: The biology of healing. In: Leaper DJ, Harding KG (eds). Wounds: Biology and Management. Oxford, New York: Oxford University Press. 1998; pp 10–22

9. Bryant WM: Wound healing. Clin Symp 1977; 29:1–36

10. Ross R, Benditt EP: Wound healing and collagen formation. 1. Sequential changes in components of guinea pig skin wounds observed in the electron microscope. J Biophys Biochem Cytol 1961; 11:677–700

11. Ross R: The fibroblast and wound repair. Biol Rev Camb Philos Soc 1968; 43:51–96

12. Clark RAF: Cutaneous tissue repair. Basic biologic considerations. I. J Am Acad Dermatol 1985; 13:701–725

13. Kanzler MH, Gorsulowsky DC, Swanson NA: Basic mechanisms in the healing cutaneous wound. J Dermatol Surg Oncol 1986; 12:1156–1164

14. Diegelmann RF, Cohen IK, Kaplan AM: The role of macrophages in wound repair: a review. Plast Reconstr Surg 1981; 68:107–113

15. Werner S, Grose R: Regulation of wound healing by growth factors and cytokines. Physiol Rev 2002; 83:835–870

16. Falanga V, Shen J: Growth factors, signal transduction and cellular responses. In: Falanga V (ed) Cutaneous Wound Healing. 1st edn. London: Martin Dunitz. 2001; pp 81–93

17. Marikovsky M, Rosenblum CI, Faltin Z, et al: Appearance of leptin in wound fluid in response to injury. Wound Rep Reg 2002; 10:302–307

18. Murad A, Nath AK, Cha ST, et al: Leptin is an autocrine/paracrine regulator of wound healing. FASEB J 2003; 17:1895–1897

19. Varghese MC, Balin AK, Carter DM, et al: Local wound environment under synthetic dressings. J Invest Dermatol 1984; 82:395–396

20. Varghese MC, Balin AK, Carter DM, et al: Local environment of chronic wounds under synthetic dressings. Arch Dermatol 1986; 122:52–57

21. Eckes B, Aumailley M, Kreig T: Collagens and the reestablishment of dermal integrity. In: Clark RAF (ed) The molecular and cellular biology of wound repair, 2nd edn. New York: Plenum Press, 1996; pp 493–512

22. Micera A, Vigneti E, Pickholtz D, et al: Nerve growth factor displays stimulatory effects on human skin and lung fibroblasts, demonstrating a direct role for this factor in tissue repair. Proc Natl Acad Sci USA 2001; 98:6162–6167,

23. Liu M, Warn JD, Fan Q, et al: Relationships between nerves and myofibroblasts during cutaneous wound healing in the developing rat. Cell Tissue Res 1999; 297:423–433

24. Smith PG, Liu M: Impaired cutaneous wound healing after sensory denervation in developing rats: effects on cell proliferation and apoptosis. Cell Tissue Res 2002; 307:281–291

25. Beer HD, Gassmann MG, Munz B, et al: Expression and function of keratinocyte growth factor and activin in skin morphogenesis and cutaneous wound repair. J Investig Dermatol Symp Proc 2000; 5:34–39

26. Gumbiner BM: Cell adhesion: the molecular basis of tissue architecture and morphogenesis. Cell 1996; 84:345–357

27. Schmitz AA, Govek EE, Bottner B, et al: Rho GTPases: signaling, migration, and invasion. Exp Cell Res 2000;261:1–12

28. Mitchison TJ, Cramer LP: Actin-based cell motility and cell locomotion. Cell 1996; 84:371–379

29. Zhao M, Song B, Pu J, et al: Direct visualization of a stratified epithelium reveals that wounds heal by unified sliding of cell sheets. FASEB J 2003; 17:397–406

30. Jacinto A, Martinez-Arias A, Martin P: Mechanisms of epithelial fusion and repair. Nat Cell Biol 2001; 3:E117–E123

31. Winter GD: Epidermal regeneration studied in the domestic pig. In: Maibach HI, Rovee DT (eds) Epidermal wound healing. Chicago: Year Book Medical Publishers, Inc. 1972; pp 71–112

32. Potten CS, Allen TD: The fine structure and cell kinetics of mouse epidermis after wounding. J Cell Sci 1975; 17:413–447

33. Garlick JA, Taichman LB: Fate of human keratinocytes during reepithelialization in an organotypic culture model. Lab Invest 1994; 70:916–924

34. Desmouliere A, Geinoz A, Gabbiani F, et al: Transforming growth factor-β 1 induces α-smooth muscle actin expression in granulation tissue myofibroblasts and in quiescent and growing cultured fibroblasts. J Cell Biol 1993; 122:103–111

35. Wrobel LK, Fray TR, Molloy JE, et al: Contractility of single human dermal myofibroblasts and fibroblasts. Cell Motil Cytoskeleton 2002; 52:82–90

36. Serini G, Gabbiani G: Mechanisms of myofibroblast activity and phenotypic modulation. Exp Cell Res 1999; 250:273–283

37. Tomasek JJ, Gabbiani G, Hinz B, et al: Myofibroblasts and mechano-regulation of connective tissue remodelling. Nat Rev Mol Cell Biol 2002; 3:349–363

38. Majno G, Gabbiani G, Hirschel BJ, et al: Contraction of granulation tissue in vitro: similarity to smooth muscle. Science 1971; 173:548–550

39. Weller R: Nitric oxide: a key mediator in cutaneous physiology. Clin Exp Dermatol 2003; 28:511–514

40. Schentker A, Billiar TR: Nitric oxide and wound repair. Surg Clin North Am 2003; 83:521–530

41. Witte MB, Barbul A: Role of nitric oxide in wound repair. Am J Surg 2002; 183:406–412

42. Efron DT, Most D, Barbul A: Role of nitric oxide in wound healing. Curr Opin Clin Nutr Metab Care 2000; 3:197–204

43. Levenson SM, Geever EF, Crowley LV, et al: The healing of rat skin wounds. Ann Surg 1965; 161:293–308

44. Cohen IK, Diegelmann RF, Yager DR, et al: Wound care and wound healing. In: Schwartz SI, Shires GT, Spencer FC, et al (eds) Principles of Surgery. 7th edn. New York: McGraw-Hill. 1999; pp 263–295

45. Verrier ED, Bossart KJ, Heer FW: Reduction of infection rates in abdominal incisions by delayed wound closure techniques. Am J Surg 1979; 138:22–28

46. Bello YM, Phillips TJ: Recent advances in wound healing. JAMA 2000; 283:716–718

47. Konig M, Peschen M, Vanscheidt W: Molecular biology of chronic wounds. In: Hafner J, Ramelet AA, Schmeller W, Brunner UV (eds) Current problems in dermatology. Management of leg ulcers. Basel: Karger. 1999; pp 8–12

48. Kloth LC, McCulloch JM: The inflammatory response to wounding. In: McCulloch JM, Kloth LC, Feedar JA (eds) Wound Healing: Alternatives in Management, 2nd edn. Philadelphia: F.A. Davis. 1995; pp 3–15

49. Rao CN, Ladin DA, Liu YY, et al: α-1-antitrypsin is degraded and non-functional in chronic wounds but intact and functional in acute wounds: the inhibitor protects fibronectin from degradation by chronic wound fluid enzymes. J Invest Dermatol 1995; 105:572–578

50. Herrick S, Ashcroft G, Ireland G, et al: Up-regulation of elastase in acute wounds of healthy aged humans and chronic venous leg ulcers are associated with matrix degradation. Lab Invest 1997; 77:281–288

51. Lauer G, Sollberg S, Cole M, et al: Expression and proteolysis of vascular endothelial growth factor is increased in chronic wounds. J Invest Dermatol 2000; 115:12–18

52. Grinnell F, Zhu M: Fibronectin degradation in chronic wounds depends on the relative levels of elastase, α1-proteinase inhibitor and α2-macroglobulin. J Invest Dermatol 1996; 106:335–341

53. Palolahti M, Lauharanta J, Stephens RW, et al: Proteolytic activity in leg ulcer exudate. Exp Dermatol 1993; 2:29–37

54. Trengove NJ, Stacey MC, MacAuley S, et al: Analysis of the acute and chronic wound environments: The role of proteases and their inhibitors. Wound Rep Reg 1999; 7:442–452

55. Bullen EC, Longaker MT, Updike DL, et al: TIMP-1 is decreased and activated gelatinases are increased in chronic wounds. J Invest Dermatol 1995; 104: 236–240

56. Mast B, Schultz GS: Interactions of cytokines, growth factors, and proteases in acute and chronic wounds. Wound Rep Reg 1996; 4:411–420

57. Peschen M, Grenz H, Grothe C, et al: Patterns of epidermal growth factor receptor, basic fibroblast growth factor and transforming growth factor-β_3 expression in the skin with chronic venous insufficiency. Eur J Dermatol 1998; 8:334–338

58. Harris IR, Yee KC, Walters CE, et al: Cytokine and protease levels in healing and non-healing chronic venous leg ulcers. Exp Dermatol 1995; 4:342–349

59. Cowin AJ, Hatzirodos N, Holding CA, et al: Effect of healing on the expression of transforming growth factor βs and their receptors in chronic venous leg ulcers. J Invest Dermatol 2001; 117:1282–1289

60. Jude EB, Blakytny R, Bulmer J, et al: Transforming growth factor-β 1,2,3 and receptor type I and II in diabetic foot ulcers. Diabet Med 2002; 19:440–447

61. Martin GM, Sprague CA, Epstein CJ: Replicative life span of cultivated human cells. Effects of donor's age, tissue and genotype. Lab Invest 1970; 23:86–92

62. Schneider EL, Mitsui Y: The relationship between *in vitro* cellular aging and *in vivo* human age. Proc Natl Acad Sci USA 1976; 73:3584–3588

63. Schneider EL, Epstein CJ: Replication rate and life span of cultured fibroblasts in Down's syndrome. Proc Soc Exp Biol Med 1972; 141:1092–1094

64. Elmore E, Swift M: Growth of cultured cells from patients with ataxia-telangiectasia. J Cell Physiol 1976; 89:429–431

65. Raffetto JD, Mendez MV, Phillips TJ, et al: The effect of passage number on fibroblast cellular senescence in patients with chronic venous insufficiency with and without ulcer. Am J Surg 1999; 178:107–112

66. Mendez MV, Stanley A, Park HY, et al: Fibroblasts cultured from venous ulcers display cellular characteristics of senescence. J Vasc Surg 1998; 28:876–883

67. Vande-Berg JS, Rudolph R, Hollan C, et al: Fibroblast senescence in pressure ulcers. Wound Repair Reg 1998; 6:38–49

68. Agren MS, Steenfos HH, Dabelsteen S, et al: Proliferation and mitogenic response to PDGF-BB of fibroblasts isolated from chronic venous leg ulcers is ulcer-age dependent. J Invest Dermatol 1999; 112: 463–469

69. Mendez MV, Raffetto JD, Phillips T, et al: The proliferative capacity of neonatal skin fibroblasts is reduced after exposure to venous ulcer wound fluid: A potential mechanism for senescence in venous ulcers. J Vasc Surg 1999; 30:734–743

70. Bucalo B, Eaglstein WH, Falanga V: Inhibition of cellular proliferation by chronic wound fluid. Wound Rep Reg 1993; 1:181–186

71. Steed DL, Donohoe D, Webster MW, et al: Effect of extensive debridement and treatment on the healing of diabetic foot ulcers. J Am Coll Surg 1996; 183: 61–64

72. Fisher JC: Skin grafting. In: Georgiades GS, Riefkohl R, Levin LS (eds) Plastic, Maxillofacial and Reconstructive Surgery, 3rd edn. Baltimore: Williams & Wilkins. 1996; pp 13–18

73. Marcusson JA, Lindgren C, Berghard A, et al: Allogeneic cultured keratinocytes in the treatment of leg ulcers: A pilot study. Acta Derm Venereol (Stockh) 1992; 72:61–64

74. Teepe RG, Roseeuw DI, Hermans J, et al: Randomized trial comparing cryopreserved cultured epidermal allografts with hydrocolloid dressings in healing chronic venous ulcers. J Am Acad Dermatol 1993; 29:982–988

75. Pham HT, Rosenblum BI, Lyons TE, et al: Evaluation of a human skin equivalent for the treatment of diabetic foot ulcers in a prospective, ramdomized, clinical trial. Wounds 1999; 11:79–86

76. Geras AJ: Dermatology: A Medical Artist's Interpretation. Sandoz Pharma Ltd. 1990

Milestones in the History of Wound Healing

3

Contents

3.1 Overview

The history of wound healing is as old as the history of medicine and probably as mankind itself. In light of its magnitude, we shall not cover the whole subject in this chapter. We shall focus rather on the principal milestones in the history of wound healing.

In the past centuries and in recent decades, there have been breakthroughs which have made significant changes in our scientific understanding of wound repair processes. These events have influenced the currently accepted approach to treating wounds and ulcers.

This historical survey is an overview of the treatment of wounds and skin lesions in general. In the medical literature, one can find historical surveys of specific types of cutaneous ulcers, especially venous leg ulcers, since they are common [1, 2].

3.2 The Ancient World

Naturally, the topic has no clear starting point. It may be attributed to that ancient father of humanity who once used leaves as a dressing and then even washed his wound in water – blissfully unaware of the fact that he was opening up new horizons in the history of medicine and of humanity.

Later, though still well prior to documentation by clear historical records, various substances were rubbed on wounds or skin lesions; natural materials were used, such as mud, various plant extracts, or honey. Throughout history, the putting together of these remedies became more complex, requiring exact notation of the mixtures that were used, as well as of just how they were to be prepared.

Magical and religious connotations were always dominant features of ancient medicine. These elements have accompanied medicine since the dawn of history, and only with the advent of modern medicine have they begun to fade.

A unique aspect in the history of medicine is the attempt to explain ancient healing rituals by relying on modern medical knowledge and technological capabilities. Thus, for example, the Greeks used to scrape the point of a lance over a wound, so that some metal powder was sprinkled on it. It has been suggested that metallic copper, when combined with vinegar, produces copper acetate, which has antibacterial properties that could help in the treatment of wounds and cutaneous ulcers [3, 4].

Similarly, inscriptions and marble carvings found in shrines to the Greek god Asklepios (or to Aesculapius, in the Roman world) associate healing with having been in contact with the oral cavity of non-poisonous serpents. Angeletti et al. [5] have suggested that salivary growth factors may have contributed to the healing process.

It is impossible to evaluate these and other suppositions today, since the ancients neither conducted nor documented strict clinical trials. It is nonetheless reasonable to assume that such magical or ritualistic treatments had significant psychological consequences.

3.2.1 Medicine in Mesopotamia

The first written historical record was found on a Sumerian clay tablet from ca. 2100 BC (Fig. 3.1). This is actually the world's oldest medical manuscript. The "three healing gestures" described in this tablet are: washing the wound, applying dressings/plasters, and bandaging the wound. These constitute the basic principles of wound treatment today.

In his book *The Healing Hand: Man and Wound in the Ancient World* [6], Guido Majno states that there were 15 prescriptions recorded on the tablet, without indication of the diseases for which they were intended. Twelve of the 15 were for external use, eight being plasters, indicating that they may have been used for local diseases. Majno presents several examples of

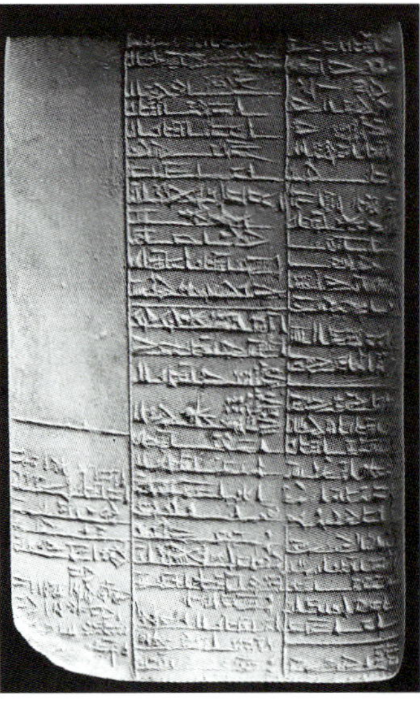

Fig. 3.1. Cuneiform medical clay tablet. (From The Wellcome Library, London)

these prescriptions, such as [6]: "Pound together: dried wine dregs, juniper and prunes, pour beer on the mixture. Then rub (the diseased part) with oil, and bind on (as a plaster)."

Beer was widely used in Sumerian treatments and it is likely that, owing to the antiseptic ingredients it contains, it did have some beneficial effect in the treatment of wounds and skin lesions [6].

However, it is impossible to assess today the beneficial effect, if any, these remedies had on the treated lesions. In fact, the Sumerians had a variety of topical agents that could have been useful. Oils may have been beneficial in soothing dry wounds. As mud and inorganic salts absorb water, they could have dried out wounds and thus prevented proliferation of bacteria. Certain plant extracts could also have had some antibacterial effect. At present, nobody knows whether the Sumerians actually made reasonable use of the materials at hand.

3.2.2 Ancient Egypt

The information we have on medicine in ancient Egypt is based on the Smith and the Ebers

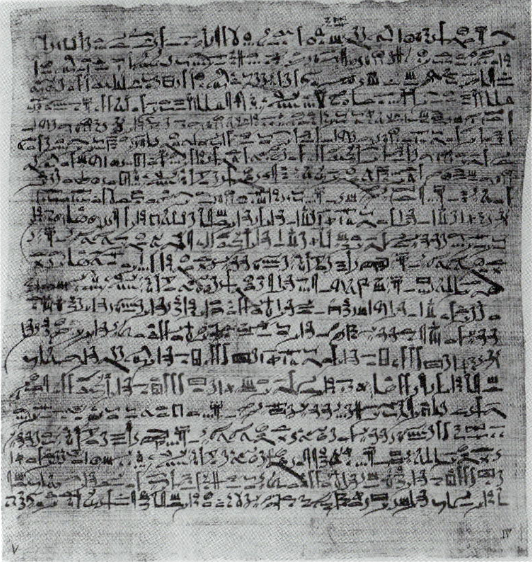

Fig. 3.2. A piece of the Edwin Smith papyrus. (From The Wellcome Library, London)

papyri, dating from around 1650 BC and 1550 BC, respectively (Fig. 3.2). The information seems to be based on older papyri that were probably written a thousand years earlier.

The ancient Egyptians made use of mixtures with substances such as honey, grease, and lint for topical application to wounds. Lint was made from vegetable fibers and apparently helped in the absorption of secretions from the wound's surface. Whether honey has a beneficial effect on the processes of wound healing is still controversial (see Chap. 17).

The Egyptian science of bandaging wounds was similar to that used in bandaging the dead during the process of mummification. Prior to bandaging, the materials were dipped in various preparations, including herbal extracts, gums, and resins. Gum applied to bandage strips was also used to draw and to approximate wound margins. This procedure can be regarded as the first adhesive bandage [7, 8].

3.3 Inflammation, Infection and the Attitude to Appearance of Purulent Discharge in the Past

The Sumerian and ancient Egyptian documents include the terms *ummu* and *shememet*, respectively, which are understood today as indicating the presence of inflammation. The Egyptians distinguished between two types of wounds: 'Good wounds' were treated according to the principles described above, including dressing with topical preparation and bandaging. On the other hand, 'bad wounds' were affected by a 'whirl of inflammation,' identified by touching the wound edge and by their tendency to secrete pus. These wounds were left open [7].

However, the earliest description of the 'four cardinal signs of inflammation' was set down by Aulus Cornelius Celsus (42? BC–37 AD), who wrote a comprehensive eight-volume compendium of medicine (*De re Medicina*). This book was based on the Hippocratic Canon and other classical sources. *De re Medicina* was forgotten some years after its writing, only to be rediscovered after a long period, in 1426. It was one of the first medical books to be printed, appearing in 1478. Thereafter, it enjoyed great success; new editions were published even in the nineteenth century [9]. It was here that Celsus first described the four cardinal signs of inflammation, namely, *rubor* (redness), *tumor* (swelling), *calor* (heat) and *dolor* (pain).

The Egyptians recognized that a suppurating wound should be drained [10]. Later, Galen indicated that when infection was localized in a wound, the discharge of pus might be followed by healing. This observation was misinterpreted in a dogmatic and rigid manner during the following 1500 years [3, 11].

During this period, pus secreted by a surgical wound was considered to be beneficial in cases where the amount of secretions gradually decreased and the patient recuperated. The presence of purulent discharge was considered to be auspicious; the ancient expression *pus bonum et laudabile* reflects this concept.

In contrast, in cases of brown, thin, and foul-smelling discharge, patients usually died. This type of discharge was, most probably, a manifestation of invasive infection.

Many topical preparations were introduced into wounds with the objective of encouraging suppuration, a mistaken treatment that could actually increase the risk of spreading infection with subsequent mortality [3, 11].

It would take until the nineteenth century for it to be understood that the presence of pus in a wound was undesirable. Not until the breakthrough discoveries of Semmelweis, Lister, and others (see below) was it possible to prevent the development of pus in surgical wounds with any degree of efficiency. These principles played a significant role in the treatment of wounds and cutaneous ulcers.

3.4 Renaissance Era

Ambroise Paré (1509–1590) was one of the greatest physicians of the Renaissance and in the entire history of medicine. His broad knowledge of medicine and surgery, stemming from his unique skills and many years of service in the French army as a military surgeon, resulted in significant changes in the medical conceptions of those times. His scientific initiatives helped to direct traditional medieval medicine towards modern medicine.

Paré was chief surgeon to four kings of France [12]: Henry II (1547–1559), Francis II (1559–1560), Charles IX (1560–1574), and Henry III (1574–1589). As a military surgeon he saved the lives of thousands of soldiers, and in so doing, changed the previous approach, which was to simply leave the wounded soldiers behind to die on the battlefield. He wrote two books: *Treatment of Gunshot Wounds* and *The Method of Treating Wounds Made by Arquebuses*, in which he summarized the surgical techniques of his era and introduced those he had developed. His books were translated into several languages from the French (Fig. 3.3).

His unique contribution to the field of wound healing prevented the suffering of many a wounded soldier. At that time, gunshot wounds were considered to be 'poisoned wounds' due to their direct contact with gunpowder. The accepted approach was to treat these wounds by

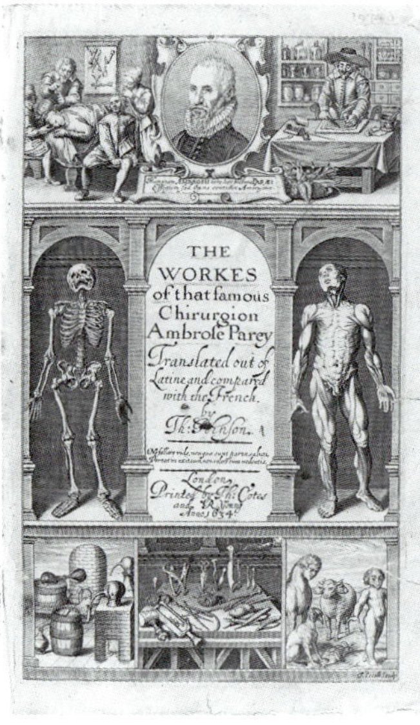

Fig. 3.3. The cover picture of Paré's book. (From The Wellcome Library, London)

cauterizing them with a red-hot iron or with boiling oil.

During a military expedition to Turin led by King Francis I (1536–1537), Paré gained important experience (Fig. 3.4). In one of the battles, the oil he used to treat gunshot wounds ran out. He had no option but to improvise a mixture that included egg yolks, oil of roses, and turpentine. When he changed their dressings on

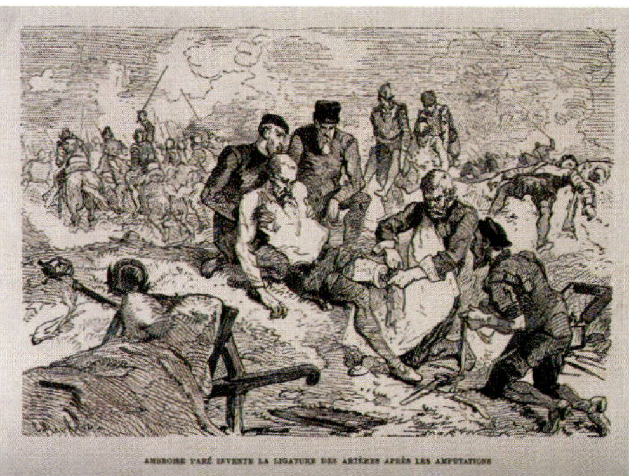

Fig. 3.4. Paré in the battlefield: A wood engraving of that period. (By C. Maurand; from The Wellcome Library, London)

the following day, he was surprised to see that the wounds treated with the improvised mixture were greatly improved, compared with those treated with the usual boiling oil. The recovery of those not cauterized with the oil was faster and with fewer complications. Of this discovery, Paré wrote [12]:

"I slept badly that night, as I greatly feared that, when I would come to examine the wounded the following morning, I should find that those whose wounds I had failed to treat with boiling oil will have died from poisoning. I arose at a very early hour, and was much surprised to discover that the wounds to which I had applied the egg and turpentine mixture were doing well: they were quite free from swelling and from all evidence of inflammatory action: and the patients themselves, who showed no signs of feverishness, said that they had experienced little or no pain and had slept quite well. On the other hand, the men to whom I had applied the boiling oil, said that they had experienced during the night, and were still suffering from, much pain at the seat of the injury; and I found that they were feverish and that their wounds were inflamed and swollen. After thinking the matter over carefully, I made up my mind that thenceforward I would abstain wholly from the painful practice of treating gunshot wounds with boiling oil."

This observation, which Paré published, yielded significant improvement in the treatment of gunshot wounds.

Paré was responsible for two further significant contributions: The first was the use of a ligature to stop bleeding, rather than cauterization. The second was the development of an artificial hand, the prosthesis. Although it was not particularly efficient, it allowed the disabled person a degree of ability to function. Paré may therefore be viewed as the father of medical rehabilitation. His most memorable statement reflects his modesty: "Je le pansay, Dieu le quarit": "I dressed him, God healed him."

3.5 Antiseptic, Identification of Bacteria and the Use of Antibiotics

A further aspect of the history of wound healing took place in parallel to that of the use of antiseptics, identification of bacteria and the development of antibiotic preparations. Breakthroughs in this field led to the prevention of serious complications in acute and chronic wounds.

3.5.1 Ignatz Phillip Semmelweis

The pioneer in this area was Ignatz Phillip Semmelweis (1818–1865). He was born in Hungary of German parentage (Fig. 3.5) and studied at the medical school in Vienna. Among his teachers were Rokitansky and Skoda [13]. At that time, 'puerperal fever' was the cause of many deaths of women after childbirth throughout Europe, and there was no reasonable explanation for this phenomenon. Some doctors believed that insufficient ventilation was responsible, and therefore many large skylights were constructed with ventilation apertures in the ceilings, still to be seen in European hospitals.

The mortality was higher in units where deliveries were carried out by obstetricians and medical students than in units where deliveries

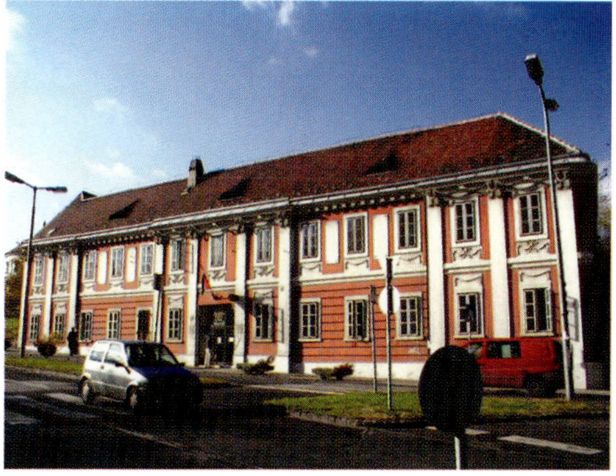

Fig. 3.5. Semmelweis house in Budapest. The building now serves as the Semmelweis Museum, Library and Archives of Medical History

were carried out by midwives. Semmelweis began to think that some substance found in corpses was being transmitted by the doctors and medical students handling autopsies to the women giving birth [13].

Because Semmelweis noticed that chlorine eliminated the smell typical of corpses, he demanded that the hands of anyone about to examine a woman after carrying out an autopsy or examining a sick woman be washed in a chlorine solution (Fig. 3.6). This policy reduced the mortality among the women giving birth in his department. However, in the early years, this approach was ignored by all the medical journals. Only in December 1847 did Von Hebra publish Semmelweis's discovery in a brief editorial in a local Viennese medical journal [14].

Throughout his life, his concept met with serious opposition. In 1858, Semmelweis published an article entitled "Etiology of Puerperal Fever" in the weekly Hungarian medical journal *Orvosi Hetilap* [13]. This was his first written article presenting his approach. His book *The Etiology, the Concept and the Prevention of Puerperal Fever* was published in 1860 [15]. However, after the book appeared, the medical establishment still failed to support his ideas.

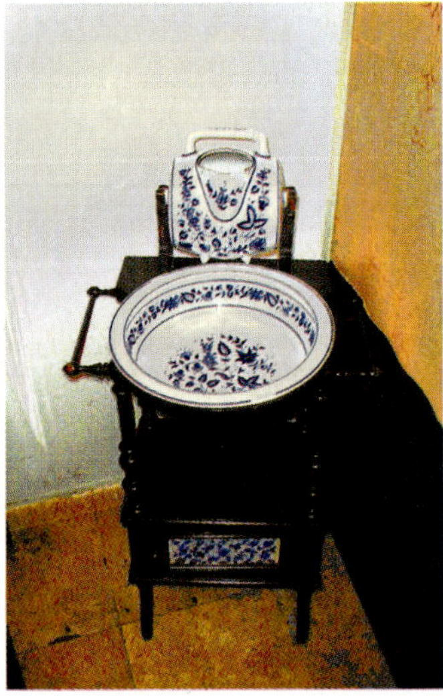

Fig. 3.6. A porcelain device for washing the hands in the Semmelweis era. (In the Semmelweis Museum of the History of Medicine, Budapest)

Towards the end of his life, Semmelweis lost his ability to reason. Researchers have found that certain characteristics of his behavior point to the Alzheimer syndrome. He died in a psychiatric hospital, and there are findings that may indicate he was beaten to death by hospital attendants.

It is noted that the possibility of transmission of some pathogenic agent causing puerperal fever was identified, at almost the same time, by Semmelweis and Oliver Wendell Holmes, Professor of Anatomy at Harvard. Holmes spoke of such matters at the Boston Society for Medical Improvement in 1843 [16]. He suspected a possible association between the mortality of mothers giving birth and the presence of physicians in autopsies, and he recommended that doctors avoid carrying out autopsies prior to treating the mothers. However, Holmes did not offer a practical solution to the problem (washing the hands in a chlorine solution) as did Semmelweis, and his statements failed to result in any response.

The scientific basis for understanding Semmelweis's observations was to be established in the years that followed by Pasteur and Joseph Lister, as described below.

3.5.2 Joseph Lister

In the middle of the nineteenth century, when Joseph Lister (Fig. 3.7) began his medical career, amputations were the most common form of surgery. However, a high percentage of the wounds became gangrenous. The mortality of patients undergoing amputation was generally higher than 40%, as a result of surgical contamination [17–19].

In 1865, Lister happened upon the work of Louis Pasteur. Pasteur had rejected the theory that had supported the spontaneous appearance of bacteria, and related the phenomena of decay and fermentation to microbial action. Lister came to the conclusion that the suppurating inflammation of wounds had a similar etiology. In contrast to the then-accepted notion that such bacteria originated in the patient's body, Lister was impressed by Pasteur's claim that they existed everywhere, including the at-

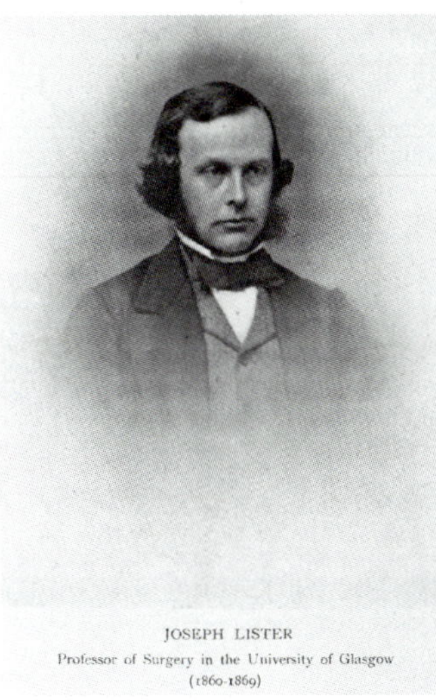

Fig. 3.7. Joseph Lister (From The Wellcome Library, London)

mosphere and the bodies and clothes of the doctors, and that they could contaminate wounds. Lister wrote [20]:

"But when it had been shown by Pasteur's researchers that the septic property of the atmosphere depended, not upon the oxygen or any gaseous constituent, but on minute organisms suspended in it, which owed their energy to their vitality, it occurred to me that decomposition of the injured part might be avoided without excluding the air, by applying as a dressing some material capable of destroying the life of the floating particles."

In order to prevent the contamination of wounds, he began to wrap them in many layers of gauze which he had first immersed in a carbolic acid solution [21]. Between the gauze layers and the wound, he would place a layer of relatively impermeable silk, which he called 'protective silk', in order to prevent damage to the tissues by the carbolic acid.

Later, he also applied these principles in the operating theater. He would cover the area of the operation in a piece of cloth dipped in carbolic acid, which he removed only when the surgical incision was made. He steeped the surgical instruments, as well as his hands, in a carbolic acid solution. Thereafter, he devised a carbolic acid spray, and the surgical area was sprayed with the solution in order to destroy the air-borne bacteria.

After a few months of carrying out these practices, the level of contamination in his unit in a Glasgow hospital dropped considerably. However, the excessive exposure to the carbolic acid was detrimental to the doctors' health. Damage to their lungs and those of the medical staff was described as being so severe that they had to stop working.

For the rest of his life, Lister tried to discover the ideal bandage that would contain antiseptic but non-irritant material – a worthy mission indeed, since papers discussing damage to the processes of wound healing caused by anti-bacterial agents are still being published today (see Chaps. 10 and 11).

Only in the 1890s, more than 20 years after the discovery that the source of contamination is external, did the use of antiseptics become universal.

3.5.3 Other Researchers

Similar to the observations of Semmelweis and Holmes, described above, a British surgeon, Spencer Wells, published an article in 1864, entitled: 'Some Causes of Excessive Mortality After Surgical Operation' [22]. Wells also referred to Pasteur's work, and in light of it proposed that bacteria settle on wounds and cause the appearance of pus and sepsis. Wells insisted on thorough washing with cold water and the use of fresh towels when operating. Only spectators who testified in writing that they had not been in an autopsy room during the preceding seven days were allowed to enter his operating theater [17]. Nevertheless, Well's conjectures caused little reverberation, and he did not apply his ideas beyond the practice noted above.

Following Pasteur's discoveries, the science of bacteriology developed. Koch noted that there was a major transfer of bacteria during surgery or treatment from the surgeon's hands, the instruments and bandages, and from the patient himself. In order to destroy such germs, he proposed the use of substances such as iodine and alcohol.

Other antiseptic preparations included sodium hypochloride, used by Alexis Carrell, and mercuric chloride, used by William Halsted [3]. A major breakthrough, however, took place later with the discovery of antibiotics.

3.5.4 Antibiotics

In 1928, Alexander Fleming discovered a blue mold growing in a Petri dish which had been accidentally exposed to its spores. He noted that all the bacteria surrounding the mold had been killed. However, this discovery found no application until it attracted the attention of Chain and Florey in 1938, an event that led directly to the isolation of penicillin in 1940 [23, 24]. The first article describing the treatment of streptococcal meningitis by penicillin was published in 1943 [25].

The development of antibiotic medicines is of primary importance in the treatment of acute wounds and chronic lesions and the prevention of possible complications such as cellulitis, osteomyelitis, and sepsis.

3.6 Investigation of Wound Healing Processes

The establishment of the unique scientific branch of histopathology by Virchow [26] in the middle of the nineteenth century is the basis for our understanding of the processes of wound healing as they are known today. The development of antiseptic preparations contributed significantly to the understanding of these processes, since this meant that it was possible for the first time to examine wounds without accompanying contamination, and thus to identify specific inflammatory characteristics.

From initial breakthroughs achieved in the works of Metchnikoff [27], our knowledge of the complex processes of wound healing has gradually increased.

3.7 The Significance of a Moist Wound Environment

In the 1950s, physicians noticed that blistered skin achieved re-epithelialization and complete healing if the blister roof was left intact, functioning as a natural biological dressing, provided that the blister content was not infected [28].

In 1962, Winter et al. [29] presented a model that changed the traditional concept of wound healing. Instead of letting a wound dry out and be covered by a dry scab, it was demonstrated that keeping the wound environment moist would yield much better clinical results. This approach was confirmed in 1963 by Hinman and Maibach [30]. They conducted a study on human subjects with superficial wounds and confirmed the beneficial effects of a moist environment on wounds, compared with wounds exposed to the air (Fig. 3.8).

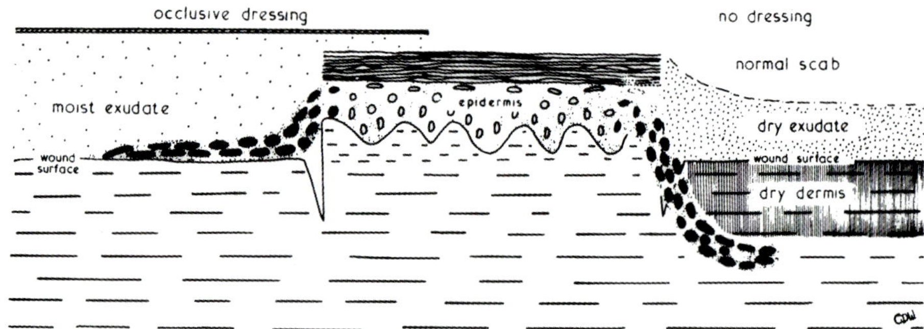

Fig. 3.8. The significance of a moist wound environment. *Left*: In a moist environment, epithelialization occurs along the wound surface. *Right*: Abnormal and prolonged course of healing under a dry scab. Epidermal cells are forced to advance under the crust; the metabolic expense is higher. (From the book *'Epidermal Wound Healing'* by Maibach & Rovee, 1972)

3.8 Keratinocyte Cultures and Advanced Skin Substitutes

In 1975, Rheinwald and Green [31] presented a method of culturing keratinocytes from single cell suspensions of human epidermal cells. Their breakthrough opened up new and challenging possibilities in the field of skin research. The technique enabled the transplantation of keratinocytes and the development of skin substitutes containing living cells. This topic is described in detail in Chap. 13.

3.9 Recent Developments

■ **Growth Factors.** There is an ever-increasing knowledge of various cytokines that function as growth factors, and the way they exert their effect on wound healing. Thus, while other currently accepted modes of therapy may provide optimal conditions for healing, preparations containing growth factors actually accelerate the wound repair process.

Epidermal growth factor was first isolated in 1962 from the submaxillary glands of adult male mice [32]. Initially, it was defined as a polypeptide hormone and was given the title of 'growth factor', since it stimulated mitosis and epidermal hypertrophy when injected subcutaneously into neonatal mice [33–35]. It was later isolated from human urine, saliva, breast milk, and amniotic fluid and, in 1975, it was the first true growth factor to be biochemically identified [36]. Pursuant to this discovery, the Nobel Prize for Physiology and Medicine was awarded to Rita Levi-Montalcini and Stanley Cohen in 1986 for the identification of nerve growth factor and epidermal growth factor.

Currently, platelet-derived growth factor (PDGF) is in practical use. One may expect that in the near future other cytokines will also become available for routine clinical purposes.

■ **Cell Senescence.** Recent research has focused on the field of cellular senescence, trying to identify the complex processes by which old cells gradually lose their proliferative capacity [37–40]. Cells from the margins and beds of chronic cutaneous ulcers become prematurely senescent [41, 42]. This topic is discussed in Chap. 2.

Research studies are currently focusing on this issue, trying to identify specific processes that lead to senescence. Identification of these processes may be followed by the development of new modes of treatment aimed at preventing senescence. These may be implemented in the field of wound repair.

3.10 Future Directions in Wound Healing

Since the 1980s, there has been a growing awareness and understanding of the subject of wound repair. A number of medical associations that specifically address the area wound healing have been established, such as the Wound Healing Society and The European Tissue Repair Society. Specialized journals are now published, such as *Wounds*, *The Journal of Wound Care*, *Advances in Wound Care*, and *Wound Repair and Regeneration*.

Future directions in this fascinating field may include the incorporation of further growth factors into clinical use and a better understanding of the conditions under which they should be utilized, e.g., the possible combination of certain growth factors and various skin substitutes, better matching and adaptation of various treatments to the etiology, healing phase, and clinical appearance of the wound.

We can also expect to have better ways to cope with infection. Moreover, the enormous progress now being made in gene therapy is opening new possibilities in the field of wound healing.

In certain respects, the significant progress in the field of wound healing is rapidly approaching the realm of science fiction. Figure 3.9 clearly illustrates this.

Fig. 3.9.
Processes of wound healing (From the book *'Dermatology: A Medical Artist's Interpretation'* by Geras AJ, 1990)

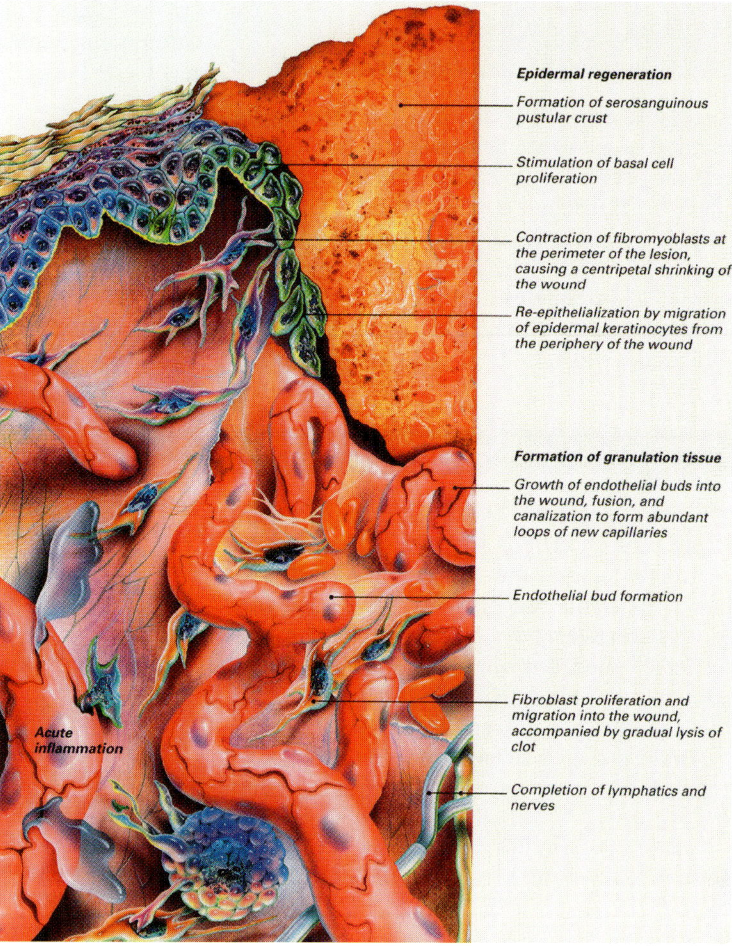

References

1. Scholz A: Historical aspects. In: Westerhof W (ed) Leg Ulcers – Diagnosis and Treatment, 1st edn. Amsterdam: Elsevier Science Publishers. 1993; pp 5–18
2. Quintal D, Jackson R: Leg ulcers: a historical perspective. Clin Dermatol 1990; 8 : 4–12
3. Caldwell MD: Topical wound therapy – an historical perspective. J Trauma 1990; 30 : S116–S122
4. The Iatros (Greece). In: Majno G: The Healing Hand. Man and Wound in the Ancient World, 2nd edn. Cambridge, Massachusetts: Harvard University Press. 1975; pp 141–205
5. Angeletti LR, Agrimi U, Curia C, et al: Healing rituals and sacred serpents. Lancet 1992; 340 : 223–225
6. The Asu (Mesopotamia). In: Majno G: The Healing Hand. Man and Wound in the Ancient World, 2nd edn. Cambridge, Massachusetts: Harvard University Press. 1975; pp 29–67
7. The Swnw (Egypt). In: Majno G: The Healing Hand. Man and Wound in the Ancient World, 2nd edn. Cambridge Massachusetts: Harvard University Press. 1975; pp 69–139
8. Witkowski JA, Parish LC: Cutaneous ulcer therapy. Int J Dermatol 1986; 25 : 420–426
9. Clendening L: Celsus. In: Clendening L. Source book of medical history. New York: Over Publications. 1960; pp 58–61
10. Ebbell B: The Ebers papyrus. The greatest Egyptian medical document. Oxford: Oxford University Press. 1937
11. Leaper DJ: History of wound healing. In: Leaper DJ, Harding KG (eds) Wounds: Biology and Management. New York: Oxford University Press. 1998; pp 5–9
12. The development of Surgery in France (continued) – Ambroise Paré. In: Buck AH: The Growth of Medicine. From the Earliest Times to About 1800. New Haven: Yale University Press. 1917; pp 499–515

13. Nuland SB: The enigma of Semmelweis – an interpretation. J Hist Med Allied Sci 1979; 34:255–272
14. Von Hebra F: Hochst wichtige Ehrfahrungen über die Aetiologie der Gebäranstalten epidemischen Puerperalfieber, KK. Ges Aerzte Wien 1847; 4:242–244
15. Semmelweis IP: Die Aetiologie, der Begriff und die Prophylaxis des Kindbettfiebers. Vienna and Leipzig,1861
16. Holmes OW: The contagiousness of puerperal fever – 1843. Medical Essays. Boston. 1895; pp 103–172
17. Lawrence G: Surgery (traditional). In: Bynum WF, Porter R (eds) Companion Encyclopedia of the History of Medicine. London New York: Routledge. 1993; vol 2, pp 961–983
18. Lyell A: Alexander Ogston, micrococci, and Joseph Lister. J Am Acad Dermatol 1989; 20:302–310
19. Godlee RJ: Lord Lister. 3rd edn. Oxford: Clarendon Press. 1924
20. Lister J: An address on the antiseptic management of wounds. Br Med J 1893; 1:161–162, 277–278, 337–339
21. Savin JA: Joseph Lister: a neglected master of investigative dermatology. Br J Dermatol 1995; 132:1003–1007
22. Wells TS: Some causes of excessive mortality after surgical operation. Medical Times and Gazette. October 1,1864; pp 349–352
23. Fleming A: On the antibacterial action of cultures of a penicillium with special reference to their use in the isolation of B. influenzae. Br J Exp Pathol 1929; 10:226–232
24. Chain E, Florey HW, Gardner AD, et al: Penicillin as a chemotherapeutic agent. Lancet 1940; 2:226–236
25. Fleming A: Streptococcal meningitis treated with penicillin. Lancet 1943; 2:434–438
26. Virchow R: Cellular Pathology. London: John Churchill. 1860; pp 283–315
27. Metchnikoff E: Immunity in Infective Diseases (translated by Binnie FG). London: Cambridge University Press. 1905
28. Gimbel NS, Kapetansky DI, Weissmen F, et al: A story of epithelization in blistered burns. Arch Surg 1957; 74:800–803
29. Winter GD: Formation of the scab and the rate of epithelization of superficial wounds in the skin of the young domestic pig. Nature 1962; 193:293–294
30. Hinman CD, Maibach H: Effect of air exposure and occlusion on experimental human skin wounds. Nature 1963; 200:377–378
31. Rheinwald JG, Green H: Serial cultivation of strains of human epidermal keratinocytes: The formation of keratinizing colonies from single cells. Cell 1975; 6:331–343
32. Cohen S: Isolation of a mouse submaxillary gland protein accelerating incisor eruption and eyelid opening in the new-born animal. J Biol Chem 1962; 237:1555–1562
33. Carpenter G, Cohen S: Epidermal growth factor. J Biol Chem 1990; 265:7709–7712
34. Cohen S, Taylor JM: Epidermal growth factor: Chemical and biological characterization. In: Maibach HI, Rovee DT (eds): Epidermal Wound Healing. Chicago: Year Book Medical Publishers, Inc. 1972; pp 203–218
35. Tranuzzer RW, Macauley SP, Mast BA, et al: Epidermal growth factor in wound healing: A model for the molecular pathogenesis of chronic wounds. In: Ziegler TR, Pierce GF, Herndon DN (eds) Growth Factors and Wound Healing. Berlin Heidelberg New York: Springer. 1997. pp 206–228
36. Starkey RH, Cohen S, Orth DN: Epidermal growth factor: Identification of a new hormone in human urine. Science 1975; 189:800–802
37. Martin GM, Sprague CA, Epstein CJ: Replicative life span of cultivated human cells. Effects of donor age, tissue and genotype. Lab Invest 1970; 23:86–92
38. Schneider EL, Mitsui Y: The relationship between *in vitro* cellular aging and *in vivo* human age. Proc Natl Acad Sci USA 1976; 73:3584–3588
39. Schneider EL, Epstein CJ: Replication rate and life span of cultured fibroblasts in Down's syndrome. Proc Soc Exp Biol Med 1972; 141:1092–1094
40. Elmore E, Swift M: Growth of cultured cells from patients with ataxia-telangiectasia. J Cell Physiol 1976; 89:429 431
41. Mendez MV, Stanley A, Park HY, et al: Fibroblasts cultured from venous ulcers display cellular characteristics of senescence. J Vasc Surg 1998; 28:876–883
42. Vande-Berg JS, Rudolph R, Hollan C, et al: Fibroblast senescence in pressure ulcers. Wound Repair Regen 1998; 6:38–49

Etiology and Mechanisms of Cutaneous Ulcer Formation

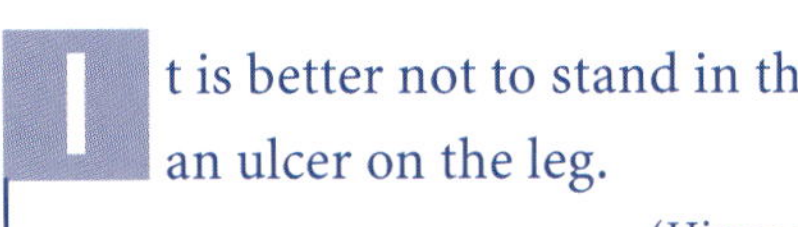

I t is better not to stand in the case of
an ulcer on the leg.

(Hippocrates)

Contents

4.1 Overview: Etiologies of Cutaneous Ulcers

Identifying the cause of a cutaneous ulcer is often a multi-staged, challenging process. Not infrequently, it requires considerable expertise in general medicine as well as in dermatology and a thorough laboratory investigation. This chapter, together with Chaps. 5 and 6, reviews etiologies of skin ulcers and discusses the basic processes underlying these mechanisms.

It is a well-known axiom in medicine that things do not always turn out to be as they first appear. A cutaneous ulcer that seems to result from venous insufficiency may, following thorough investigation, turn out to be a manifestation of carcinoma or the outcome of an occult infectious process. In some cases, the underlying disease is rare, requiring considerable clinical experience for its identification.

Etiologies of cutaneous ulcers are presented in Table 4.1. Note that in many patients, there are several co-existing etiologies. Moreover, in certain conditions, such as venous insufficiency, lymphedema, peripheral arterial disease, or diabetes, the skin is much more vulnerable. In these cases, development of a cutaneous ulcer is not necessarily 'spontaneous' – the skin tends to ulcerate following various triggers such as penetrating injury, blunt trauma, or contact dermatitis. One should distinguish between underlying conditions that gradually affect the quality of the skin and actual triggers that result directly in ulceration [1].

4.2 Mechanisms of Ulcer Formation

As Table 4.1 indicates, there is a wide array of possible etiologies of cutaneous ulcers. However, in many cases, it is not sufficient to merely 'label' or classify an ulcer as being caused by a specific disease. In a given disease, or for any given 'etiology', the ulcer may be formed by a series of complex mechanisms. Hence, the exact mechanism by which the ulcer was formed should also be considered.

One may assume that the main mechanism of ulceration in an infectious process is a direct

Table 4.1. Etiologies of cutaneous ulcers

Following injury

Trauma (including self-inflicted ulcers)
Burns
Injection sites (e.g., heroin, cocaine, steroids)
Severe contact dermatitis (e.g., chrome ulcers)
Cold exposure: frostbite; chillblain (perniosis); Raynaud's phenomenon
Radiation dermatitis
Bites (spider, scorpion, snake)

Pressure ulcers (presented here as a model of ongoing injury)

Infections

Bacterial

In the course of bullous erysipelas (or cellulitis)
Necrotising fasciitis
Skin over a bone affected by osteomyelitis

Ecthyma
Ecthyma gangrenosum

Meleney's ulcer (progressive bacterial synergistic gangrene)

Noma (chancrum oris)
Tropical ulcer (tropical sloughing phagedena)

Mycobacterial
    Tuberculosis (M. tuberculosis)
    Swimming pool granuloma (M. marinum)
    Buruli ulcer (M. ulcerans)

Leprosy (M. leprae)

Spirochetal
    Syphilis
    Yaws

Tularemia (Francisella tularensis)
Anthrax (Bacillus anthracis)

Viral

Herpes genitalis
CMV
Ecthymatous varicella zoster

Fungal

Deep fungal infections

Protozoal

Leishmaniasis

Venereal ulcers

Syphilis
Chancroid
Lymphogranuloma venereum
Granuloma inguinale
Herpes genitalis

Table 4.1. Etiologies of cutaneous ulcers *(Continued)*

Vascular

Venous

Arterial
Peripheral arterial disease
Thromboangiitis obliterans (Buerger's disease)
Embolus: atheromatous,
                cholesterol,
                cardiac origin

Lymphedema

Vasculitis

Leukocytoclastic vasculitis
Nodular vasculitis (erythema induratum)
Serum sickness
Cryoglobulinemia (mixed, type II & III)
Erythema elevatum diutinum

Connective tissue/multisystem diseases

Rheumatoid arthritis
Systemic lupus erythematosus
Dermatomyositis
Polyarteritis nodosa
Wegener's granulomatosis
Churg-Strauss syndrome
Systemic sclerosis
Behçet's disease
Sjögren's syndrome
Temporal arteritis
Takayasu disease

Anti phospholipid syndrome

Dysproteinemias

Cryoglubulinemia (monoclonal, type 1)
Cryofibrinogemia
Waldenstrom's macroglubulinemia

Hypercoagulable states

Coumarin-induced necrosis
Heparin necrosis
Disseminated intravascular coagulation
Purpura fulminans

Protein C deficiency
Activated protein C resistance
Protein S deficiency
Anti-thrombin III deficiency
Hyperhomocystinemia

Table 4.1. Etiologies of cutaneous ulcers *(Continued)*

Hematologic abnormalities

Hemolytic anemia

Hemoglobinopathies
   Sickle cell anemia
   Thalassemia

Hereditary spherocytosis
Pyruvate kinase deficiency
Paroxysmal nocturnal hemoglobinuria

Myeloproliferative diseases

   Polycythemia vera
   Essential thrombocytosis

Tumoral/malignant diseases

Lymphoproliferative diseases

B-cell lymphoma
Mycosis fungoides

Leukemia

Acute and chronic leukemia

Epithelial tumors

Basal cell carcinoma
Squamous cell carcinoma
Keratoacanthoma

Other epidermal tumors

Malignant melanoma
Merkel cell carcinoma
Tumors of skin appendages
   (i.e., sebaceous carcinoma)

Lymph vessel/Vascular tumors

Hemangioma
Lymphangioma

Sarcomas

Kaposi's sarcoma and other sarcomatous tumors

Other soft tissue tumors

Histiocytosis syndromes
Malignant peripheral nerve tumors

Other tumors (non-cutaneous) that may affect skin

By direct invasion into the skin
Skin metastases originating from an internal malignant tumor

Table 4.1. Etiologies of cutaneous ulcers *(Continued)*

Neuropathic ulcers

Diabetes mellitus
Leprosy
Tabes dorsalis
Syringomyelia
Poliomyelitis
Hereditary peripheral sensory neuropathy type 4 (insensitivity to pain)

Metabolic disorders

Diabetes mellitus
Prolidase deficiency
Calciphylaxis

Ulcerating panniculitis

Pancreatic fat necrosis
Weber-Christian disease
Histiocytic cytophagic panniculitis
α 1 anti-trypsin deficiency panniculitis
Nodular vasculitis

Nutritional disorders

Noma (chancrum oris)
Tropical ulcer (Tropical sloughing phagedena)
Vitamin C deficiency

Others

Pyoderma gangrenosum

Metastatic Crohn's disease

Necrobiosis lipoidica diabeticorum

Atrophie blanche

Kawasaki syndrome

Klinefelter's syndrome

Insect infestation

Drugs

Drugs that induce ulceration directly

Drugs that interfere with normal mechanisms of wound healing

Drugs that adversely affect the quality of the skin

       (detailed in chapter 16)

toxic effect and its subsequent abnormal local inflammatory processes [2, 3]. However, some infectious diseases may result in ulcers by other mechanisms. For example, hepatitis B may induce leukocytoclastic vasculitis, cryoglobulinemia, or periarteritis nodosa, all of which may lead to the development of cutaneous ulcers. Moreover, in certain infectious diseases such as syphilis, tuberculosis, and leprosy, there are unique pathways by which cutaneous ulcers may appear, as detailed below.

Similarly, several pathways may lead to ulceration in connective-tissue diseases. Ulcers may be caused by vasculitis, Raynaud's phenomenon, secondary anti-phospholipid syndrome, or other mechanisms, as discussed below.

4.3 Mechanisms of Formation of Specific Types of Cutaneous Ulcers

Since the subject of cutaneous ulcer formation is extensive, this section limits the discussion to the mechanisms of formation in certain types of cutaneous ulcers, with reference to the data presented in the table above. We shall concentrate here on those topics particularly important for establishing an etiologic diagnosis clinically.

4.3.1 Ulceration Following Injury/ External Damage to the Skin

4.3.1.1 Trauma and Ulcers

Mechanical trauma or some other injury may result in a cutaneous ulcer. In some cases, the external trauma may be minor. Although the patient may consider it to be the cause of the ulcer, the skin may have been previously affected by some underlying process (e.g., deep fungal infection or malignancy) which may well be the actual cause of the ulcer and should be identified.

Note that a skin injury may become a portal of entry for bacterial or fungal infection, with subsequent ulceration. Even a superficial erosion due to trauma may become an ulcer following bacterial infection. The chances of this occurring are much higher when there is an underlying problem such as diabetes or peripheral arterial disease.

■ **Self-Inflicted Ulcers.** In most cases, self-inflicted ulcers are induced by continuous scratching, rubbing, or cutting of the skin. Once an ulcer exists, the continuing 'fiddling' with it by the patient interferes with its normal healing process.

The clinical appearance of such ulcers depends on the way in which they were created. For example, they may present sharp angular borders as a result of the device or instrument that was used. In some cases, self-inflicted ulcers are induced by injecting foreign material into the skin. This issue is discussed in Chap. 16.

4.3.1.2 Contact Dermatitis

Patients with leg ulcers often suffer from contact dermatitis. Leg ulceration has been reported following exposure to numerous topical preparations applied to cutaneous ulcers such as topical antibiotics, certain vehicles (e.g., lanolin), or preservatives [4–6]. In these patients, the application of such preparations may significantly aggravate the ulcers. Be aware of this possibility; topical treatment should be re-evaluated and patch tests performed when needed. Moreover, skin areas affected by contact dermatitis may be secondarily infected, with the subsequent formation of cutaneous ulcers.

In addition, the following should be noted with regard to cutaneous ulcers and contact dermatitis:
- A few substances such as chromates [7, 8] or sodium silicate [9] are well-known inducers of contact dermatitis. They have a highly irritant and corrosive effect, and patients may present with severe dermatitis characterized by the appearance of cutaneous ulcers. Skin ulceration has al-

so been documented following the use of povidone iodine [10].

- The scrotal skin is highly vulnerable. Certain topical preparations that would not normally cause contact dermatitis elsewhere may induce severe irritant contact dermatitis with ulceration when applied to the scrotal skin [11].
- Jacquet's erosive diaper dermatitis has been attributed to the presence of various chemicals used in home diapering. This problem is much less common these days due to the widespread use of disposable diapers [12].

4.3.1.3 Pressure Ulcers

Pressure ulcers are presented here as a model of continuous injury. The prevalence of pressure ulcers varies from population to population. Elderly patients, or patients who are bed-ridden or bound to a wheelchair, are particularly prone to pressure ulcers. They may occur in an immobilized or bed-ridden patient of any age [13–15]. For example, among patients admitted to hospital following spinal cord injury, the prevalence, 1 5 years after the initial injury, is between 20% and 30% [16].

Two other commonly accepted terms for pressure ulcers are 'pressure sores' and 'decubitus ulcers'.

■ **Mechanism of Formation.** Local pressure on the affected site is the most important etiologic factor, with the degree of pressure and its duration being the most significant variables [14, 17]. Pressure ulcers tend to develop in areas where soft tissues are compressed for prolonged periods between a bony prominence and any external object, but they may also evolve over any cutaneous region that is exposed to continuous pressure. Pressures exceeding normal capillary pressure result in reduced oxygenation and impair the microcircu-

lation of the affected tissue. Garfin et al. [18] determined that 30 mmHg was the critical value for ischemia. However, high pressures of 70 mmHg or more, which may occur when a patient lies on a standard hospital mattress, may induce tissue death within a few hours [14, 19–21]. Most of the potential damage may be prevented by relieving the pressure intermittently [22, 23]. Therefore, prolonged immobilization is a significant risk factor [24, 25]. This emphasizes the importance of frequently moving and repositioning immobilized patients in order to prevent the formation of pressure ulcers.

Apart from pressure, there are other mechanical factors such as shearing forces and friction which may enhance ulceration [14, 26–29]. Significant topical factors include excessive moisture and exposure to irritant substances. Both the general condition and nutritional status of the patient play a major role in the formation of pressure ulcers.

■ **Location.** More than 90% of pressure ulcers appear on the lower parts of the body – 65% in the pelvic region and 30% on the lower legs. Heels and malleoli are also frequently affected [14, 30].

■ **Clinical Appearance.** The clinical appearance of a pressure ulcer depends on its severity. Several gradation scales have been proposed. A commonly accepted system was developed in the USA in 1987 by The National Pressure Ulcer Advisory Panel (NPUAP) (see Chap. 1) [31].

Pressure ulcers are characterized by peripheral undermining. At any stage, the initial impression of the depth of a pressure ulcer may be misleading and the ulceration of the tissue may be much deeper and more extensive than originally thought.

4.3.2 Infections

Mild injuries may be aggravated when they become secondarily infected by bacteria such as *Staphylococci* or *Streptococci*. In some cases, an ulcer caused by a relatively minor trauma may become deeper as a result of infection.

As described below, legs affected by venous insufficiency, peripheral arterial disease, or diabetes are at a particularly high risk of developing ulcers following trivial trauma, which may be associated with infection. By the same token, erosions of bullous diseases may deepen in the case of a secondary infection, resulting in the formation of cutaneous ulcers. We discuss below classical examples of cutaneous infectious processes: cellulitis, necrotizing fasciitis, and ecthyma.

4.3.2.1 Erysipelas and Cellulitis

Erysipelas and cellulitis may cause leg ulcers. The main mechanism of ulcer formation in these cases is the direct effect of bacterial toxins. Presumably, the associated edema also interferes with lymphatic and venous return and further contributes to the ulceration.

Approximately 3% of bullous erysipelas may result in ulceration [32] (Fig. 4.1). Other (less frequent) cases of ulceration in erysipelas or cellulitis are due to abscess formation, or concomitant trauma. Note that cellulitis or erysipelas can be associated with a pre-existing ulcer.

Repeated episodes of cellulitis or erysipelas cause cumulative tissue damage, which almost certainly further compromises lymphatic and venous return. Following an episode of cellulitis there is some degree of damage to the limb

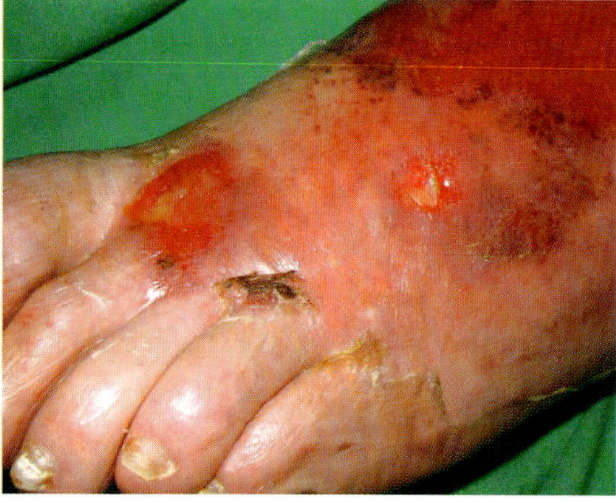

Fig. 4.1. Bullous erysipelas with erosions. In many cases, chronic leg ulcers may evolve

tissue, which increases the likelihood of recurrent local infection.

4.3.2.2 Necrotizing Fasciitis

Necrotizing fasciitis is an extreme example of an ulcerative process caused by bacterial infection. It is defined as a deep-seated infection of the subcutaneous tissue, causing invasive destruction of the fascia and subcutaneous fat, with or without overlying cellulitis [33]. In cases where the genitalia are involved, the preferred term is Fournier's gangrene.

In the past two decades there has been a noticeable increase in reports of invasive group A streptococcal infections, leading to necrotizing fasciitis. Other types of bacteria, such as *Clostridium perfringes* or *Clostridium septicum*, may also cause necrotizing fasciitis. In addition, it may be caused by a synergistic combination of organisms such as anaerobes with aerobic gram-negative bacteria. Mixed infections tend to occur in children, in diabetic patients, or in patients with an open wound exposed to bowel content [34, 35].

The course of necrotizing fasciitis is extremely severe, frequently with a fatal outcome. This quality has earned it the science-fiction-like name, 'flesh-eating bacterium'. It can occur in normally healthy people, sometimes following a relatively minor trauma. A high incidence of necrotizing fasciitis has been reported in people with diabetes, malnutrition, obesity, and malignancy, and in drug addicts [36, 37].

Its severe pathogenicity is attributed to bacterial toxins such as exotoxin A in the case of group A Streptococcus. Delay in the diagnosis or treatment of this disease can have fatal consequences. It requires radical debridement, high-dose antibiotic therapy, and intensive supportive care.

In view of the unique, severe character of this condition, it may be regarded as a separate category, different from the various types of cutaneous ulcers described in this chapter. However, even after the invasive process has been arrested, it may leave a residue of chronic, difficult-to-heal ulcers.

4.3.2.3 Ecthyma

Ecthyma (Fig. 4.2) is a classic example of an ulcer caused by *Streptococcal* toxins (*Staphylococci* may also be identified within a lesion). Such a lesion begins as a vesicle or a pustule that undergoes ulceration. It occurs most commonly on the lower extremities. Ecthyma usually occurs following minor trauma in children or elderly people under poor hygienic conditions. It is frequent in warm, moist, tropical regions [38].

In other infectious diseases and pathologic processes the mechanisms of ulcer formation are more complex. As described below, ulcers may develop in certain specific or unique forms of certain diseases.

4.3.2.4 Syphilis

Apart from the primary chancre (detailed in the section 'Venereal Ulcers' in Chap. 5), other types of ulcerated lesions may evolve in the course of syphilis:

- Ulcerated skin lesions may occur in the nodulo-ulcerative type of late/tertiary syphilis. Syphilitic gummata, appearing as pink/red painless nodules in late/tertiary syphilis, may also undergo ulceration [39, 40].
- In addition, cutaneous ulcers may appear in 'malignant' syphilis (*lues maligna, rupial syphilid*) in the context of secondary syphilis. Typical papulopustules, located mainly on the face and scalp, gradually become necrotic, with subsequent formation of 'rupioid' ulcers. The adjective 'rupioid' is derived from the appearance of the crusts that cover the ulcers, which are thick and dark in color and resemble an oyster shell [39, 41]. Recently, cases of malignant syphilids have been reported in HIV patients [42].

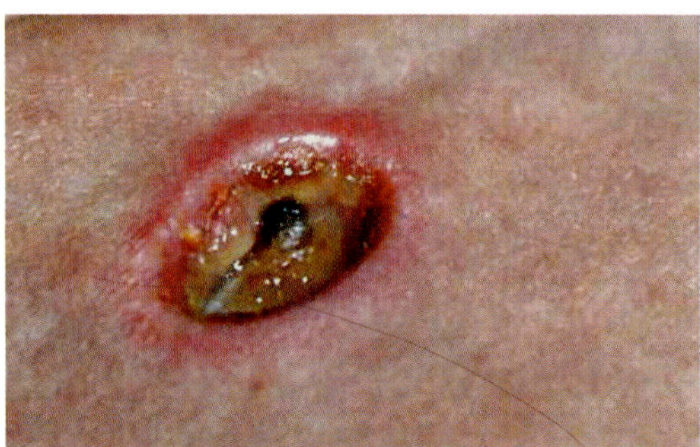

Fig. 4.2. Ecthyma

4.3.2.5 Tuberculosis

Ulcers may occur in several types of tuberculosis:

- Lupus vulgaris: Plaques of lupus vulgaris may ulcerate. Most commonly, the lesions appear in the head and neck region, i.e., on the nose, cheeks, and earlobes. Ulcerative and mutilating forms of lupus vulgaris are characterized by ulceration that may be severely invasive [43].
- Tuberculous chancre: This may appear as a ragged ulcer with undermined margins [43].
- Scrofuloderma: The lesion begins as a bluish-red nodule that may ulcerate. It is situated over an infected lymph node or over an infected joint.
- Papulo-necrotic tuberculid: In this form, symmetrically distributed reddish papules, usually located on the extensor regions of the extremities, back, and buttocks, may break down and form ulcers.
- Tuberculous gumma: In this form of tuberculosis, also called 'metastatic tuberculous abscess', a subcutaneous nodule may ulcerate. Lesions may occur in malnourished children [43, 44]
- Miliary tuberculosis: Lesions of miliary tuberculosis may ulcerate [43, 45].

4.3.2.6 Leprosy

The classical form of ulcers in leprosy is the 'neuropathic ulcer'. Infiltration of peripheral nerves of the lower limbs by *Mycobacterium leprae* is followed by the development of cutaneous ulcers due to sensory and motor neuropathy. The former results in anesthesia of the sole with subsequent loss of protective sensation, while the latter leads to difficulty in activating certain muscle groups and to inadequate distribution of pressure on the sole while walking [46–50].

In addition, cutaneous nodules infiltrated by the bacteria may ulcerate. This occurs more often in areas exposed to trauma.

One should identify other conditions that may develop in the course of leprosy, where cutaneous ulcers may develop:
- Lesions of **erythema nodosum leprosum** may ulcerate [51, 52].
- A relatively rare complication of diffuse lepromatous leprosy is known as **'Lucio's phenomenon'**. This is a cutaneous vasculitis manifested by the appearance of pink-to-red plaques, located mainly on the buttocks and lower limbs, which may undergo severe ulceration [51, 53, 54].

4.3.2.7 Infections in Immuno-compromised Patients

In immune deficiency states, organisms which usually do not cause ulceration may result in the development of ulcerated lesions:
- In HIV patients, varicella infection may result in ecthymatous varicella zoster.
- Perianal ulcerated lesions have been documented in immunocompromised patients due to the herpes virus or CMV [55, 56] (Fig. 4.3).
- Ecthyma gangrenosum is a typical lesion appearing in immunocomprom-

ised patients (Fig. 4.4). It begins as a hemorrhagic vesicle or pustule that undergoes ulceration. In more than 80% of cases, it occurs in the perineal region or on the extremities. Ecthyma gangrenosum lesions are usually caused by *Pseudomonas*. However, *Klebsiella* and other bacteria have also been isolated. It may occur in the course of bacteremia, when it is considered to be a marker of poor prognosis [57].
- Fungal infections tend to be more aggressive in immunocompromised patients [58]. In rare cases, atypical fungal ulcerating lesions have been documented in patients with no known immune system disorder [59, 60].

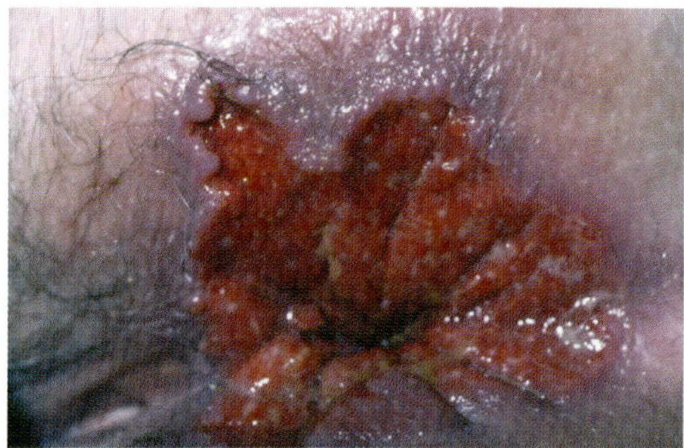

Fig. 4.3. Perianal ulceration in a leukemic patient; herpes virus was cultured from the lesion

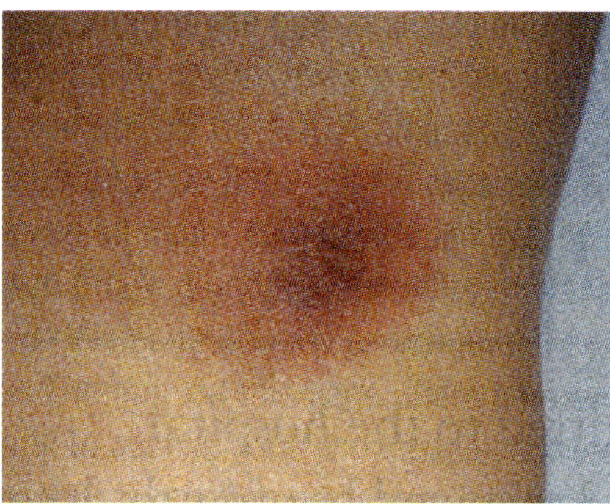

Fig. 4.4. Ecthyma gangrenosum, initial lesion

4.3.3 Vascular Disease

4.3.3.1 Venous Ulcers

Around 70% of leg ulcers are venous in origin [61–63] (Fig. 4.5). Older sources of data may present a higher percentage. However, in modern medicine, the prevalence of venous ulcers is declining. This is attributed to the higher standards of medical care currently practiced. The significance of compression therapy is well recognized nowadays; the use of low-molecular-weight heparins prevents venous thromboembolism in high-risk situations. In addition, vein surgery has become minimally invasive. Venous insufficiency may coexist with peripheral arterial disease in 10–15% of patients with leg ulcers [63, 64]. In many cases, the direct trigger for ulceration is some external physical injury [1, 65]. Whereas in a healthy person mild injury does not cause significant damage, in patients with venous insufficiency the skin runs a much higher risk of developing ulceration.

Histologically, microvessels in areas subjected to chronic venous hypertension become dilated and coiled; i.e., they have a glomerular appearance in intravital capillaroscopy. In the advanced disease, the number of functioning, perfused capillaries is markedly reduced [66–69]. The severity of cutaneous microangiopathy has been found to correlate closely to the development of clinical cutaneous trophic changes [66, 70].

■ **Mechanisms of Formation.** At present, the exact mechanism leading to the histologic picture and tissue damage in venous insufficiency remains uncertain. Nevertheless, in recent years we have acquired an increased understanding of certain physiological mechanisms involved in this process.

In chronic venous insufficiency, the venous pressure (or venous hypertension) in the deep venous system may be transmitted to the superficial system. Partsch [71] suggested that venous insufficiency is characterized by peaks of pressure occurring with every muscle contraction and transmitted to the capillary network. It is suggested that these pressure peaks have a progressive, gradual, destructive effect on the capillaries in the skin and subcutaneous tissues [72–74].

In addition, leakage of fluids from within the capillaries into the interstitium of the dermis and subcutaneous tissues results in edema. Whatever the mechanisms leading to edema, edema in itself has been shown to affect the quality of the skin. It induces sclerotic changes in subcutaneous tissue, with consequent interference of metabolic and gas exchange [75]. Moreover, due to the presence of edema, lymphatic vessels and their valves are subjected to fibrotic changes, with a further reduction in normal lymphatic function and drainage of the tissues, which sets up a vicious cycle of edema [76, 77].

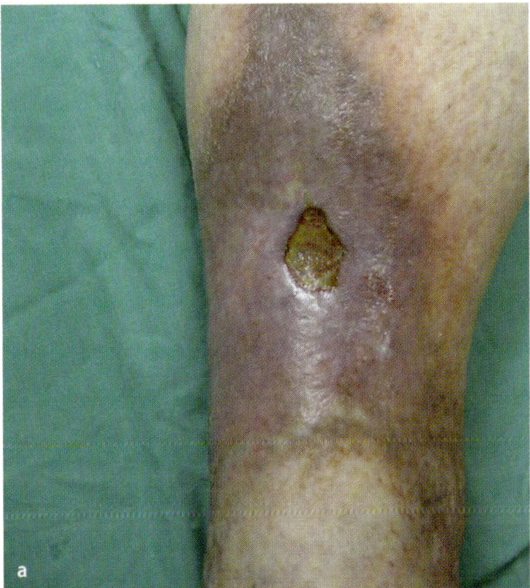

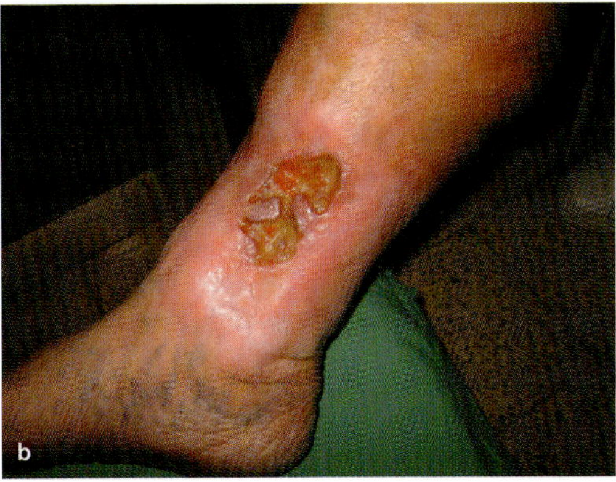

Fig. 4.5 a, b. Venous ulcers. a. Brown pigmentation of stasis dermatitis around the ulcer. b. Lipodermatosclerotic leg; varicosities are seen in the medial area of the foot

Endothelial damage, therefore, is the result of edema with subsequent impaired oxygenation and interference of metabolic activity (and, perhaps, peaks of venous pressure). Intercellular adhesion molecules seem to play a significant role in the pathologic process, as reflected by their expression on endothelial cells [78–81]. This process is followed by endothelial-leukocyte adhesion and the trapping of white cells within the capillaries. Loss of endothelial integrity, together with the increasing presence of white blood cells, may lead to the destruction of adjacent tissue, protracted inflammation, and fibrosis [82–86].

In addition to the above, numerous hypotheses have been put forward to explain the exact mechanism of skin damage and the development of ulceration in the presence of venous insufficiency.

Two presented below are worth mentioning:
- Pericapillary fibrin cuffs are a prominent histological feature of venous insufficiency. In 1982, Browse and Burnard [87, 88] suggested that venous hypertension, transmitted to the capillary network, results in the distention of capillary walls and the widening of capillary pores. Subsequently, fibrinogen molecules leak into the extracellular fluid, forming complexes of fibrin around the capillaries. The pericapillary fibrin layer is claimed to form a mechanical barrier, which prevents the transfer of oxygen and nutrients, leading to progressive damage to the skin and subcutaneous tissues. However, other researchers have indicated that the fibrin cuffs do not function as a barrier for oxygen transport [89]. If so, these cuffs only seem to reflect abnormal microcirculation with transmural deposition of plasmatic macromolecules.

- Falanga and Eaglstein [90] have suggested that growth factors may be trapped by certain macromolecules leaking through the capillary pores into the dermis. Therefore, growth factors are unable to participate and function in the processes of tissue repair.

■ **Location.** The above discussion may help to explain the distribution of venous ulcers. Since venous pressure and the subsequent detrimental effect on tissue is maximal distally, venous ulcers tend to occur in the lower calf. The medial malleolus is more commonly affected than the lateral. This finding is attributed to the anatomy of the venous system, in which a larger mass of venous vessels is located medially. Therefore, the medial aspects of the legs are subjected to higher venous pressures. Nevertheless, not infrequently these ulcers may appear above the lateral malleolus as well [91]. Lateral venous ulcers usually reflect the presence of an incompetent lesser saphenous vein, with or without deep venous insufficiency. Other characteristics of venous ulcers are detailed in Chap. 5.

4.3.3.2 Ulcers in Peripheral Arterial Disease

Most patients with peripheral arterial disease are over the age of 70. In contrast to venous ulcers, arterial ulcers are increasing in number. People live longer nowadays, and peripheral arterial disease is becoming more prevalent. Arterial ulcers are estimated to constitute about 10% of leg ulcers [64]. Mixed ulcers, of arterial and venous disease, are said to affect approximately 10–15% of patients with leg ulcers [63, 64].

■ **Mechanisms of Formation.** In many cases, so-called 'arterial' ulcers develop following physical trauma [65]. The trauma may be minor, but it affects vulnerable, poorly vascular-

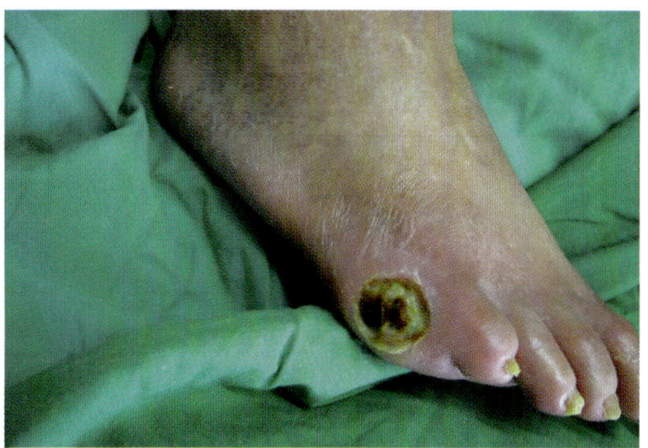

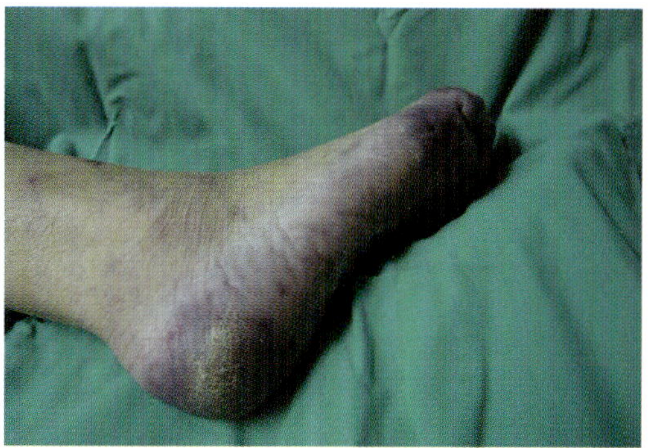

Fig. 4.6. An ulcer in peripheral arterial disease

Fig. 4.7. Arterial occlusion with significant ischemia, pending ulceration

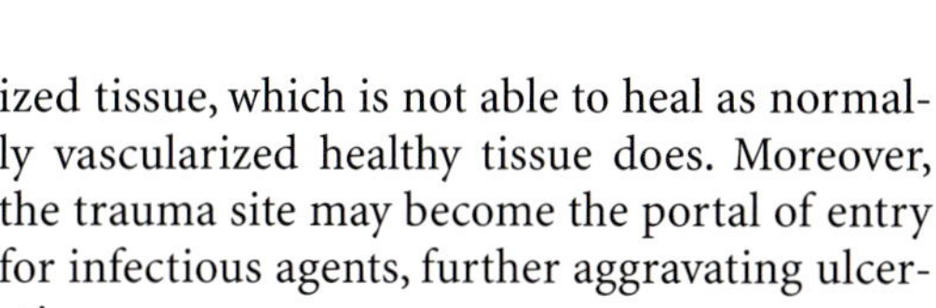

ized tissue, which is not able to heal as normally vascularized healthy tissue does. Moreover, the trauma site may become the portal of entry for infectious agents, further aggravating ulceration.

In other cases, arterial ulcers may appear without trauma, when critical limb ischemia has developed. Beyond a certain degree of ischemia, there is a complex chain of events that may end in necrosis.

The definition of critical limb ischemia, according to the Trans-Atlantic Inter-Society Consensus Document on the Management of Peripheral Arterial Disease (The TASC Working Group 2000), is based on a patient having chronic ischemic rest pain, ulcers, or gangrene attributable to objectively proven arterial occlusive disease [92, 93]. The suggested inclusion criteria in TASC for critical leg ischemia were absolute ankle pressure below 50–70 mmHg or reduced toe pressure (<30–50 mmHg).

Atherosclerosis of large arteries is the fundamental process in the pathogenesis of chronic critical limb ischemia. It results in occlusion or severe narrowing of vessels, with subsequent reduction of blood flow and decreased perfusion to distal regions. Other parameters such as low blood pressure or the presence of anemia may influence the degree of ischemia, and hence the likelihood of progression to necrosis.

■ **Location.** Since a high percentage of arterial ulcers are caused by trauma, arterial ulceration (above the threshold of critical limb ischemia)

may develop anywhere on the lower calves. Ulcers tend to appear in the lateral or pretibial area of the leg or on the dorsum of the foot (Fig. 4.6). Note that they may appear in the malleolar region as well.

If critical limb ischemia has developed, it may be manifested by distal necrosis of the toes or forefoot (Fig. 4.7). This condition has a poor prognosis, and amputation may be required. The dorsum of the feet and heels may be affected as well.

Other characteristics of arterial ulcers are detailed in Chap. 5.

4.3.3.3 Peripheral Arterial Disease and Hypertensive Ulcers

Hypertensive ulcers were described by Martorell in 1945 as ulcers located in the pretibial or lateral area of the leg. These ulcers were said to occur mainly in hypertensive women above the age of 60 [94]. Some suggest that the so-called Martorell's ulcer represents a special variant of an arterial leg ulcer, which should not be regarded as a separate entity. Others doubt the validity of this clinical term, based on nonspecific histologic features in leg ulcers clinically diagnosed as 'Martorell's ulcers' [95, 96]. In any case, the elderly population is prone to developing hypertension, as well as atherosclerotic changes within blood vessels.

4.3.3.4 Embolus

An acute, rapid development of limb ischemia is caused by emboli. An atheromatous plaque that becomes detached from a blood vessel wall is a relatively large embolus that occludes a large vessel and generally affects a specific anatomic region. Cholesterol emboli, on the other hand, are microemboli composed of cholesterol crystals, 100–200 μm, which may occlude many small arteries with the induction of multiple lesions [97, 98].

4.3.4 Leukocytoclastic Vasculitis

Note that leukocytoclastic vasculitis may be induced by several types of infections, most commonly *Streptococcus group A*, *Mycobacterium leprae*, and the hepatitis B and C virus [99]. Sometimes leukocytoclastic vasculitis may appear following the use of certain drugs (see Chap. 16).

4.3.5 Connective Tissue and Multisystem Diseases

Cutaneous ulcers appear in connective tissue diseases and multisystem diseases. A classical example is systemic lupus erythematosus (SLE), which may present in several forms. In most cases, ulcers in connective tissue diseases are attributed to vasculitis. For example, the incidence of cutaneous ulcers in idiopathic SLE patients is about 5%. The ulcers are usually located in malleolar or pretibial areas [100, 101] due to the vasculitic process. Vasculitis may also result in gangrene of the finger tips. However, SLE may also lead to a secondary form of anti-phospholipid syndrome with the subsequent development of cutaneous ulcers. Similarly, the presence of cryoglobulins in SLE may lead to the formation of cutaneous ulcers located in the extremities.

In rheumatoid arthritis, various forms of cutaneous ulcers may be seen: leg ulcers or digital necrosis, due to the vasculitic process, similar to those of SLE; ulceration of subcutaneous nodules; and pyoderma gangrenosum, which may be found in rheumatoid arthritis. Prolonged glucocorticoid therapy may be detrimental to the quality of the skin in these cases, thus further hindering the repair of cutaneous ulcers.

Vasculitic involvement may induce ulceration in other connective tissue diseases, such as dermatomyositis, Sjögren's syndrome, or scleroderma. However, there may be other reasons for ulceration in connective tissue disease. For example, Raynaud's phenomenon, which may be associated with connective tissue diseases, may result in digital ulceration. Similarly, the gradual damage to the quality of the skin in scleroderma predisposes to ulceration.

4.3.6 Hypercoagulable States

Some of the 'hypercoagulable' conditions listed in Table 4.1, such as coumadin-induced necrosis, heparin necrosis, or disseminated intravascular coagulation, are characterized by the development of micro-thrombi [102]. The histologic hallmark of these cases is the presence of fibrin thrombi (see Chap. 6). The occlusion of blood vessels by fibrin thrombi may manifest clinically as cutaneous ulceration.

Other conditions listed in Table 4.1, i.e., protein C deficiency, activated protein C resistance, protein S deficiency, and anti-thrombin III deficiency, classified under the heading 'thrombophilia', may lead to vascular thrombosis. In many cases, the mechanism leading to ulceration is not direct. Thrombophilia may result in deep vein thrombosis which, in itself, predisposes to chronic venous ulceration [103, 104]. However, fibrin thrombi have been described in such cases as well [105]. Most of these cases have been associated with coumadin or heparin therapy.

Conditions such as hyperhomocystinemia have been implicated in the formation of deep venous thrombosis with the subsequent development of venous ulcers [106]. To the best of our knowledge, it has never been described in the literature as having directly caused a cutaneous ulcer through the formation of fibrin thrombi.

4.3.7 Metabolic Disorders: Diabetes Mellitus

Diabetic ulcers are included in Table 4.1 under the term 'metabolic ulcers'. The metabolic abnormalities in diabetes may lead to the formation of ulcers by several mechanisms, as detailed below.

4.3.7.1 Peripheral Arterial Disease and Atherosclerosis (Macroangiopathy)

Peripheral vascular disease is more common in people with diabetes than in the rest of the population. In the presence of additional risk factors such as smoking, hyperlipidemia, or hypertension, the incidence is even higher.

The prevalence of peripheral arterial disease in diabetic patients is between 20% and 40%, and it is regarded as a sign of premature aging of blood vessels [107–109]. A distinguishing feature of diabetes is that the ulcers tend to occur more distally than they do in non-diabetic patients with peripheral arterial disease [110].

Diabetic ulcers due to peripheral arterial disease may therefore appear anywhere on the lower calves, usually on the lateral or pretibial aspect of the leg, dorsum of the foot, or malleolar region. As in peripheral arterial disease, necrosis of a distal toe or foot may develop if there is severe ischemia of a diabetic limb. In advanced cases, widespread calcification may develop along the length of the media of the arterial wall. Hence, Doppler measurement of ankle blood pressure (and consequently ABI measurement) may indicate high pressures, which does not accurately reflect the true degree of ischemia of the limb [110, 111].

4.3.7.2 Neuropathy

Neuropathy in diabetes affects sensory, motor, and autonomic fibers. It is estimated that almost 30% of type-2 diabetic patients have neuropathy, while it affects 50% of patients over the age of 60 years [112]. Ulceration of the soles of diabetic patients is, in most cases, attributed to neuropathy [113, 114].

The detrimental effects of sensory, motor, and autonomic neuropathy are as follows:

- Sensory neuropathy results in anesthesia and loss of protective sensation.
- Motor neuropathy results in difficulty in activating certain muscle groups, resulting in inadequate distribution of pressure on the sole while walking. Areas subjected to repetitive focal pressure may ulcerate or, alternatively, may develop a callus, which predisposes to ulceration. The consequences of motor neuropathy are reflected in the presence of typical foot deformities seen in diabetic neuropathy, such as protrusion of the metatarsal heads. *Mal perforant* is a common neuropathic ulcer of the sole, which appears over the metatarsal heads [110].
- Autonomic neuropathy is associated with dry skin and further contributes to fissuring and callus formation. In addition, it leads to arteriovenous shunting which, although accompanied by increased blood flow, reduces nutritive cutaneous capillary flow [115, 116].

The above-mentioned processes may mislead the physician, due to the following phenomena:

- Sensory neuropathy may conceal symptoms of intermittent claudication and rest pain.
- An ischemic foot may nevertheless be warm and pink on clinical examination, due to autonomic neuropathy [115, 117, 118].

The neuropathic process leads to the formation of ulcers on the sole or on the lateral and medial regions of the foot in diabetic patients (Fig. 4.8). Typically, a neuropathic ulcer of the sole is surrounded by circumscribed callus formation. Neuropathy and decreased sensation render the patient even more prone to trauma and subsequent ulceration, which may occur anywhere in the distal regions of the limbs. In some cases, the presence of neuropathy prevents early identification of an ulcer by the affected person, and appropriate intervention, therefore, is not carried out.

4.3.7.3 Microangiopathy in Diabetes

Diabetic microangiopathy is characterized by the thickening of basal membranes and increased capillary permeability. In its advanced stages, it results in compromised gas exchange, a decrease in cutaneous pO_2, and ischemia [110, 119].

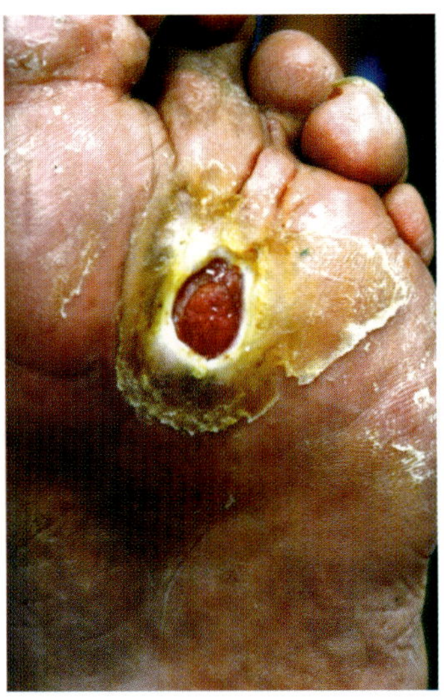

Fig. 4.8. A neuropathic ulcer in diabetes

The main clinical implications of microangiopathy with respect to skin ulcers are as follows:

— The ischemic changes described above (together with macroangiopathy) cause additional damage to the skin, thereby increasing the probability of ulceration. The combination of macroangiopathy and microangiopathy seems to be the reason why diabetic ulcerations tend to be located more distally, compared with ulceration in non-diabetic peripheral arterial disease.

— Microangiopathic involvement of the vasa nervosum results in diabetic neuropathy.

Note: The effect of microangiopathy is most obvious in the kidneys and the retina. The possible influence of these vascular changes on ulcer formation in the diabetic leg is questionable and has not yet been fully evaluated. It is reasonable to assume that they affect capillary function [111, 120].

4.3.7.4 Other Factors: Osteoarthropathy, Cheiroarthropathy

Charcot's osteoarthropathy describes a destructive process of the joints, occurring in diabetic neuropathy. It creates excessive focal pressure on the sole of the foot, predisposing it to ulcer formation. Another process is known as cheiroarthropathy, in which there is a thickening of the skin with limitation of joint mobility and an abnormal gait, with subsequent inappropriate weight distribution on the sole of the foot [121, 122].

4.3.7.5 Reduced Resistance to Infections

Infection is a frequent complication of diabetes, which aggravates tissue damage. Diabetes is associated with decreased phagocytic activity and decreased function of leukocytes

[123]. Chemotaxis of leukocytes and phagocytosis are impaired in poorly controlled diabetes [110]. Hyperglycemia has been found to inhibit the cellular transport of vitamin C into fibroblasts and leukocytes, with reduced chemotaxis of leukocytes [124].

4.3.7.6 Location of Ulcers in Diabetes

In view of the above-mentioned pathologic characteristics of diabetes, even minor trauma or otherwise negligible superficial infection may be sufficient to induce ulceration.

In a diabetic patient, ulcers may be located as follows:

- Lateral or pretibial regions of the leg, dorsum of the foot, or malleolar regions, due to peripheral arterial disease and subsequent damage to the skin and subcutaneous tissue
- Distal toes (Fig. 4.9) or distal forefoot, due to the severe ischemia of peripheral arterial disease
- Neuropathy predisposes to ulceration mainly on the sole. Nevertheless, the decreased sensation combined with increased susceptibility to trauma may occur anywhere on the distal limb. Osteoarthropathy further contributes to the formation of plantar ulcers.

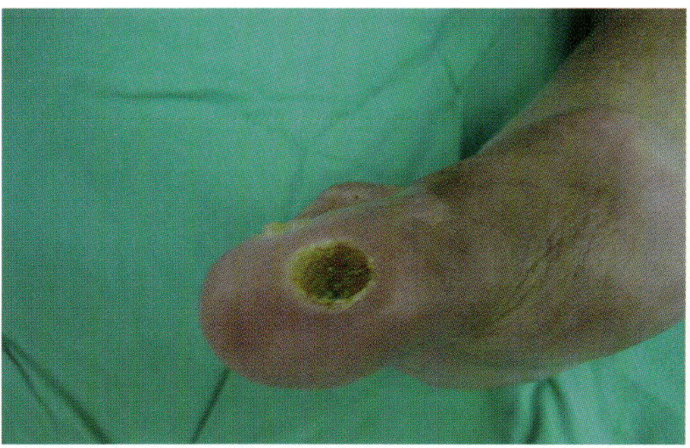

Fig. 4.9. An ulcer on the toe of a diabetic patient

In summary, the classical diabetic ulcer appears on the sole. However, in view of the combination of several detrimental factors including macroangiopathy, microangiopathy, neuropathy, and reduced resistance to infections, ulcers in diabetes can, in fact, occur anywhere on the lower leg.

4.3.8 Hematologic Abnormalities

4.3.8.1 Hemolytic Anemia and Cutaneous Ulcers

Most of the literature in the field of hemolytic anemia and cutaneous ulcers relates to sickle cell disease. Blood vessels occluded by the sludging of sickled erythrocytes are the histologic hallmark of an ulcer in sickle cell anemia.

Sickle cells are relatively rigid, with a reduced ability to alter their shape. It seems that the reduced deformability of sickled erythrocytes is a major factor leading to vascular occlusion and ulceration [125]. These features of sickled erythrocytes may significantly decrease blood flow, especially in capillary beds subjected to venous stasis [126]. Below a certain level of blood flow, there is a clumping of sickled erythrocytes with subsequent obstruction of blood vessels [125, 127]. The vascular occlusion leads to ulceration. When the level of oxygen is reduced, these processes are more pronounced.

The causes of ulceration in other types of anemia such as thalassemia, hereditary spherocytosis, or pyruvate kinase deficiency are not fully understood. For example, leg ulcers are rare in α-thalassemia, but relatively common in severe β-thalassemia [128]. It is reasonable to assume that, in these cases, there is also a diminished deformability of abnormal erythrocytes. The tendency for ulcers to appear in the gaiter area of the lower limbs suggests that there is an element of venous stasis that contributes to a reduction in blood flow.

In certain types of hemolytic anemia such as hereditary spherocytosis, cutaneous ulcers have been reported to improve and heal following a splenectomy [129, 130]. In other cases of anemia, such as in β-thalassemia, no beneficial effect of a splenectomy has been observed [131]. A possible explanation for the above observation regarding hereditary spherocytosis has been suggested: During their passage through the spleen, red blood cells may lose a membrane lipid. This change may lead to the entrapment of cells in the microvasculature, resulting in stasis with impaired oxygenation and the formation of cutaneous ulcers. A splenectomy prevents this sort of damage to red blood cells; their improved function and increased capacity of deformability leads to healing of the ulcers [125, 132].

4.3.9 Nutritional Disorders

In most cases, malnutrition is not a *direct* cause of ulceration. However, malnutrition does interfere with wound healing and has a detrimental effect on the general condition of the patient. This issue is discussed in detail in Chap. 18.

> Conditions in which malnutrition may induce ulceration directly are:
> - Vitamin C deficiency
> - Noma (cancrum oris, necrotizing ulcerative gingivitis)
> - Tropical ulcer (tropical sloughing phagedena)

Vitamin C deficiency results in impaired collagen synthesis with subsequent poor wound healing. The classical clinical descriptions of scurvy by Lind [133] documented the appearance of ulcers on affected skin, induced mostly by minor trauma. Boulinguez et al. [134] documented three patients with scurvy presenting with ecchymotic purpura and hemorrhagic ulcers of the lower limbs.

However, vitamin C is an important factor not only in those relatively rare patients whose ulcers are caused directly by vitamin C deficiency. It is also very important to identify patients with cutaneous ulcers (caused by other etiologies) who happen to be deficient in vitamin C. In these cases, vitamin C supplementation may improve wound healing.

In the latter two conditions, i.e., noma and tropical ulcer, the specific mechanisms leading to ulceration have not yet been identified, but it appears that opportunistic infection, related to the state of malnutrition, plays a significant role in their pathogenesis.

4.3.10 Other Causes

Epithelial tumors and leg ulcers are discussed in Chap. 6, and a detailed review of drugs and cutaneous ulcers is presented in Chap. 16.

References

1. Shai A, Halevy S: Direct triggers for ulceration in patients with venous insufficiency. Int J Dermatol (in press)
2. Reed BR, Clark RAF: Cutaneous tissue repair. Practical implications of current knowledge. II. J Am Acad Dermatol 1985; 13 : 919–941
3. Robson MC, Stenberg BD, Heggers JP: Wound healing alterations caused by infection. Clin Plast Surg 1990; 17 : 485–492
4. Rietchel RL, Fowler JF: The role of age, sex and color of skin in contact dermatitis. In: Rietchel RL, Fowler JF (eds) In: Fisher's Contact Dermatitis, 4th edn. Baltimore: Williams & Wilkins.1995; pp 41–65
5. Dooms-Goossens A, Degreef H, Parijs M, et al: A retrospective study of patch test results from 163 patients with stasis dermatitis or leg ulcers. Dermatologica 1979; 159 : 93–100
6. Wilson CL, Cameron J, Powell SM, Cherry G, Ryan TJ: High incidence of contact dermatitis in leg-ulcer patients-implications for management. Clin Exp Dermatol 1991; 16 : 250–253
7. Rietchel RL, Fowler JF: Contact dermatitis and other reactions to metals. In: Rietchel RL, Fowler JF (eds) In: Fisher's Contact Dermatitis, 4th edn. Baltimore. Williams & Wilkins.1995; pp 808–885
8. Lee HS, Goh CL: Occupational dermatosis among chrome platers. Contact Dermatitis 1988; 18 : 89–93
9. Tanaka T, Miyachi Y, Horio T: Ulcerative contact dermatitis caused by sodium silicate. Coexistence of primary irritant contact dermatitis and contact urticaria. Arch-Dermatol 1982; 118 : 518–520
10. Mochida K, Hisa T, Yasunaga C, et al: Skin ulceration due to povidone-iodine. Contact Dermatitis 1995; 33 : 61–62
11. Fisher AA: Unique reactions of scrotal skin to topical agents. Cutis 1989; 44 : 445–447
12. Krafchik BR: Eczematous dermatitis. In: Schachner LA, Hansen RC (eds) Pediatric Dermatology, 2nd edn. New York: Churchill Livingstone. 1995; pp 704–705

13. Rijswijk LV: Epidemiology. In: Morison MJ: The prevention and treatment of pressure ulcers. 1st edn. Edinburgh: Mosby. 2001; pp 7–15

14. Kanj LF, Wilking SV, Phillips TJ: Pressure ulcers. J Am Acad Dermatol 1998; 38:517–536

15. Allman RM: Epidemiology of pressure sores in different populations. Decubitus 1989; 2:30–33

16. Young JS, Burns PE, Bowen AM, et al: Spinal cord injury statistics: experience of the regional spinal cord injury systems. National Spinal Cord Injury Data Research Center. Phoenix. 1982

17. Nixon J: The pathophysiology and aetiology of pressure ulcers. In: Morison MJ (ed) The prevention and treatment of pressure ulcers, 1st edn. Edinburgh: Mosby. 2001; pp 17–36

18. Garfin SR, Pye SA, Hargens AR, Akeson WH: Surface pressure distribution of the human body in the recumbent position. Arch Phys Med Rehabil 1980; 61:409–413

19. Kosiak M: Etiology and pathology of ischemic ulcers. Arch Phys Med Rehabil 1959; 40:62–69

20. Daniel RK, Priest DL, Wheatley DC: Etiologic factors in pressure sores: an experimental model. Arch Phys Med Rehabil 1981; 62:492–498

21. Falanga V: Chronic wounds: pathophysiologic and experimental considerations. J Invest Dermatol 1993; 100:721–725

22. Kosiak M: Etiology of decubitus ulcers. Arch Phys Med Rehabil 1961; 42:19–29

23. Dinsdale SM: Decubitus ulcers: role of pressure and friction in causation. Arch Phys Med Rehabil 1974; 55:147–152

24. Exton-Smith AN, Sherwin RW: The prevention of pressure sores: significance of spontaneous bodily movements. Lancet 1961; 2:1124–1126

25. Barbenel JC, Jordan MM, Nicol SM, et al: Incidence of pressure sores in the Greater Glasgow Health Board Area. Lancet 1977; 2:548–550

26. Reuler JB, Cooney TG: The pressure sore: pathophysiology and principles of management. Ann Intern Med 1981; 94:661–666

27. Bennet L, Bok YL: Pressure versus shear in pressure sore causation. In: Lee BY: Chronic Ulcers of the Skin, 1st edn. New York: McGraw-Hill. 1986; pp 39–56

28. Bennett L, Kavner D, Lee BK, et al: Shear vs pressure as causative factors in skin blood flow occlusion. Arch Phys Med Rehabil 1979; 60: 309–314

29. Reichel SM: Shearing force as a factor in decubitus ulcers in paraplegics. JAMA 1958; 166:762–763

30. Agris J, Spira M: Pressure ulcers: prevention and treatment. Clin Symp 1979; 31:1–32

31. The National Pressure Ulcer Advisory Panel. Pressure ulcers prevalence, cost and risk assessment: consensus development conference statement. Decubitus 1989; 2:24–28

32. Crickx B: Erysipelas: evolution under treatment, complications. Ann Dermatol Venereol 2001; 128: 358–362

33. Ahrenholz DH: Necrotizing soft-tissue infections. Surg Clin North Am 1988; 68:199–214

34. Fustes-Morales A, Gutierrez-Castrellon P, Duran-Mckinster C et al: Necrotizing fasciitis: Report of 39 pediatric cases. Arch Dermatol 2002; 138:893–899

35. Stevens DL: The flesh-eating bacterium: What's next? J Infect Dis 1999; 179 [Suppl 2]:S366–S374

36. Bosshardt TL, Henderson VJ, Organ CH Jr: Necrotizing soft tissue infections. Arch Surg 1996; 131: 846–852

37. Umbert IJ, Winkelmann RK, Oliver GF, et al: Necrotizing fasciitis: a clinical, microbiologic, and histopathologic study of 14 patients. J Am Acad Dermatol 1989; 20:774–781

38. Lee PK, Zipoli MT, Weinberg AN, Swartz MN, Johnson RA: Pyodermas: staphylococcus aureus, streptococcus and other gram-positive bacteria. In: Freedberg IM, Eisen AZ, Wolff K, Austen KF, Goldsmith LA, Katz SI (eds) Fitzpatrick's Dermatology in General Medicine, 6th edn. New York: McGraw-Hill. 2003; pp 1856–1878

39. Sanchez MR: Syphilis. In: Freedberg IM, Eisen AZ, Wolff K, Austen KF, Goldsmith LA, Katz SI (eds) Fitzpatrick's Dermatology in General Medicine, 6th edn. New York: McGraw-Hill. 2003; pp 2163–2188

40. Varela P, Alves R, Velho G, et al: Two recent cases of tertiary syphilis. Eur J Dermatol 1999; 9:371–373

41. Merkert R: Generalized ulcers. Noduloulcerative syphilis (malignant syphilis, lues maligna). Arch Dermatol 1997; 133:1027–1028, 1030–1031

42. Don PC, Rubinstein R, Christie S: Malignant syphilis (lues maligna) and concurrent infection with HIV. Int J Dermatol 1995; 34:403–407

43. Gawkrodger DJ: Mycobacterial infections. In: Champion RH, Burton JL, Burns DA, Breathnach SM (eds) In: Rook/Wilkinson/Ebling Textbook of Dermatology, 6th edn. Oxford: Blackwell Scientific Publications. 1998; pp 1181–1214

44. Lantos G, Fisher BK, Contreras M: Tuberculous ulcer of the skin. J Am Acad Dermatol 1988; 19: 1067–1072

45. Marechal V, Maradeix S, Pouaha J, et al: Cas pour diagnostic: Ulceration atone de la cheville. Ann Dermatol Venereol 2002; 129:439–440

46. Rao PT, Jena SK: Surgical treatment of plantar ulcers in leprosy. Int Orthop 1986; 10:75–78

47. Cross H, Kulkarni VN, Dey A, et al: Plantar ulceration in patients with leprosy. J Wound Care 1996; 5: 406–411

48. Mitchell PD: The threshold for protective sensation that prevents neuropathic ulceration on the plantar aspect of the foot: a study of leprosy patients in a rural community in India. Lepr Rev 2001; 72: 143–150

49. Boucher P, Sebille A: Frequency of the association of perforating plantar leprotic lesions and truncal involvement of the posterior tibial nerve. Acta Leprol 1983; 1:177–182

50. Feenstra W, Van de Vijver S, Benbow C, et al: Can people affected by leprosy at risk of developing plantar ulcers be identified? A field study from central Ethiopia. Lepr Rev 2001; 72:151–157

51. Morton RS: The treponematoses. In: Champion RH, Burton JL, Burns DA, Breathnach SM (eds) In: Rook/Wilkinson/Ebling Textbook of Dermatology. 6th edn. Oxford: Blackwell Scientific Publications. 1998; pp 1237–1275

52. Ramesh V, Saxena U, Mukherjee A, et al: Multiple ulcers in an elderly man. Necrotizing erythema nodosum leprosum (ENL) (necrotizing ENL). Arch Dermatol 1992; 128:1643, 1646

53. Bernadat JP, Faucher JF, Huerre M: Diffuse lepromatous leprosy disclosed by cutaneous vasculitis. The Lucio phenomenon. Ann Dermatol Venereol 1996; 123:21–23

54. Souza CS, Roselino AM, Figueiredo F, et al: Lucio's phenomenon: clinical and therapeutic aspects. Int J Lepr Other Mycobact Dis 2000; 68:417–425

55. Barbarulo AM, Metha N, Bucalo B, et al: Recurrent disseminated herpes zoster and cytomegalic perianal ulcer: a case report and review of the literature. Cutis 2001; 67:43–46

56. Pariser RJ: Histologically specific skin lesions in disseminated cytomegalovirus infection. J Am Acad Dermatol 1983; 9:937–946

57. Rodot S, Lacour JP, van Elslande L, et al: Ecthyma gangrenosum caused by Klebsiella pneumoniae. Int J Dermatol 1995: 34:216–217

58. Cohen PR, Grossman ME: Recognizing skin lesions of systemic fungal infections in patients with AIDS. Am Fam Physician 1994; 49:1627–1634

59. Ginter G, Rieger E, Soyer HP, et al: Granulomatous panniculitis caused by Candida albicans: a case presenting with multiple leg ulcers. J Am Acad Dermatol 1993; 28:315–317

60. Orem J, Mpanga L, Habyara E, et al: Disseminated aspergillus fumigatus infection: case report. East Afr Med J 1998; 75:436–438

61. Phillips TJ, Dover JS: Leg ulcers. J Am Acad Dermatol 1991; 25:965–987

62. Nelzen O, Bergqvist D, Lindhagen A: Venous and non-venous leg ulcers: clinical history and appearance in a population study. Br J Surg 1994; 81:182–187

63. Baker SR, Stacey MC, Singh G, et al: Aetiology of chronic leg ulcers. Eur J Vasc Surg 1992; 6:245–251

64. Hafner J: Management of arterial leg ulcers and combined (mixed) venous-arterial leg ulcers. Curr Probl Dermatol 1999; 27:211–219

65. Husni EA: Skin ulcers secondary to arterial and venous disease. Lee BY: Chronic Ulcers of the Skin, 1st edn. New York: McGraw-Hill. 1986; pp 93–101

66. Junger M, Hahn M, Klyscz T, et al: Microangiopathy in the pathogenesis of chronic venous leg ulcers insufficiency. Curr Probl Dermatol 1999; 27:124–129

67. Incandela L, Belcaro G, Cesarone MR, et al: Microangiopathy and venous ulceration: Topical treatment with Essaven gel. A placebo-controlled, randomized study. Angiology 2001; 52 [Suppl 3]: S17–S21

68. Bollinger A, Leu AJ, Hoffmann U, et al: Microvascular changes in venous disease: An update. Angiology 1997; 48:27–32

69. Nicolaides AN: Investigation of chronic venous insufficiency. A consensus statement. Circulation 2000; 102:e126–e163

70. Bollinger A, Jager K, Geser A, et al: Transcapillary and interstitial diffusion of Na-fluorescein in chronic venous insufficiency with white atrophy. Int J Microcirc Clin Exp 1982; 1:5–17

71. Partsch H: Pathogenesis of the venous leg ulcer. Hautarzt 1985; 36:196–202

72. Junger M, Steins A, Hahn M, et al: Microcirculatory dysfunction in chronic venous insufficiency (CVI). Microcirculation 2000; 7:S3–S12

73. Fagrell B: Microcirculatory disturbances – The final cause for venous leg ulcers? Vasa 1982; 11:101–103

74. Leu AJ, Yanar A, Pfister G, et al: Microangiopathy in chronic venous insufficiency. Dtsch Med Wochenschr 1991; 116:447–453

75. Pierard-Franchimont C, Letawe C, Fumal I, et al: Gravitational syndrome and tensile properties of skin in the elderly. Dermatology 1998; 197:317–320

76. Olszewski W: Pathophysiology and clinical observations of obstructive lymphedema of the limbs. In: Clodius L (ed) Lymphedema. Stuttgart: Georg Thieme Verlag. 1977; pp 79–102

77. Casley-Smith JR, Casley-Smith JR: Pathology of oedema – effect of oedema. In: Casley-Smith JR, Casley-Smith JR (eds) Modern Treatment for Lymphoedema, 5th revised edn. Adelaide: The Lymphoedema Association of Australia, Inc. 1997; pp 60–73

78. Peschen M: Cytokines in progressing stages of chronic venous insufficiency. Curr Probl Dermatol 1999; 27:13–19

79. Hahn TL, Whitfield R, Salter J, et al: Evaluation of the role of intercellular adhesion molecule 1 in a rodent model of chronic venous hypertension. J Surg Res 2000; 88:150–154

80. Peschen M, Lahaye T, Hennig B, et al: Expression of the adhesion molecules ICAM-1, VCAM-1, LFA-1 and VLA-4 in the skin is modulated in progressing stages of chronic venous insufficiency. Acta Derm Venereol 1999; 79:27–32

81. Junger M, Steins A, Hahn M, et al: Microcirculatory dysfunction in chronic venous insufficiency. Microcirculation 2000; 7:S3–S12

82. Valencia IC, Falabella A, Kirsner RS, et al: Chronic venous insufficiency and venous leg ulceration. J Am Acad Dermatol 2001; 44:401–421

83. Coleridge-Smith PD, Thomas P, Scurr JH, et al: Causes of venous ulceration: a new hypothesis? Br Med J 1988; 296:1726–1727

84. Thomas PR, Nash GB, Dormandy JA: White cell accumulation in dependent legs of patients with venous hypertension: a possible mechanism for trophic changes in the skin. Br Med J (Clin Res Ed) 1988; 296:1693–1695

85. Scott HJ, Coleridge Smith PD, Scurr JH: Histological study of white blood cells and their association with lipodermatosclerosis and venous ulceration. Br J Surg 1991; 78:210–211

86. Bradbury AW, Murie JA, Ruckley CV: Role of the leukocyte in the pathogenesis of vascular disease. Br J Surg 1993; 80: 1503–1512

87. Browse NL, Burnand KG: The cause of venous ulceration. Lancet 1982; 2:243–245

88. Burnand KG, Whimster I, Naidoo A, et al: Pericapillary fibrin in the ulcer-bearing skin of the leg: the cause of lipodermatosclerosis and venous ulceration. Br Med J 1982; 285:1071–1072

89. Neumann HA, van den Broek MJ, Boersma IH, et al: Transcutaneous oxygen tension in patients with and without pericapillary fibrin cuffs in chronic venous insufficiency, porphyria cutanea tarda and non-venous leg ulcers. Vasa 1996; 25:127–133

90. Falanga V, Eaglstein WH: The "trap" hypothesis of venous ulceration. Lancet 1993; 341:1006–1008

91. Wienert V: Epidemiology of leg ulcers. Curr Probl Dermatol 1999; 27:65–69

92. Dormandy JA, Rutherford RB: Management of peripheral arterial disease (PAD). TASC Working Group. J Vasc Surg 2000; 31 [Suppl 1]: S1–S296

93. de Graaff JC, Ubbink DT, Legemate DA, et al: Evaluation of toe pressure and transcutaneous oxygen measurements in management of chronic critical leg ischemia: A diagnostic randomized clinical trial. J Vasc Surg 2003; 38:528–534

94. Martorell F: Las ulceras supramaleolares par arteriolitis de los grandes hypertensos. Actas Inst Policlinico (Barcelona) 1945; 1:6–9

95. Hafner J, Schaad I, Schneider E, et al: Leg ulcers in peripheral arterial disease (arterial leg ulcers): Impaired wound healing above the threshold of chronic critical limb ischemia. J Am Acad Dermatol 2000; 43:1001–1008

96. Leu HJ: Hypertensive ischemic leg ulcer (Martorell's ulcer): a specific disease entity? Int Angiol 1992; 11:132–136

97. Falanga V, Fine MJ, Kapoor WN: The cutaneous manifestations of cholesterol crystal embolization. Arch Dermatol 1986; 122:1194–1198

98. Kalter DC, Rudolph A, McGavran M: Livedo reticularis due to multiple cholesterol emboli. J Am Acad Dermatol 1985; 13:235–242

99. Soter NA: Cutaneous necrotizing venulitis.In: Freedberg IM, Eisen AZ, Wolff K, Austen KF, Goldsmith LA, Katz SI (eds) Fitzpatrick's Dermatology in General Medicine, 6th edn. New York: McGraw-Hill. 2003; pp 1727–1735

100. Goslen JB: Autoimmune ulceration of the leg. Clin Dermatol 1990; 8:92–117

101. Rowell NR, Goodfield MJD: The'connective tissue diseases'. In: Champion RH, Burton JL, Burns DA, Breathnach SM (eds) Rook/Wilkinson/Ebling Textbook of Dermatology, 6th edn. Oxford: Blackwell Scientific Publications. 1998; pp 2437–2575

102. Ackerman AB, Chongchitnant N, sanchez Y, Guo Y, Benin B, Reichel M, Randall MB (eds) Proceeding to specific diagnoses. Basic patterns and analysis of them. In: Histologic Diagnosis of Inflammatory Skin Diseases: An Algorithmic Method Based on Pattern Analysis, 2nd edn. Baltimore: Williams & Wilkins. 1997; pp 107–144

103. Bradbury AW, MacKenzie RK, Burns P, et al: Thrombophilia and chronic venous ulceration. Eur J Vasc Endovasc Surg 2002; 24:97–104

104. MacKenzie RK, Ludlam CA, Ruckley CV, et al: The prevalence of thrombophilia in patients with chronic venous leg ulceration. J Vasc Surg 2002; 35: 718–722

105. Barnhill RL, Busam KJ: Vascular diseases. In: Elder D, Elenitsas R, Jaworsky C, Johnson B (eds) Lever's Histopathology of the Skin; 8th edn. Philadelphia: Lippincott-Raven. 1997; pp 185–208

106. den Heijer M, Keijzer MB: Hyperhomocysteinemia as a risk factor for venous thrombosis. Clin Chem Lab Med 2001; 39:710–713

107. Schaper NC, Nabuurs-Franssen MH, Huijberts MS: Peripheral vascular disease and type 2 diabetes mellitus. Diabetes Metab Res Rev 2000; 16 [Suppl 1]: S11–S15

108. Osmundson PJ, O'Fallon WM, Zimmerman BR, et al: Course of peripheral occlusive arterial disease in diabetes. Vascular laboratory assessment. Diabetes Care 1990; 13:143–152

109. Beach KW, Bedford GR, Bergelin RO, et al: Progression of lower-extremity arterial occlusive disease in type II diabetes mellitus. Diabetes Care 1988; 11: 464–472

110. Zinnagl N: Conservative therapy of diabetic foot. Curr Probl Dermatol 1999; 27:235–241

111. Krone W, Muller-Wieland D: Special problems of the diabetic patient. In: Dormandy JA, Stock G (eds) Critical leg ischemia: its pathophysiology and management. Berlin Heidelberg New York: Springer-Verlag. 1990; pp 145–157

112. Young MJ, Boulton AJM, MacLeod AF, et al: A multicentre study of the prevalence of diabetic peripheral neuropathy in the United Kingdom hospital clinic population. Diabetologia 1993; 36:150–154

113. Murray HJ, Boulton AJ: The pathophysiology of diabetic foot ulceration. Clin Podiatr Med and Surg 1995; 12:1–17

114. Boulton AJ: Peripheral neuropathy and the diabetic foot. Foot 1992; 2:67–72

115. Boulton AJ: The diabetic foot. Med Clin North Am 1988; 72:1513–1530

116. Boulton AJ, Scarpello JH, Ward JD: Venous oxygenation in the diabetic neuropathic foot: evidence of arteriovenous shunting? Diabetologia 1982; 22:6–8

117. Slater R, Ramot Y, Rapoport M: Diabetic foot ulcers: Principles of assessment and treatment. Isr Med Assoc J 2001; 3:59–62

118. Sykes MT, Godsey JB: Vascular evaluation of the problem diabetic foot. Clin Podiatr Med Surg 1998; 15:49–83

119. Incandela L, Belcaro G, Cesarone MR, et al: Microvascular alterations in diabetic microangiopathy: Topical treatment with Essaven gel. A placebo-controlled, randomized study. Angiology 2001; 52 [Suppl 3]:S35–S41

120. LoGerfo FW, Coffman JD: Vascular and microvascular disease of the foot in diabetes. N Engl J Med 1984; 311:1615–1619

121. Frykberg RG, Mendeszoon E: Management of the diabetic Charcot foot. Diabetes Metab Res Rev 2000; 16 [Suppl 1]:S59–S65

122. Delbridge L, Perry P, Marr S, et al: Limited joint mobility in the diabetic foot. Relationship to neuropathic ulceration. Diabet Med 1988; 5:333–337

123. Ehrlichman RJ, Seckel BR, Bryan DJ, et al: Common complications of wound healing: prevention and management. Surg Clin North Am 1991; 71:1323–1351

124. Barbul A, Purtill W: Nutrition in wound healing. Clin Dermatol 1994; 12:133–140

125. Peachey RD: Leg ulceration and haemolytic anaemia: an hypotheses. Br J Dermatol 1978; 98:245–249

126. Gabuzda TG: Sickle cell leg ulcers: current pathophysiologic concepts. Int J Dermatol 1975; 14:322–325

127. Richards RS, Bowen CV, Glynn MF: Microsurgical free flap transfer in sickle cell disease. Ann Plast Surg 1992; 29:278–281

128. Daneshmend TK, Peachey RD: Leg ulcers in α-thalassaemia (haemoglobin H disease). Br J Dermatol 1978; 98:233–235

129. Lawrence P, Aronson I, Saxe N, et al: Leg ulcers in hereditary spherocytosis. Clin Exp Dermatol 1991; 16:28–30

130. Peretz E, Hallel-Halevy D, Grunwald M, Halevy S: Hereditary spherocytosis with leg ulcers which healed after splenectomy. Eur J Dermatol 1997; 7:527–528

131. Gimmon Z, Wexler MR, Rachmilewitz EA: Juvenile leg ulceration in β-thalassemia major and intermedia. Plast Reconst Surg 1982; 69:320–325

132. Palek J: Hereditary spherocytosis. In: Williams JW, Beutler E, Erslev AJ, et al (eds): Hematolgy, 4th edn. New York: McGraw-Hill. 1990; pp 558–569

133. Hirschmann JV, Raugi GJ: Adult scurvy. J Am Acad Dermatol 1999; 41:895–906

134. Boulinguez S, Bouyssou-Gauthier M, De-Vencay P, et al: Scurvy presenting with ecchymotic purpura and hemorrhagic ulcers of the lower limbs. Ann Dermatol Venereol 2000; 127:510–512

Determining Etiology: History and Physical Examination

Contents

5.1 Diagnostic Approach: Overview

This chapter focuses on the clinical determination of an ulcer's etiology, based on history and physical examination. As mentioned in the previous chapter, determining the cause of a cutaneous ulcer can be a somewhat complex, multistaged process, demanding a high level of expertise in medicine and dermatology.

The correlation between an ulcer and its underlying cause is sometimes apparent. For example, when a cutaneous ulcer appears in a patient with ulcerative colitis or rheumatoid arthritis, a physician is expected to consider the possibility of pyoderma gangrenosum. Similarly, the rapid spreading of cutaneous ulcers in a patient with chronic renal insufficiency should alert the clinician to the possibility of calciphylaxis.

Yet, in some cases, a cutaneous ulcer may be the presenting sign of diseases such as systemic lupus erythematosus (SLE) and SLE-like syndromes [1–3], systemic scleroderma [4], or Wegener's granulomatosis [5–7]. A cutaneous ulcer may also appear as a presenting sign in hemolytic anemia [8].

The underlying disease is not always evident or 'handed to the physician on a silver platter'. However, in many cases the information may be readily obtained from the patient's history or physical examination.

It would be difficult to build an algorithmic flow-chart to establish an ulcer's etiology, since too many parameters are involved. Nevertheless, we will present here a systematic approach, based on data obtainable from the patient's history and physical examination.

The clues to follow are:
- Clue 1 — Incidence by age
- Clue 2 — Typical location of various cutaneous ulcers
- Clue 3 — The ulcer's appearance and its surroundings
- Clue 4 — The primary lesion from which the ulcer originates
- Clue 5 — Incidence of infectious ulcers in various geographic regions
- More clues — Additional points to consider

5.2 Incidence by Age: Common Causes of Ulcers in Adults and Children

5.2.1 Adults

There are certain diseases (see below) that cause more than 95% of cutaneous ulcers in the general adult population.

It is therefore reasonable, as a first step, to check whether the ulcer belongs to one of the following diagnoses:
- Venous ulcers
- Ulcers due to peripheral arterial disease
- Diabetic ulcers
- Livedoid vasculitis (atrophie blanche)
- Ulcers developing in the course of cellulitis
- Pressure ulcers

In most cases, it is highly recommended that clinical diagnoses be supported by an ancillary laboratory investigation (e.g., Doppler flowmeter examination of leg arteries; Doppler ultrasonography of the lower-limb venous system). If the diagnosis is doubtful, other possibilities should be explored.

Note that even in cases where the etiology seems to be obvious, but the ulcer does not heal within a reasonable period (up to 3–4 months), the diagnosis should be reconsidered and a thorough investigation should be undertaken. This should follow the schemes recommended in Chap. 6.

5.2.2 Children

The differential diagnosis of cutaneous ulcers in children is presented below in Table 5.1. In contrast to adults, the etiology of cutaneous ulcers in children is quite different. For example, diabetic ulcers in long-standing diabetes mellitus type I are extremely rare in childhood [9]. Similarly, venous ulcers are rare in childhood; when present, they are associated with venous-lymphatic malformations.

In most cases, cutaneous ulcers in children reflect an infectious process, the nature of which is often related to the geographic region (see Sect. 5.6). Ecthyma appearing in warm, humid areas or leishmaniasis are classical examples of the above concept. Infected insect bites

Table 5.1. Causes of cutaneous ulcers in children

Infection

Ecthyma
Infected insect bite
Leishmaniasis
Tuberculosis and atypical mycobacterium
    infections
Buruli ulcer
Sexually transmitted diseases[a] [11]

Physical injuries

Traumatic wounds
Burns
Cold injuries (frost bites and pernio)[b] [12]
Jaquet's erosive diaper dermatitis [13]
Extravasation injury[c] [14]
Artifactual injury[d] [12]

Hemolytic anemia [8, 15–20]

Sickle cell anemia
Thalassemia
Hereditery spherocytosis

Connective tissue diseases/ multi-system diseases[e] [5, 6, 21–23]

Systemic lupus erythematosus
Scleroderma
Dermatomyositis
Periarteritis nodosa

Others

Pressure ulcers[f]
Spider bites, scorpion bites

a. Sexually transmitted diseases may be acquired by children by one of the following [11]:
   - Sexual activity (in adolescents)
   - Sexual abuse
   - Transplacental infection or infection following passage through birth canal
b. While lesions of pernio appear to be more common in children, they rarely ulcerate in this age group [12].
c. Extravasation injury is relatively common in neonatal intensive care units [14].
d. In contrast to adults, artifactual ulcers in young children may be caused by a parent or a care giver, and not always by the patients themselves [12].
e. Raynaud's phenomenon and cryoglobulinemia may also result in cutaneous ulcers in children [24], usually as a finding associated with a connective tissue disease.
f. Pressure ulcers may occur in bed-ridden children, or in cases where the child is subjected to another sort of continous pressure; e.g. improperly-fitted prosthesis [12].

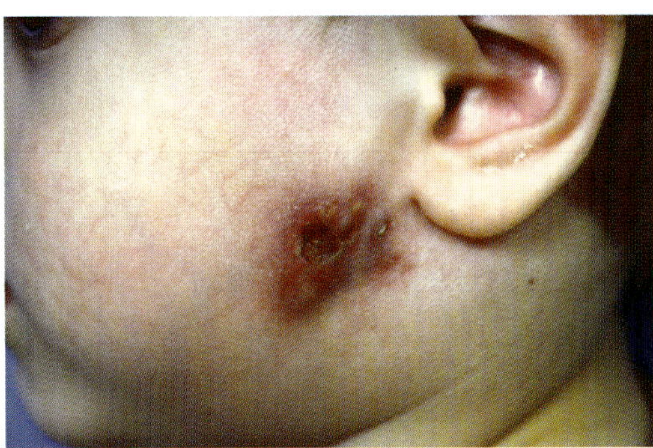

Fig. 5.1. A cutaneous ulcer appearing on the cheek of a 3-year-old child; *Mycobacterium avium intracellulare* was isolated from the ulcer

not infrequently, result in ulceration in children. Other infectious processes, such as tuberculosis and atypical mycobacterium infections (Fig. 5.1), or Buruli ulcers should be considered, depending on the circumstances and clinical findings.

Table 5.1 presents infectious diseases that commonly affect children; other infectious processes, less common, are not mentioned in Table 5.1. Certain diseases may affect both adults and children without having any particular predilection for a specific age group; etiologies of cutaneous ulcers are presented in Table 4.1.

Another group of ulcers in pediatrics are those caused by physical injuries, including burns and cold injuries. In a healthy child, traumatic ulcerations tend to recover rapidly.

An ulcer in a child that does not heal within a few weeks may be a manifestation of a systemic disorder such as hemolytic anemia or a connective tissue disease. Periarteritis nodosa results in peripheral gangrene more frequently in children than in adults [10].

In addition to the above, other conditions should be considered when dealing with ulcerations in the pediatric age group. These conditions, while relatively uncommon, include Kawasaki disease, pyoderma gangrenosum (PG), and hypercoagulability states such as protein C deficiency or protein S deficiency. In addition, cutaneous metastases of malignancies occurring during childhood (such as neuroblastoma, leukemia, or lymphoma) may ulcerate [25].

■ **Kawasaki Disease.** Kawasaki disease may manifest as severe peripheral ischemia with subsequent gangrene. It is more common in infants under seven months [25].

■ **Pyoderma Gangrenosum.** Powell and Perry [26] documented eight (4%) of 180 cases of PG in which the lesions appeared before the age of 15 years. There are isolated reports of PG occurring in infants [26, 27].

■ **Prolidase Deficiency.** Prolidase deficiency is a rare metabolic disease causing chronic cutaneous ulcers. This possibility should be considered when dealing with children who develop chronic ulcers [28, 29].

5.3 Typical Location of Various Cutaneous Ulcers

The location of an ulcer may provide valuable information. Table 5.2 presents some of the pathologic processes that tend to affect specific locations. Note that ulcers may occur in 'unexpected' sites, so not all possibilities are introduced in the table.

5.3.1 Lower Legs

Venous, diabetic, and arterial ulcers, as discussed in the previous chapter, appear on the lower legs. Not infrequently, there is a tendency to label cutaneous ulcers of lower legs as 'venous' or 'arterial'. In some cases, the correct diagnosis can be revealed only following a thorough investigation.

It is reasonable to assume that the component of hydrostatic pressure, which plays a major role in ulcerations of venous insufficiency, may also be a significant factor in various other ulcerative conditions, such as connective tissue diseases, vasculitis, and hypercoguability states. Ulcers in hemoglobinopathies (sickle cell anemia, thalassemia) also tend to appear on the lower third of the tibia [15–18], most probably for the same reason.

As a region generally exposed to trauma and infection, the lower legs tend to be more prone to ulcers attributed to infection as well.

■ **Cutaneous Ulcers of Lower Legs in Connective Tissue/Multi-System Diseases.** Cutaneous ulcers in systemic lupus erythematosus (SLE) tend to appear in the malleolar region [4]. Similar leg ulcers may be seen in rheumatoid arthritis.

In periarteritis nodosa, cutaneous or subcutaneous nodules which may undergo ulceration appear along the course of superficial arteries, i.e., around the knee, the anterior and distal shin, and the dorsum of the foot [10].

In Wegener's granulomatosis, nodules that may ulcerate tend to appear most commonly in crops along the extensor surface of extremities. The lower extremities have been found to be the most common location affected in Wegener's granulomatosis, involved in more than 70% of cases [6].

■ **Hypercoagulable States.** Hypercoagulable states, such as protein C deficiency, protein S deficiency, or activated protein C resistance, may present as leg ulcers [37–40]. In contrast, coumarin necrosis tends to occur in regions with increased subcutaneous fat, such as the thighs, breasts, and buttocks [68, 69].

■ **Pyoderma Gangrenosum.** The lower extremity is a common site of involvement of pyoderma gangrenosum; particularly the anterior tibial surface. Nevertheless, pyoderma gangrenosum may appear anywhere [42].

■ **Epitheliomatous Tumors.** Basal cell carcinoma or squamous cell carcinoma may develop on the legs [43–47]. Such an ulcer may pose a diagnostic challenge. As will be discussed in Chap. 6, a biopsy should be considered in the case of any cutaneous ulcer that does not heal within a reasonable time.

■ **Pressure Ulcers.** Pressure ulcers usually develop over bony prominences. In about 30% of cases they are located on the lower legs [70, 71].

Table 5.2. Locations of cutaneous ulcers

Lower legs	Fingers and toes
Most common causes	**Cold exposure**
Venous ulcers	Frost bite, perniosis [48]
Peripheral arterial disease	Raynaud's phenomenon
Diabetic ulcers	Cryoglobulinemia
Infectious	**Connective tissue/multi-system diseases** [4, 10]
Ulcers developing in the course of cellulitis	Systemic lupus erythematosus
Ecthyma [30]	Dermatomyositis
Yaws [31]	Periarteritis nodosa
Tropical ulcer [32]	Systemic scleroderma
Connective tissue diseases	**Arterial occlusion**
Systemic lupus erythematosus [4]	Peripheral arterial disease
Rheumatoid arthritis	Embolus [49, 50]
Periarteritis nodosa [33]	Diabetes
Wegener's granulomatosis [6]	
Temporal arteritis [34]	**Infectios diseases**
Anti-phospholipid syndrome [35]	Venereal diseases (such as syphilis) [51]
	Tularemia,
Hemolytic anemia [15–18, 36]	Swimming pool granuloma
Hemoglobinopathies	
Sickle cell anemia	**Malignancy**
Thalassemia	Essential thrombocytosis
	Polycytemia vera
Leukocytoclastic vasculitis	Leukemia, Lymphoma [52]
Drugs	
Infections	
Malignancy	
Hypercoagulabale state	
Protein S deficiency [37]	
Protein C deficiency [38]	
Activated protein C resistance [39, 40]	
Others	
Atrophie blanche: [41]	
Kaposi sarcoma (classic type)	
Pressure sores	
Pyoderma gangrenosum [42]	
Basal cell carcinoma [43–45]	
Squamous cell carcinoma [45, 46]	
Malignant melanoma	

Table 5.2. Locations of cutaneous ulcers *(Continued)*

Genital ulcers; Perianal ulcers	Soles

Classical venereal diseases

Syphilitic chancre
Chancroid
Lymphgranuloma venereum
Granuloma inguinale
Herpes genitalis
Herpetic or CMV infection
    in immunocompromised patients [56, 57]

Other infections

Infected insect bite
Leishmania
Ecthyma gangrenosum [58]
Fournier's gangrene [59, 60]

Following injury/dermatitis

Trauma
Papaverine injections [61]
Contact dermatitis [64]
Jaquet's erosive diaper dermatitis [13]

Malignancy

Tumor located on the genital area
Ucerations of the scrotum, or vagina
in leukemik patients [65, 66]

Others

Erosive/ulcerative lichen planus
Behçet's disease [67]
Suppositories containing ergotamine [62, 63]

Neuropathic ulcers

Diabetes
Leprosy

Deformities of the foot

e.g. prominent metatarsal head

Others

Ulcerative lichen planus [53–55]

Ulcers on the face

Epithelial tumors

Basal cell carcinoma
Squamous cell carcinoma

Cold exposure

Frost bite

Infections

Infected insect bites
Leishmania
Tularemia
Anthrax
Tuberculosis (Lupus vulgaris)

Others

Pyoderma gangrenosum
    (In the form of malignant pyodermia)
Noma
Malignant melanoma

5.3.2 Fingers and Toes

When ulcers appear on the fingers or toes, two main points should be clarified: (a) Is there a history of exposure to cold? (b) Are there other characteristics of connective tissue diseases?

■ **Exposure to Cold.** Frostbite and pernio (chilblains) are associated with exposure to cold. Frostbite usually affects fingers, toes, ears, cheeks, and nose. In pernio, the proximal phalanges of the fingers and toes and the plantar surface of the toes are usually involved [48].

In addition, Raynaud's disease and cryoglubulinemia, which can manifest as ulceration following exposure to cold, may be secondary to collagen diseases or malignancy.

■ **Connective Tissue/Multi-system Diseases.** SLE, dermatomyositis, systemic scleroderma, and periarteritis nodosa may be associated with necrosis of the fingers or toes, occasionally as the presenting sign. Other characteristics of connective tissue disease, such as a butterfly rash or arthritis, may point to a diagnosis.

■ **Arterial Pathology.** Angiopathy due to peripheral arterial disease, embolus, or diabetes, may result in necrotic toes. Abrupt appearance of a blue toe (even prior to necrosis and ulceration), may be a manifestation of embolization that may require limb-salvaging surgery. Cholesterol emboli may result from surgical interventions such as angiography, bypass surgery, and vascular injuries [49, 50].

■ **Venereal Diseases.** In some venereal diseases the primary lesion may appear on a finger [51]. In addition, in some infectious diseases (e.g., tularemia, swimming pool granuloma) the primary inoculation site may be an exposed cutaneous area such as fingers or hands.

■ **Malignancy.** Digital ulceration may occur in lymphoma or leukemia. In some cases the ulceration is attributed to the presence of cryoglobulins [52]. Digital ulceration may also occur in thrombocythemia and polycythemia vera due to stasis of the blood and secondary thrombosis.

5.3.3 Soles

When ulcers develop on the soles, the most common etiologies are neuropathy or deformities of the foot (see Chap. 4, sect. 4.3.7.2, on diabetic neuropathy). For example, a prominent metatarsal head produces excessive pressure on tissues at a specific site, with subsequent formation of a cutaneous ulcer. Typical clinical features of neuropathic ulcer, such as callus formation around the ulcer, should be sought. Deformities of the foot should be looked for on physical examination and by X-ray.

5.3.4 Facial Ulcers

The face, as a highly exposed region of the human body, is subjected to ulcerations originating from infectious processes, such as leishmaniasis (Fig. 5.2). Tularemia and anthrax are also documented as occurring on the face. Insect bites, if they become infected, may cause cutaneous ulcers.

Solar exposure and actinic damage may induce formation of basal cell carcinoma or squamous cell carcinoma. Severe exposure to cold may affect the ears and nose and may cause frostbite ulcerations.

Other unique clinical conditions that affect the face are noma and pyoderma gangrenosum (in the form of malignant pyodermia).

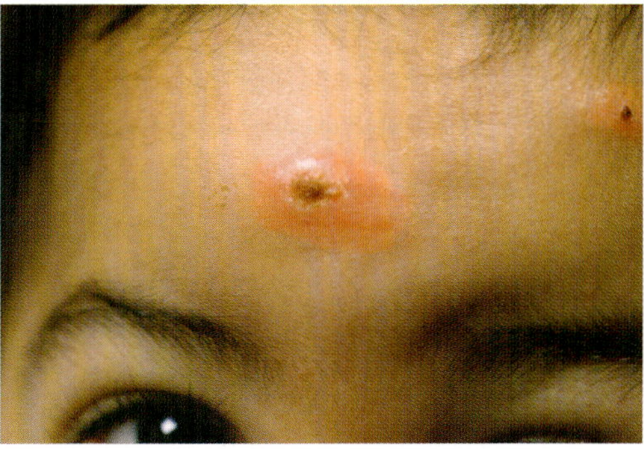

Fig. 5.2. An ulcerated lesion of leishmaniasis

5.3.5 Genital Ulcers

Classical venereal diseases, manifested by genital ulcers are syphilitic chancre, chancroid, lymphogranuloma venereum, granuloma inguinale, and herpes genitalis. Note, however, that venereal diseases may involve extragenital areas. Common sites are lips, fingers, and the perianal region. Syphilitic chancres, for example, have been reported to appear on the tongue, a tonsil, or a nipple; they may in fact occur anywhere on the abdomen, trunk, or extremities [51].

Not infrequently, venereal diseases may also affect the perianal region. Other conditions mentioned in Table 5.2 may induce both genital ulcers, perianal ulcers, or both.

Cutaneous ulcers that usually affect other regions in the body may also occur in the genital area. Thus, other etiologies should be considered, such as trauma, malignancy, and even less likely conditions such as infected insect bite or leishmaniasis [72]. As mentioned in Sect. 5.2, sexually transmitted diseases may also affect children.

5.3.5.1 Further Comments

Fournier's gangrene is an extensive fulminant infection of the genital area, anorectal area, and perineum which may extend to the abdominal wall. Rapid progression of tissue necrosis of these areas necessitates prompt antibiotic treatment together with debridement of necrotic tissue.

Ulcerations of the scrotum and vaginal ulcers have been reported in leukemic patients [65, 66].

Behçet's disease is commonly characterized by the presence of genital ulcers. In men they tend to appear on the scrotum (rarely on the penis); in women they are located on the labia, vulva, and vaginal wall [67].

Ulcerations may develop in diaper dermatitis due to secondary infection. A unique form of diaper dermatitis appears in children, as Jacquet's erosive diaper dermatitis. It consists of erosions and ulcers appearing on the labia or penis. Jacquet's erosive diaper dermatitis has been attributed to home diapering, accompanied by the use of various chemicals for washing. It is less frequent nowadays, with the increasing use of disposable diapers [13].

5.3.5.2 Differential Diagnosis of Venereal Ulcers

The typical syphilitic chancre lesion begins as a red macule that gradually evolves into an inflammatory papule. It may undergo further changes and become (not necessarily) an indurated ulceration, described in the literature as 'button-like' and approximately 1–2 cm in diameter. A typical chancre is slightly elevated, well defined, and surrounded by a red margin. In more than 20% of cases there is more than one chancre [51].

The diagnosis may be supported by the patient's reporting having had sexual intercourse within a period of time that fits the clinical diagnosis.

Note that lesions of late/tertiary syphilis may undergo ulceration. *Pseudo chancre redux* is a gummatous lesion on the penis.

Other clues for the diagnosis of venereal ulcers are:
- Level of pain
- Consistency of the ulcer
- Clinical characteristics of draining lymph nodes

■ **Level of Pain.** A primary chancre is typically painless, whereas chancroid and genital herpes are characterized by particularly painful ulcers. Granuloma inguinale and lymphogranuloma venereum do not tend to cause pain [73, 74].

■ **Consistency of the Ulcer.** A syphilitic chancre is firm at its margin (ulcus durum), whereas ulcers in chancroid are soft (ulcus molle).

■ **Draining Lymph Nodes.** Lymph nodes in chancroid and lymphogranuloma venereum are tender and painful. They may undergo suppuration. Lymph nodes tend not to be painful in syphilis. Granuloma inguinale is not characterized by lymphadenopathy.

The **groove sign** has been described in lymphogranuloma venereum. The enlarged inguinal and femoral nodes are separated by a depression caused by the presence of Poupart's ligament.

5.4 The Ulcer's Appearance and Its Surroundings

One should distinguish between morphological features that can be used as diagnostic clues and those that are irrelevant to proper identification of the ulcer's cause. The general appearance of the ulcer surface and its depth are less relevant with respect to etiology.

■ **Surface Area.** The presence of a purulent discharge or a crust on the ulcer's surface, in most cases, does not contribute to the diagnostic process. Any cutaneous ulcer may become secondarily infected irrespective of the underlying disease causing it and produce a purulent or seropurulent discharge. Similarly, cutaneous ulcers of any origin may become crusted.

A pale pink surface is characteristic of ulcers caused by arterial peripheral disease. The paleness is attributed to decreased vascularization. These ulcers do not present healthy, red-to-purple granulation tissue.

■ **Depth of Ulcer.** Ulcers of the same cause may appear at different degrees of severity (due to secondary infection, patient's immune status etc.). Thus, information regarding the ulcer's depth does not usually help the physician trying to determine the etiology.

In most cases, the clinical appearance of the ulcer itself does not contribute valuable information to the diagnostic process. The main morphological characteristics that may direct the physician to the underlying cause are (a) the appearance of the ulcer's margin and (b) the appearance of the skin around the ulcer.

5.4.1 The Ulcer's Margin

■ **Peripheral Discoloration.** The search for peripheral discoloration and the presence of undermining is of utmost importance. Peripheral purple discoloration, i.e., a purple halo around the ulcer's margin, classically appears in pyoderma gangrenosum. It is also documented in infectious ulcers, such as ecthyma gangrenosum [74], or Meleny's ulcer [75]. Pyoderma gangrenosum-like ulcers may also appear in vasculitis [76, 77], connective tissue/multi-system diseases [78–80], anti-phospholipid syndrome [81], lymphocytic leukemia [82], and cutaneous cryptococcosis [83].

It is reasonable to assume that the blue, purple, and red discoloration around the ulcer margin is the end result of a combination of certain processes:
- Damage to blood vessels; decreased perfusion with subsequent impaired oxygenation of blood within the ulcer's margin
- Level of inflammation, accompanied by dilatation of blood vessels

Peripheral bluish/violet discoloration may also be seen in ulcers appearing in peripheral arterial disease (Fig. 5.3).

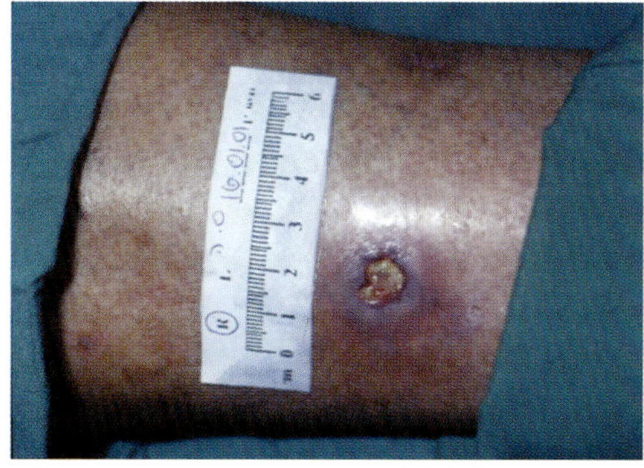

Fig. 5.3. Bluish discoloration around an ulcer caused by peripheral arterial disease

■ **Undermining.** Undermining is defined as the spread of the ulceration with involvement and destruction of tissue, located deep but peripheral to the ulcer margin, beyond the apparently normal skin. Pressure ulcers are commonly undermined in stages III or IV. Pyoderma gangrenosum ulcers are typically undermined as well. Yet undermined margins are known to develop in other types, such as steroid ulcer [84] and Buruli ulcer [85]. Tuberculous chancre is described as undermined [86]. Meleney's ulcer is also known as a 'chronic undermining burrowing ulcer'.

There are other features that may help to identify the ulcer's etiology. Self-inflicted ulcers have angular margins and an 'artificial' shape (Fig. 5.4); they often present a geometric outline, clearly demarcated from its surroundings. Circumscribed callus formation around the ulcer is the hallmark of a neuropathic ulcer (Fig. 5.5).

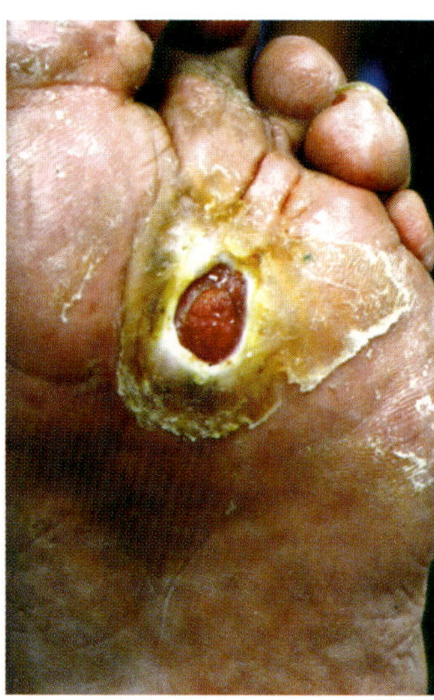

Fig. 5.5. A neuropathic ulcer surrounded by callus formation

5.4.2 The Skin that Surrounds the Ulcer

The appearance of the skin around the ulcer may provide valuable information regarding etiology. For example, vasculitic ulcers can be identified by their being surrounded by areas of palpable purpura.

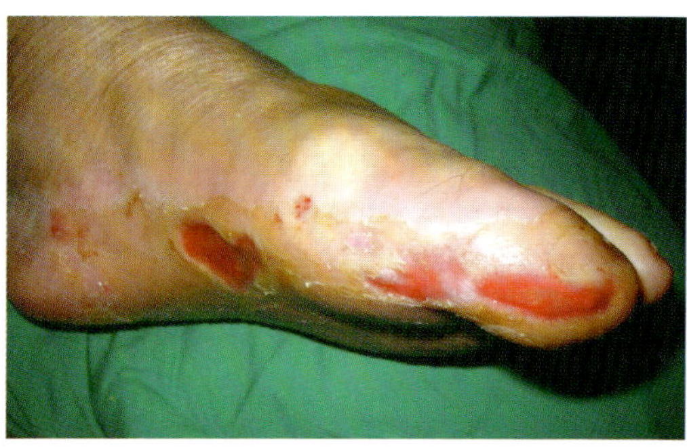

Fig. 5.4. A self-inflicted ulcer. Note the artificial, linear margin

Other clinical clues are:

- Atrophy: Atrophic skin, with hair loss, accompanied by pallor or cyanosis, may imply the presence of peripheral arterial disease.
- Stasis dermatitis: Venous ulcers are usually surrounded by stasis dermatitis with brown to purple pigmentation and varicose veins.
- Livedo reticularis: This may appear in vasculitis, connective tissue diseases, atrophie blanche, anti-phospholipid syndrome, thrombocythemia and polycythemia vera. Livedo

reticularis has also been documented in bacterial infections such as syphilis and tuberculosis [87] and in three patients with multiple cholesterol emboli [88].
- Dermatitis and excoriations: Dermatitis and excoriations around an ulcer may suggest the possibility that the ulcer developed because of a bacterial infection, following repeated scratching of the skin.

- Erythema: In the case of an ulcer surrounded by an inflammatory erythematous area, one should determine which component developed first: If the redness appeared following the development of the ulcer, it suggests that the ulcer area underwent secondary infection. On the other hand, ulcers may develop in the course of cellulitis, when the infectious process itself results in ulceration of the skin.
- Ivory plaque: In atrophie blanche, the ulcer is located within ivory white plaque, ranging from less than one cm to a few centimeters in size. The scar-like plaques are commonly described in the literature as 'star-like' (Fig. 5.6). Telangiectases and areas of hyperpigmentation are found peripherally.

5.5 The Primary Lesion from Which the Ulcer Originates

A cutaneous ulcer is not a primary lesion. An ulcer does not develop *de novo*, from an intact normal skin; it is preceded by an initial lesion from which it evolves.

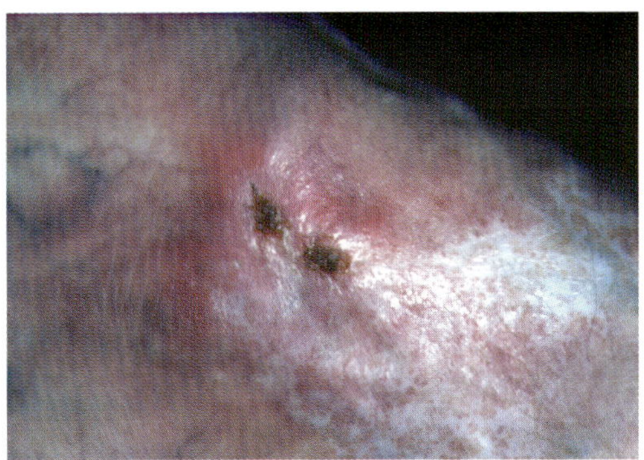

Fig. 5.6. Scar-like plaque around an atrophie blanche ulcer

Knowing the identity of the primary lesion from which the ulcer developed may be an important clue in the diagnostic process. The primary lesion can be identified by (a) examining the affected area, on which one of the primary lesions or its remnant can be recognized, and (b) asking the patient how the ulcer began.

Three categories can thus be discerned:
- A plaque or nodule
- A vesicle or pustule
- A cutaneous infarct, which begins as a pink to dusky red macule, progressively becoming a black necrotic area

5.5.1 Ulcers Originating from a Plaque or a Nodule

Plaques and nodules may develop in the course of certain inflammatory diseases (e.g., panniculitis), infectious diseases (e.g., deep fungal infections), or other pathologic processes (see Table 5.3). The lesions may ulcerate due to a gradual obliteration of small blood vessels in the course of the basic pathologic process.

5.5.2 Ulcers that May Originate from a Vesicle or a Pustule

In most cases, an ulcer that develops from a vesicle or pustule is due to an infectious process (see Table 5.3). However, pyoderma gangrenosum ulcer may also appear initially as a small pustule (Fig. 5.7)

5.5.3 Erythematous Area that Gradually Darkens

The finding of an erythematous, ecchymotic area that gradually becomes darker, developing

Table 5.3. The primary lesion from which the ulcer originates

Ulcers originating from a plaque or a nodule

- Ulcerating panniculitis
- Some connective tissue diseases (e.g. ulcerating rheumatoid nodule of rheumatoid arthritis)
- Ulcers developing in malignant lesions such as lymphoma (and mycoses fungoides), leukemia, skin metastases, or Kaposi sarcoma.
- Deep fungal infections
- In some bacterial infections such as ayphilis, yaws, tuberculosis, atypical mycobacterial infections and leprosy.
- Leishmaniasis

Ulcers that may originate from a vesicle or a pustule

Infections
- Ecthyma
- Ecthyma gangrenosum
- Tularemia
- Anthrax
- Tropical ulcer
- Ecthymateous varicella zoster

Pyoderma gangrenosum
Spider bites

Erythematotic area that gradually darken

- Vasculitis and connective tissue diseases
- Livedoid vasculitis (atrophie blanche)
- Hypercoagulabile states
- Arterial occlusion; e.g., in peripheral arterial disease or embolus; it may occur in diabetes as well, due to vascular damage
- Spider bites
- Pressure ulcers

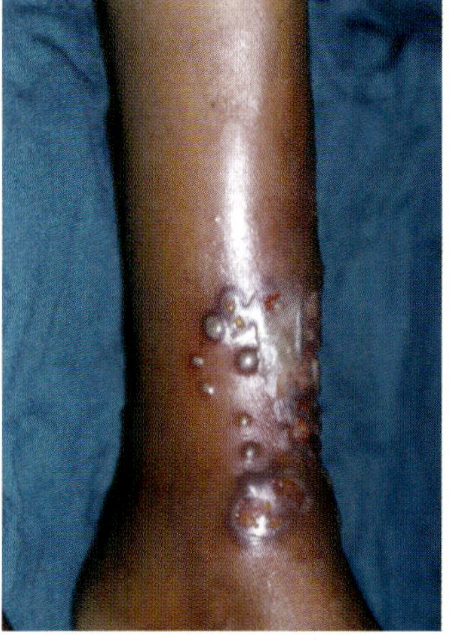

Fig. 5.7. Ulcerated pyoderma gangrenosum. Note initial pustular lesions

a black eschar-like covering, is the hallmark of blood vessel occlusion and a cutaneous infarct. The black eschar represents devitalized tissue, similar to that of deep burn wounds.

Note that certain medical conditions such as spider bites or relatively severe cutaneous infections may manifest initially as a vesicle or a pustule (Fig. 5.8), but later the involved area may become black and necrotic as a result of the destructive vascular process.

5.6 Infectious Ulcers in Various Geographical Areas

The occurrence of ulcerative lesions of infectious etiology varies according to the geo-

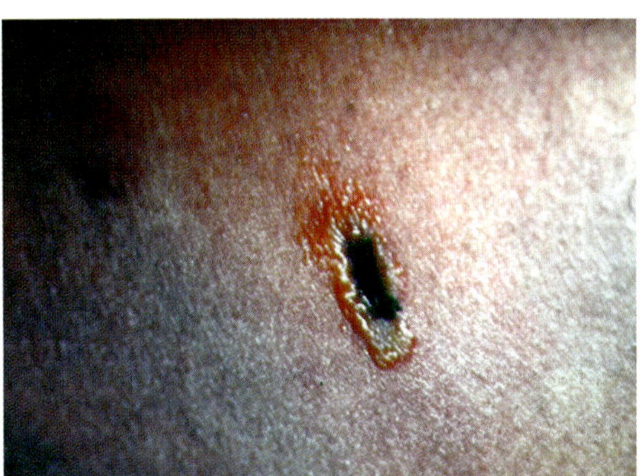

Fig. 5.8. Remnants of a blister surrounding an ulcerated spider bite

graphical region, both in children and adults. A full history should include information regarding overseas travel.

Bacterial diseases such as Buruli ulcer and yaws appear in warm tropical regions with high humidity. Nowadays yaws appears mainly in Africa, although there are sporadic reports from Asia and Central America. It usually appears in children; 70% of yaws infections appear before the age of 15 [31]. (Subcutaneous nodules may ulcerate in late yaws.)

Ecthyma is more frequent in humid areas, especially among children (or elderly populations).

The geographic distribution of leprosy varies. It is endemic only in certain tropical and subtropical regions of Asia, Africa, and Central America [89].

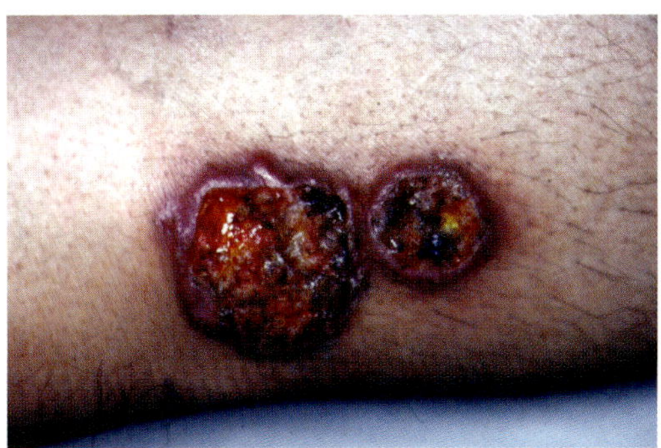

Fig. 5.9. Ulcerated lesions of leishmaniasis developing from a nodule (seen peripherally)

The possibility of certain infectious diseases, such as certain types of deep fungi or leishmaniasis (Fig. 5.9), should be considered according to the geographic location.

Tropical ulcer and noma develop mainly in malnourished children, in geographical areas subject to hunger; they have been documented in Africa and the Far East.

5.7 Additional Points

■ **Severity of Pain.** Severely painful ulcers occur in peripheral arterial disease, thromboangiitis obliterans (Buerger's disease). Ulcers caused by embolus, atrophie blanche, vasculitis, and connective tissue diseases are also painful. Pyoderma gangrenosum tends to be painful.

Neuropathic ulcers are painless. Venous ulcers are usually not associated with significant pain. If an ulcer labeled as venous causes severe pain, the diagnosis should be reconsidered.

In infectious ulcers the level of pain varies. Buruli ulcer is typically painless, while Meleney's ulcers are reported to be painful.

■ **Splenomegaly and Cutaneous Ulcers**

Splenomegaly and cutaneous ulcers tend to appear in the following conditions:
- Hemolytic anemia
- Felty's syndrome
- Malignant diseases (lymphoma, leukemia)
- Disseminated infectious disease
- Prolidase deficiency: splenomegaly appears in 30% of patients

■ **Ulcers in Linear Distribution.** Certain conditions are characterized by a linear distribution of cutaneous ulcers. The classical descriptions of a linear distribution of lesions are associated with sporotrichosis (where the distribution is determined by lymphatic drainage); hence, a linear pattern of distribution may also be referred to as a 'sporotrichoid pattern'.

Other conditions characterized by linear distribution are:

- Periarteritis nodosa: Cutaneous or subcutaneous nodules, that may undergo ulceration, appear along the course of superficial arteries: around the knee, anterior and distal shins, and dorsum of the foot.
- Wegener's granulomatosis: Nodules which may ulcerate tend to appear in crops, most commonly along extensor surface of extremities.
- Leishmaniasis or insect bites (secondarily infected): along the track of the 'hostile' insect (Fig. 5.10)
- Atypical mycobacterial infections: Such lesions may also appear in linear distribution.

■ Ulcers with Marked/Painful Lymphadenopathy

Lymphadenopathy characterizes ulcers in:
- Tuberculosis and atypical mycobacterial infections
- Tularemia
- Certain deep fungal infections (e.g., sporotrichosis)

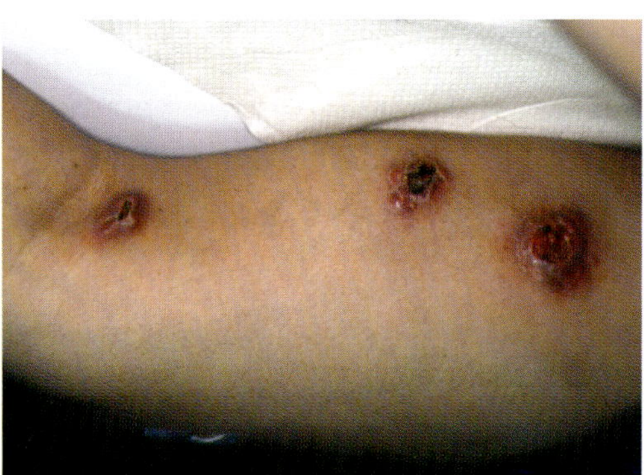

Fig. 5.10. Ulcers of leishmaniasis in linear distribution

The breaking down of lymph nodes and subsequent ulceration is characteristic of scrofuloderma. It occurs in the supraclavicular, parotidal, and submandibular areas and on the lateral aspect of the neck, due to the presence of lymph nodes in those areas. It is often bilateral. Scrofuloderma may occur on the extremities or the trunk, when the tuberculous process involves bones, joints, phalanges, ribs, or the sternum.

Suppuration of lymph nodes may also occur in chancroid and lymphogranuloma venereum.

■ Rapid Progression of Ulcerative Lesions

Rapid progression of multiple ulcerative lesions may appear in the following conditions:
- Vasculitis
- Multiple emboli
- Calciphylaxis
- Various infections (related to virulence of the offending micro-organism and the host's defense mechanisms

■ Corymbiform Pattern. A larger central lesion surrounded by smaller lesions is said to have a corymbiform pattern. It may occur in syphilitic chancres, leishmaniasis, and pyoderma gangrenosum.

5.8 Addendum: Details Regarding Venous and Arterial Ulcers

Since venous and arterial ulcers are relatively common, we shall discuss here more details regarding the history and physical examination of these ulcers.

5.8.1 Venous Ulcers

Patients with venous insufficiency frequently complain of dull pain and heaviness associated with standing, usually accompanied by swelling of the legs. These symptoms are relieved by walking and by elevating the legs; night cramps occur not infrequently. (In the presence of severe or excruciating pain, other diagnoses should be considered.)

■ **Skin Around the Ulcer.** Eczematous changes of varying degree of severity may appear. There are usually varicose veins. Purple to brown pigmentation is attributed to extravasation of red blood cells and sedimentation of hemosiderin in the surrounding tissues. The edema becomes more and more indurated as the process advances. Lipodermatosclerosis appears in long-standing disease, manifested by highly indurated skin on the lower third of the leg, which looks relatively thin compared with the edematous upper part.

■ **Location of Venous Ulcers.** The discussion on mechanisms of venous ulcer formation in Chap. 4 may help to explain the distribution of venous ulcers. Since venous pressure and its detrimental effect on tissues is maximal distally, venous ulcers occur on the lower calf. The medial malleolus is more commonly affected. This finding is attributed to the anatomy of the venous system; a larger mass of venous vessels is located medially. Therefore, the medial aspects of the legs are subjected to higher venous pressures. Nevertheless, not infrequently, these ulcers may appear above the lateral malleolus as well.

5.8.2 Arterial Ulcers

The initial complaint in peripheral arterial disease is intermittent claudication: a cramping pain, primarily affecting the calf muscles, that appears on walking and is relieved by rest. Note that a patient whose mobility is limited may not complain of intermittent claudication. In the advanced stage of the disease, pain appears at rest; it tends to appear in the foot region and can be excruciating, disturbing the patient's sleep. Lowering of the legs may relieve the pain to some degree.

■ **Physical Examination.** Peripheral pulses are decreased or absent on physical examination. The limbs tend to be cold; they are pale or cyanotic, but a red hue may be present, especially on the foot. Capillary filling time tends to be prolonged. When there is a significant degree of ischemia, elevation of the legs causes pallor; lowering the legs again causes delayed and exaggerated hyperemia, prominent in the dorsum of the foot.

The skin tends to be dry and a little scaly, with hair loss. It may be atrophic. The nails appear brittle, distorted, and thickened.

■ **Location of Arterial Ulcers.** In view of the fact that a high percentage of arterial ulcers are caused by trauma, arterial ulceration may develop anywhere on the lower calves. Ulcers tend to appear on the lateral or pretibial aspects of the leg, or on the dorsum of the foot. Note that they may appear in the malleolar region as well.

When critical limb ischemia has developed, it may be manifested by distal necrosis of the toes or forefoot necrosis; this condition has a poor prognosis, and amputation may be necessary.

References

1. Wenzel HC, Wollina U: Systemic lupus erythematosus presenting as pyoderma gangrenosum. J Eur Acad Dermatol Venereol 1995; 4:20–25
2. Cheah JS: Systemic lupus erythematosus in a Chinese woman presenting with gangrene of the fingers. Aust N Z J Med 1973; 3:197–199
3. Kissin MW, Williamson RC: Hydralazine-induced SLE-like syndrome presenting as a leg ulcer. Br Med J 1979; 2:1330
4. Rowell NR, Goodfield MJD: The 'connective tissue diseases'. In: Champion RH, Burton JL, Ebling FJG (eds) Rook/Wilkinson/Ebling Textbook of Dermatology, 5th edn. Oxford: Blackwell Scientific Publications. 1992; pp 2163–2294
5. Brazzelli V, Vassallo C, Baldini F, et al: Wegener granulomatosis in a child: Cutaneous findings as the presenting signs. Pediatr Dermatol 1999; 16:277–280
6. Daoud MS, Gibson LE, DeRemee RA, et al: Cutaneous Wegener's granulomatosis: Clinical histopathologic, and immunopathologic features of thirty patients. J Am Acad Dermatol 1994; 31:605–612

7. Chyu JY, Hagstrom WJ, Soltani K, et al: Wegener's granulomatosis in childhood: cutaneous manifestations as the presenting signs. J Am Acad Dermatol 1984; 10:341–346

8. Odom BO, James WD, Berger TG (eds) Cutaneous vascular diseases. In: Andrews' Diseases of the Skin: Clinical Dermatology, 9th edn. Philadelphia: WB Saunders. 2000; pp 1052–1053

9. Lucky AW: Cutaneous manifestations of endocrine, metabolic and nutritional diorders.In: Schachner LA, Hansen RC (eds) Pediatric Dermatology, 2nd edn. New York: Churchill Livingstone. 1995; pp 1043–1104

10. Ryan TJ: Cutaneous vasculitis. Champion RH, Burton JL, Ebling FJG (eds) In: Rook/Wilkinson/Ebling Textbook of Dermatology, 5th edn. Oxford: Blackwell Scientific Publications. 1992; pp 1893–1961

11. Krause W, Happle R: Sexually transmitted diseases. In: Schachner LA, Hansen RC (eds) Pediatric Dermatology, 2nd edn. New York: Churchill Livingstone. 1995; pp 1393–1444

12. Raimer S, Raimer BG, Lane AT: Physical injury and enviromental hazards. In: Schachner LA, Hansen RC (eds) Pediatric Dermatology, 2nd edn. New York: Churchill Livingstone. 1995; pp 1475–1499

13. Krafchik BR: Eczematous dermatitis. In: Schachner LA, Hansen RC (eds) Pediatric Dermatology, 2nd edn. New York: Churchill Livingstone. 1995; pp 704–705

14. Wagner AM, Hansen RC: Neonatal skin and skin disorders. In: Schachner LA, Hansen RC (eds) Pediatric Dermatology, 2nd edn. New York: Churchill Livingstone. 1995; pp 263–346

15. Pearson H: Sickle cell diseases: diagnosis and management in infancy and childhood. Pediatr Rev 1987; 9:121–130

16. Wethers DL: Problems and complications in the adolescent with sickle cell disease. Am J Pediatr Hematol Oncol 1982; 4:47–53

17. Koshy M, Entsuah R, Koranda A, et al: Leg ulcers in patients with sickle cell disease. Blood 1989; 74:1403–1408

18. Gimmon Z, Wexler MR, Rachmilewitz EA: Juvenile leg ulceration in β-thalassemia major and intermedia. Plast Recontr Surg 1982; 69:320–325

19. Peretz E, Hallel-Halevy D, Grunwald MH: Hereditary spherocytosis with leg ulcers healed after splenectomy. Eur J Dermatol 1997; 7:527–528

20. Muller-Soyano A, Tovar de Roura E, Duke PR: Pyruvate kinase deficiency and leg ulcers. Blood 1976; 47:807–813

21. Sills EM, Barnett NK, Provost TT: Collagen vascular and connective tissue diseases. In: Schachner LA, Hansen RC (eds) Pediatric Dermatology, 2nd edn. New York: Churchill Livingstone. 1995; pp 1105–1150

22. Hurowitz S: Vasculitic disorders. In: Clinical Pediatric Dermatology, 2nd edn. Philadelphia: W B Saunders. 1993; pp 539–557

23. Sheth AP, Olson JC, Esterly NB: Cutaneous polyarteritis nodosa of childhood J Am Acad Dermatol 1994; 31:561–566

24. Navon P, Yarom A, Davis E: Raynaud's features in childhood. Clinical, immunological and capillaroscopic study. J Mal Vasc 1992; 17:273–276

25. Tredwell PA: Selected systemic diseases with skin manifestations. In: Schachner LA, Hansen RC (eds) Pediatric Dermatology, 2nd edn. New York: Churchill Livingstone. 1995; pp 1151–1168

26. Powell FC, Perry HO: Pyoderma gangrenosum in childhood. Arch Dermatol 1984; 120:757–761

27. Dick DC, MacKie RM, Patrick WJ, et al: Pyoderma gangrenosum in infancy. Acta Derm Venereol (Stockh) 1982; 62:348–350

28. Bissonnette R, Friedmann D, Giroux JM et al: Prolidase deficiency: a multisystemic hereditary disorder. J Am Acad Dermatol 1993; 29:818–821

29. Paquet P, Lapiere CM: Causes of delayed wound healing and optimization of the patient's condition. In: Westerhof W (ed) Leg Ulcers: Diagnosis and Treatment, 1st edn. Amsterdam: Elsevier. 1993; pp 281–292

30. Lee PK, Zipoli MT, Weinberg AN, Swartz MN, Johnson RA: Pyodermas: staphylococcus aureus, streptococcus and other gram-positive bacteria. In: Freedberg IM, Eisen AZ, Wolff K, Austen KF, Goldsmith LA, Katz SI (eds) Fitzpatrick's Dermatology in General Medicine, 6th edn. New York: McGraw-Hill 2003; pp 1856– 1878

31. Engelkens HJ, Judanarso J, Oranje AP, et al: Endemic treponematoses. Int J Dermatol 1991; 30:77–83

32. Robinson DC, Adriaans B, Hay RJ, et al: The clinical and epidemiologic features of tropical ulcer (tropical phagedenic ulcer). Int J Dermatol 1988; 27:49–53

33. Mandell BF, Hoffman GS: Systemic necrotizing arteritis. Freedberg IM, EisenAZ, Wolff K, AustenKF, Goldsmith LA, Katz SI (eds) In Fitzpatrick's Dermatology in General Medicine, 6th edn. New York: McGraw-Hill. 2003; pp 1718–1727

34. Bridges AJ, Porter J, England D: Lower extremity peripheral neuropathy and ischemic ulcers associated with giant cell arteritis. J Rheumatol 1989; 16:1366–1369

35. Gibson GE, Su WP, Pittelkow MR: Antiphospholipid syndrome and the skin. J Am Acad Dermatol 1997; 36:970–982

36. Vanscheidt W, Leder O, Vanscheidt E, et al: Leg ulcers in a patient with spherocytosis: a clinicopathological report. Dermatologica 1990; 181:56–59

37. Kulthanan K, Krudum T, Pintadit P, et al: Chronic leg ulcers associated with hereditary protein S deficiency. Int J Dermatol 1997; 36:210–212

38. Falanga V, Bontempo FA, Eaglstein WH: Protein C and Protein S plasma levels in patients with lipodermatosclerosis and venous ulceration. Arch Dermatol 1990; 126:1195–1197

39. Hafner J, von Felten A: Resistance to activated protein C in patients with venous leg ulcers. Dermatology 1997; 195:413–414

40. Maessen-Visch MB, Hamulyak K, Tazelaar DJ, et al: The prevalence of factor V Leiden mutation in patients with leg ulcers and venous insufficiency. Arch Dermatol 1999; 135:41–44

41. Maessen-Visch MB, Koedam MI, Hamulyak K, et al: Atrophie blanche. Int J Dermatol 1999; 38:161–172

42. Schwaegerle SM, Bergfeld WF, Senitzer D, et al. Pyoderma gangrenosum: a review. J Am Acad Dermatol 1988; 18:559–568

43. Phillips TJ, Salman SM, Rogers GS: Nonhealing leg ulcers: A manifestation of basal cell carcinoma. J Am Acad Dermatol 1991; 25:47–49

44. Harris B, Eaglstein WH, Falanga V: Basal cell carcinoma arising in venous ulcers and mimicking granulation tissue. J Dermatol Surg Oncol 1993; 19:150–152

45. Brodell RT, Wagamon K: The persistent nonhealing ulcer. Could it be basal cell carcinoma? Postgrad Med 2001; 109:29–32

46. Blank AA, Schnyder UW: Squamous cell carcinoma and basal cell carcinoma within the clinical picture of a chronic venous insufficiency in the third stage. Dermatologica 1990; 181:248–250

47. Ackroyd S, Young AE: Leg ulcers that do not heal. Br Med J 1983; 286:207–208

48. Pierard G, Fumal I, Pierard-Franchimont C: Cold injuries. In: Freedberg IM, Eisen AZ, Wolff K, Austen KF, Goldsmith LA, Katz SI (eds) Fitzpatrick's Dermatology in General Medicine, 6th edn. New York: McGraw-Hill. 2003; pp 1211–1220

49. Karmody AM, Powers SR, Monaco VJ, et al: 'Blue toe' syndrome: An indication for limb salvage surgery. Arch Surg 1976; 111:1263–1268

50. Freund NS: Cholesterol emboli syndrome following cardiac catheterization. Postgrad Med 1990; 87:55–60

51. Morton RS: The treponematoses. In: Champion RH, Burton JL, Burns DA, Breathnach SM (eds) Rook/Wilkinson/Ebling Textbook of Dermatology, 6th edn. Oxford: Blackwell Scientific Publications. 1998; pp 1237–1275

52. Ohtsuka T, Yamakage A, Yamazaki S: Digital ulcers and necroses: novel manifestations of angiocentric lymphoma. Br J Dermatol 2000; 142:1013–1016

53. Russwurm R, Hagedorn M: Lichen ruber ulcerosus. Hautarzt 1989; 40:233–235

54. Parodi A, Ciulla P, Rebora A: An old lady with scarring alopecia and an ulcerated sole. Ulcerative lichen planus. Arch Dermatol 1991; 127:407–410

55. Micalizzi C, Tagliapietra G, Farris A: Ulcerative lichen planus of the sole with rheumatoid arthritis. Int J Dermatol 1998; 37:862–863

56. Barbarulo AM, Metha N, Bucalo B, et al: Recurrent disseminated herpes zoster and cytomegalic perianal ulcer: a case report and review of the literature. Cutis 2001; 67:43–46

57. Pariser RJ: Histologically specific skin lesions in disseminated cytomegalovirus infection. J Am Acad Dermatol 1983; 9:937–946

58. Rodot S, Lacour JP, Elslande L, et al: Ecthyma gangrenosum caused by Klebsiella pneumoniae. Int J Dermatol 1995; 34:216–217

59. Eke N: Fournier's gangrene: a review of 1726 cases. Br J Surg 2000; 87:718–728

60. Vick R, Carson CC 3rd: Fournier's disease. Urol Clin North Am 1999; 26:841–849

61. Borgstrom E: Penile ulcer as complication in self induced papaverine erections. Urology 1988; 32:416–417

62. Brandt O, Abeck D, Breitbart E, Ring J: Perianal ergotismus gangraenosus. Hautarzt 1997; 48:199–202

63. Baptista AP, Mariano A, Machado A: Peranal ulcers caused by ergotamine-containing suppositories. Acta Med Port 1992; 5:39–41

64. Fisher AA: Unique reactions of scrotal skin to topical agents. Cutis 1989; 44:445–447

65. Zax RH, Kulp-Shorten CL, Callen JP: Leukemia cutis presenting as a scrotal ulcer. J Am Acad Dermatol 1989; 21:410–413

66. Senti G, Schleiffenbaumb B, Dummera R: Vaginal ulcers as initial presentation of subacute myelomonocytic leukemia. Dermatology 1999; 199:346–348

67. Magro CM, Crowson AN: Cutaneous manifestations of Behçet's disease. Int J Dermatol 1995; 34:159–165

68. Slutzki S, Bogokowsky H, Gilboa Y, et al: Coumadin-induced skin necrosis. Int J Dermatol 1984; 23:117–119

69. Defranzo AJ, Marasco P, Argenta LC: Warfarin-induced skin necrosis of the skin. Ann Plast Surg 1995; 34:203–208

70. Kanj LF, Wilking SVB, Phillips TJ: Pressure ulcers. J Am Acad Dermatol 1998; 38:517–536

71. Agris J, Spira M: Pressure ulcers: prevention and treatment. Clin Symp 1979; 31:1–32

72. Grunwald MH, Amichai B, Trau H: Cutaneous leishmaniasis on an unusual site – the glans penis. Br J Urol 1998; 82:928

73. Hay RJ, Adriaans B: Bacterial infections. In: Champion RH, Burton JL, Burns DA, Breathnach SM (eds) Rook/Wilkinson/Ebling Textbook of Dermatology, 6th edn. Oxford: Blackwell Scientific Publications. 1998; pp 1097–1179

74. Odom BO, James WD, Berger TG (eds) Bacterial infections. In: Andrews' Diseases of the Skin: Clinical Dermatology, 9th edn. Philadelphia: WB Saunders. 2000; pp 307–357

75. Tsao H, Swartz MN, Weinberg AN, Johnson RA: Soft tissue infections; erysipelas, cellulitis and gangrenous cellulitis. In: Freedberg IM, Eisen AZ, Wolff K, Austen KF, Goldsmith LA, Katz SI, Fitzpatrick TB (eds) Fitzpatrick's Dermatology in General Medicine, 5th edn. New York: McGraw-Hill. 1999; pp 2213–2231

76. Irvine AD, Bruce IN, Walsh M, et al: Dermatological presentation of disease associated with antineutrophil cytoplasmic antibodies: a report of two contrasting cases and a review of the literature. Br J Dermatol 1996; 134:924–928

77. Weninger W, Kain R, Tschachler E, et al: Microscopic polyangiitis with eosinophilia- an overlap syndrome or separate disease entity? A case report and review of the literature. Hautarzt 1997; 48:332–338

78. Peterson LL: Hydralazine-induced systemic lupus erythematosus presenting as pyoderma gangreno-

sum-like ulcers. J Am Acad Dermatol 1984; 10: 379–384

79. Skaria AM, Ruffieux P, Piletta P, et al: Takayasu arteritis and cutaneous necrotizing vasculitis. Dermatology 2000; 200:139–143

80. Frances C: Dermato-mucosal manifestations of Behçet's disease. Ann Med Interne (Paris) 1999; 150: 535–541

81. Schlesinger IH, Farber GA: Cutaneous ulceration resembling pyoderma gangrenosum in the primary antiphospholid syndrome: a report of two additional cases and review of the literature. J La State Med Soc 1995; 147:357–361

82. Helm KF, Peters MS, Tefferi A, et al: Pyoderma gangrenosum-like ulcer in a patient with large granular lymphocytic leukemia. J Am Acad Dermatol 1992; 27:868–871

83. Massa MC, Doyle JA: Cutaneous cryptococcosis simulating pyoderma gangrenosum. J Am Acad Dermatol 1981; 5:32–36

84. Ryan TJ, Burnand KG: Diseases of the veins and arteries – leg ulcers. In: Champion RH, Burton JL, Ebling FJG (eds) Rook/Wilkinson/Ebling Textbook of Dermatology, 5th edn. Oxford: Blackwell Scientific Publications. 1992; pp 1963–2013

85. Weinberg AN, Swartz MN: Miscellaneous bacterial infections with cutaneous manifestations. In: Freedberg IM, EisenAZ, Wolff K, Austen KF, Goldsmith LA, Katz SI and Fitzpatrick TB (eds) Fitzpatrick's Dermatology in General Medicine, 5th edn. New York: McGraw-Hill. 1999; pp 2257–2273

86. Gwakrodger DJ: Mycobacterial infections. In: Champion RH, Burton JL, Burns DA, Breathnach SM (eds) Rook/Wilkinson/Ebling Textbook of Dermatology, 6th edn. Oxford: Blackwell Scientific Publications. 1998; pp 1181–1214

87. Dowd PM: Reactions to cold. In: Champion RH, Burton JL, Burns DA, Breathnach SM (eds) Rook/Wilkinson/Ebling Textbook of Dermatology, 6th edn. Oxford: Blackwell Scientific Publications. 1998; pp 957– 972

88. Kalter DC, Rudolph A, McGavran M: Livedo reticularis due to multiple cholesterol emboli. J Am Acad Dermatol 1985; 13:235–242

89. Ramos-e-Silva M, Rebello PF: Leprosy. Recognition and treatment. Am J Clin Dermatol 2001; 2:203–211

Determining Etiology: Biopsy and Laboratory Investigation

6

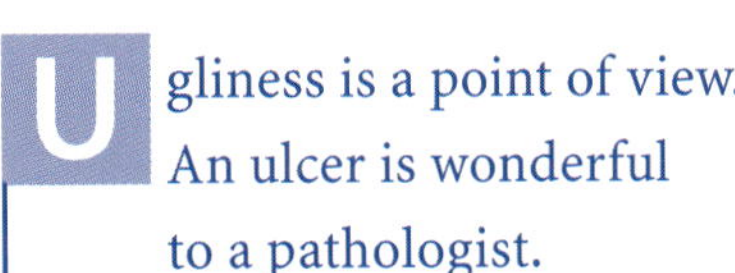

gliness is a point of view.
An ulcer is wonderful
to a pathologist.

(Austin O'Malley)

Contents

6.1 Overview

The etiology of a cutaneous ulcer is determined essentially by history and physical examination. When these do not suffice to establish the diagnosis, laboratory investigation, including histologic sampling, is required.

In most cases, routine blood tests should be performed for every patient presenting with a cutaneous ulcer where the diagnosis is not established. These routine workups, which generally include tests such as erythrocyte sedimentation rate, complete blood count, and blood chemistry, may direct the physician towards the etiology in certain cases. In many other situations with cutaneous ulcers, the anamnesis and physical examination may suggest the need for a more specific and focused investigation.

For example, an ulcer suspected of being related to hemolytic anemia requires the performance of a blood smear, which may reveal sickled cells, spherocytes, etc.

Similarly, when a connective-tissue disease is suspected, the workup should include laboratory parameters such as anti-nuclear factor, rheumatoid factor, cryoglobulin level, or anti-neutrophil cytoplasmic antibody (ANCA).

In cases of cutaneous ulcers, histologic specimens may provide valuable information regarding their etiology. The histologic hallmark of a cutaneous ulcer is dictated by its medical definition, namely, *the absence of epidermis and the partial or complete absence of dermis.* Yet the question is not whether there is an ulcer but what the underlying pathology is. Therefore, the biopsy should not be taken from the ulcer itself, but rather from an area adjacent to the ulcer margin, covered by dermis and epidermis; where specific histologic features may be identified.

In order to cover all the clinical possibilities that may derive from the histology of a cutaneous ulcer, a broad knowledge of dermatopathology is required. Nevertheless, our purpose here is not to review the entire gamut of currently available dermatopathological knowledge, but to relate only the most practical clinical implications arising from histologic features of cutaneous ulcers.

A biopsy should be considered from an ulcer's margin under the following conditions:

- **An ulcer in which the clinical diagnosis is not established:** when history, physical examination and the ulcer's appearance do not provide a concrete diagnosis i.e., when there is no clinical clue, or when one wants to confirm a suspected/doubtful diagnosis.
- **A non-healing ulcer:** Biopsy should be considered when dealing with an ulcer that does not heal within three to four months of optimal treatment. This is subject to the clinical set-up (see below).
- **Suspected malignancy:** when the ulcer is suspected of being malignant/cancerous. Under these circumstances, a biopsy should be performed as early as possible.

Each of the above possibilities is discussed below.

6.2 A Cutaneous Ulcer in Which the Clinical Diagnosis Is Not Established

6.2.1 Possibilities of Histologic Picture

Sometimes, neither the history nor the physical examination provides any clues to assist in arriving at a diagnosis. A biopsy from an area adjacent to the ulcer margin should be done, in order to obtain diagnostic clues.

This chapter deals with those topics that are specifically relevant to the histopathology of skin ulcers, such as intravascular occlusion or vasculitis. In addition, we shall discuss the steps to be taken if the histologic specimen does not provide sufficient diagnostic information.

6.2.2 Intravascular Occlusion

Intravascular occlusion may manifest in several forms, depending on the pathologic process leading to occlusion. Conditions characterized by intravascular occlusion are listed in Table 6.1.

Coagulopathies are common forms of intravascular occlusion [1, 2]. In these cases, intravascular occlusion is reflected histologically by the presence of fibrin thrombi within the lumen of blood vessels (Fig. 6.1). Fibrin thrombi appear as amorphous eosinophilic material in hematoxylin and eosin (H&E) stain; they may be more obvious in a periodic acid-Schiff (PAS) stain. In severe forms of coagulopathy, areas of cutaneous necrosis may be observed [2].

Fibrin thrombi may be accompanied by unique features such as cholesterol clefts in cholesterol emboli (Fig. 6.2) or calcium deposition in calciphylaxis (Fig. 6.3). Other histologic features may also be involved in intravascular occlusion. For example, in sickle cell anemia, blood vessels are occluded by the sludging of sickled erythrocytes [3, 4] (Fig. 6.4).

Note that intravascular occlusion and the presence of fibrin thrombi within the lumen of blood vessels may variably appear in vasculitic processes as well. Yet, vasculitis also has unique characteristics, such as the infiltration of white blood cells within the wall of blood vessels or actual signs of damage to the vessel wall (see Sect. 6.2.3). In this section, we present conditions of intravascular occlusion which are *not* accompanied by vasculitis.

In some cases, the clinical diagnosis is straightforward and the histology simply complements the history and physical examination.

Table 6.1. Intravascular occlusion

Coagulopathies [1, 2, 5–7]

- Coumarin-induced necrosis[a]
- Heparin necrosis
- Disseminated intravascular coagulation
- Purpura fulminans
- Protein C deficiency[b]
- Activated protein C resistance[b]
- Protein S deficiency[b]
- Anti-thrombin III deficiency[b]

Hemolytic anemia [3, 4, 11, 12]

- Sickle cell anemia
- Hereditary spherocytosis
- Paroxysmal nocturnal hemoglobinuria

Dysproteinemia [1, 2, 8–10]

- Cryoglobulinemia (monoclonal, type 1)
- Waldenstrom's macroglobulinemia
- Cryofibrinogenemia

Others [1, 2, 13–22]

- Atrophie blanche
- Anti-phospholipid syndrome
- Calciphylaxis
- Cholesterol emboli
- Other embolic phenomena

a. Although coumarin is usually associated with fibrin thrombi, certain cases of vasculitis (with ulceration) following its use have been reported [23, 24].
b. In most cases, these conditions result in leg ulcers via the formation of deep vein thrombosis which, in itself, predisposes to venous ulceration. However, fibrin thrombi have been described in such cases as well [2]. Most of these cases have been associated with coumarin or heparin therapy.

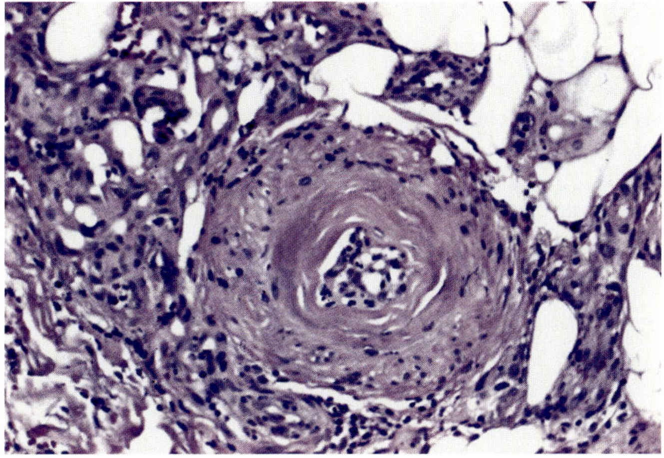

Fig. 6.1.
A fibrin thrombus within
the lumen of a blood vessel

Fig. 6.2.
Cholesterol clefts

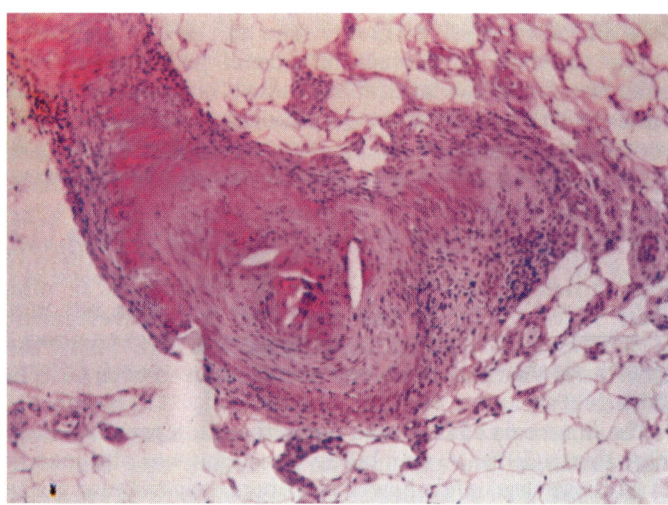

Fig. 6.3.
An occluded blood vessel
in calciphylaxis

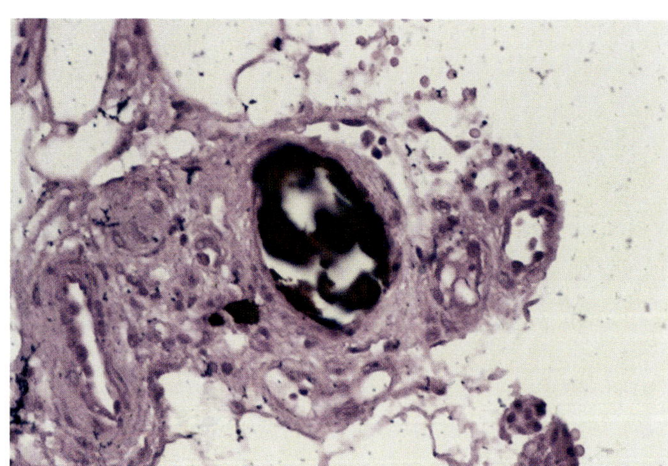

For instance, the diagnosis of coumarin necrosis may be reached when anamnesis confirms intake of the drug a few days before ulceration. Similarly, cutaneous ulcers and splenomegaly in a young patient raise the possibility of hemolytic anemia.

6.2.2.1 Histologic Features

In conditions such as coagulopathies, dysproteinemias, or anti-phospholipid syndrome, the histopathologic features may be similar, and an accurate diagnosis cannot be established by biopsy alone. On the other hand, in other conditions, specific histologic features may assist in determining the ulcer's etiology.

Fig. 6.4.
Sickled erythrocytes occluding
blood vessels

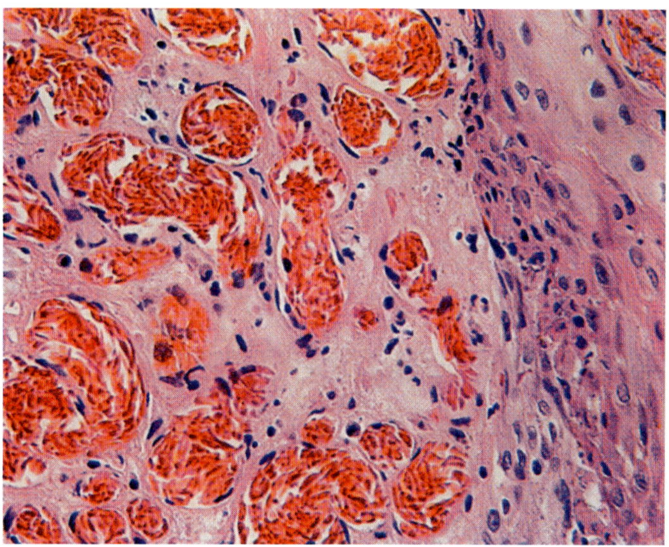

Histologic clues such as those mentioned below should be sought (presented in Schema 6.1):

- **Microcalcifications in small to medium sized vessels:** This histologic finding appears in calciphylaxis. It is well demonstrated by a Von Kossa stain [17–19].
- **Bizarre forms of red blood cells:** Bizarre forms of red blood cells such as sickled erythrocytes or spherocytes may be found within capillaries in ulcers caused by hemolytic anemia; extravasation of red blood cells may be seen [3, 4, 11].
- **Cholesterol clefts:** Cholesterol emboli are characterized by the presence of cholesterol clefts within the fibrinous material [20–22]. Note that the absence of typical cholesterol clefts does not necessarily rule out the diagnosis of cholesterol emboli [25, 26]. It may be difficult to locate and identify cholesterol emboli, and a deep biopsy may be needed [2].

6.2.2.2 Other Histologic Clues

■ **Atrophie Blanche.** In the initial stages of atrophie blanche, the entity might still not be identified by histology; i.e., fibrin thrombi within blood vessels may be the sole finding. However, more severe cases may present features such as infarction with hemorrhage or an inflammatory infiltrate. In late atrophic lesions, a thin epidermis is usually seen, and the dermis becomes sclerotic [2, 13].

■ **Stain Type.** The type of stain used may give and clues for diagnosis: Precipitated cryoglobulins appear bright red with PAS stain, while other fibrinoid depositions, caused by other processes, tend to stain lighter [2]. As mentioned above, deposition of calcium within blood vessels, as appears in calciphylaxis, may be identified by using the Von Kossa stain [19].

6.2.2.3 Blood Tests

When fibrin thrombi are seen and the diagnosis is not established, certain blood tests should be considered:

Anti-phospholipid syndrome
- Anti-cardiolipin antibodies
- Lupus anticoagulant
- β 2 glycoprotein 1

Impaired coagulability
- Protein S level
- Protein C level
- Anti-thrombin III level
- Resistance to activated protein C
- Analysis of DNA to factor V Leiden

Deposition of paraprotein
- Cryoglobulin
- Cryofibrinogen
- Protein electrophoresis
- Quantitive immunoglobulins

Although the scheme for histological identification shown in Fig. 6.5 is quite comprehensive, we have encountered isolated cases of cutaneous ulcers with fibrin thrombi in which, following thorough investigation, a definite etiology could not be identified.

6.2.3 Vasculitis

Fully developed vasculitis is characterized by the following histologic features [1] (see Fig. 6.6):
- Infiltration of white blood cells within the wall of blood vessels
- Deposits of fibrin within the wall and lumen of blood vessels
- Extravasation of red blood cells – secondary to injury of the blood vessels

Other signs of damage to the wall may be present, such as the degeneration of collagen fibers, and the necrosis of endothelial cells and smooth muscle cells.

A special type of vasculitis that manifests unique features is **leukocytoclastic vasculitis**, the hallmark of which is the presence of polymorphonuclear cells and fragmented nuclei, usually termed 'nuclear dust'.

Note that when vasculitis results in the formation of cutaneous ulcers, we expect to identify a form of **necrotizing vasculitis** in the histologic specimen, showing necrotic areas with

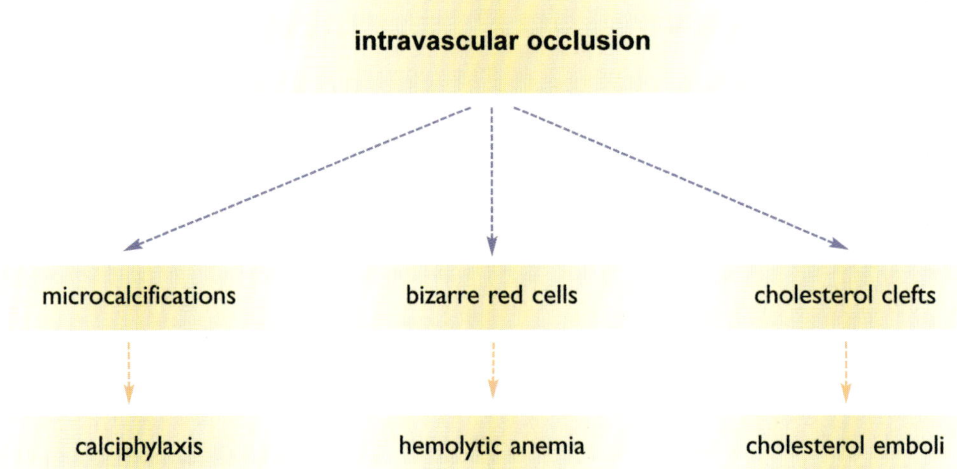

Fig. 6.5. Histological identification of certain conditions characterized by intravascular occlusion

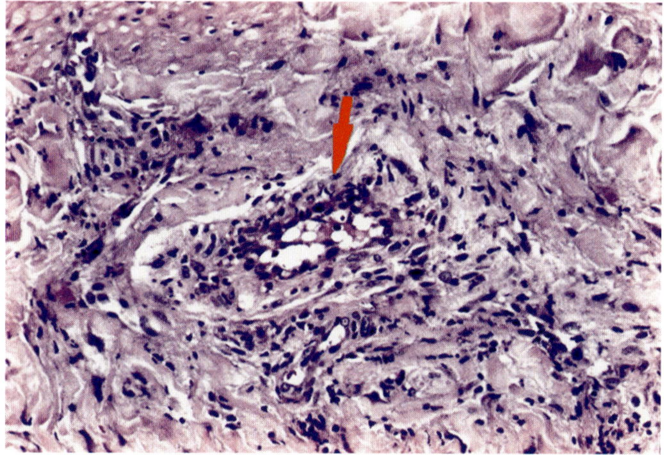

Fig. 6.6.
Vasculitis: note the damaged vessel wall, infiltrated by inflammatory cells

significant damage to blood vessels and surrounding tissues.

The literature is replete with a wide range of different classifications of vasculitic lesions, and there is no one accepted classification. Most authors present differing specific classifications.

Tables 6.2, 6.3, and 6.4 present a reasonable and convenient classification of types of vasculitis that tend to be associated with ulceration. These tables are based, in part, on the following:
1. Classification of vasculitis, as presented by A.B. Ackerman [1]
2. Classification of the vasculitis syndromes, as presented by A.S. Fauci [27] in *Harrison's Principles of Internal Medicine*
3. The definitions of vasculitis as delineated by the *Chapel Hill Consensus Conference* in 1992 [28, 29]

Accurate identification of the subtype of vasculitis is determined by the following data:
- Type of vessel involved (arterial system versus venous system)
- Size of vessel involved (e.g., postcapillary venule)
- Type of infiltrate: neutrophilic? lymphocytic?
- Presence or absence of leukocytoclasis (fragmented neutrophilic nuclei)

Table 6.3 presents conditions associated with small-vessel leukocytoclastic vasculitis.

In some cases of vasculitis, the pathology will not be obvious in a given histologic specimen. The lesion may be in its early stages, when the vasculitic process may not yet be evident. In other cases, the specific site from which the biopsy was taken will not reflect the pathology accurately. Therefore, if a histologic specimen is not diagnostic, the biopsy should be repeated.

Grunwald et al. [33] have shown that direct immunofluorescence is a very sensitive test, which may confirm the presence of vasculitis in conditions where routine histologic specimens sometimes fail to do so (e.g., in the early and resolving stages of the vasculitic process).

Where there is histologic evidence of vasculitis, the following laboratory workup should be considered, depending on the clinical setup:
- Erythrocyte sedimentation rate
- Complete blood count
- Blood chemistry
- Anti-nuclear factor
- Rheumatoid factor
- Cryoglobulin level
- Hepatitis C
- Hepatitis B
- c-antineutrophil cytoplasmic antibody (cANCA)

- p-antineutrophil cytoplasmic antibody (pANCA)
- Serum markers for malignancy
- Chest X-ray
- Abdominal ultrasound
- Fecal occult blood testing

In some cases, even after extensive investigation, no definite explanation for the vasculitis can be found. Such cases remain defined as idiopathic vasculitis, in which a specific disease may become apparent at a later date.

Table 6.2. Cutaneous ulcers characterized by vasculitis

Vasculitis induced by an exogenous stimulus:

- Drug-induced vasculitis[a]
- Serum sickness
- Infectious agent[b]

As an expression of a connective tissue disease/ multi-system diseases[c]:

- Rheumatoid arthritis
- Systemic lupus erythematosus
- Dermatomyositis
- Scleroderma
- Sjögren's disease
- Cryoglobulinemia (mixed, type II & III)[d]
- Periarteritis nodosa
- Wegener's granulomatosis
- Allergic angiitis and granulomatosis (Churg-Strauss syndrome)
- Behçet's disease
- Temporal arteritis
- Takayasu disease

Other vasculitic processes

- Vasculitis associated with malignancy
- Nodular vasculitis (erythema induratum)
- Erythema elevatum diutinum
- Kawasaki disease
- Pyoderma gangrenosum
- Idiopathic vasculitis

a. Many drugs may induce vasculitis. Drugs commonly associated with vasculitis include penicillin, sulfonamides, thiazides, allopurinol and non-steroidal anti-inflammatory agents [30].

b. Leukocytoclastic vasculitis may be induced by several types of infections, most commonly *Streptococcus* group A and *Mycobacterium leprae*; hepatitis B and C are also well-known inducers of leukocytoclastic vasculitis [30].

c. In some of the conditions presented above, ulceration may develop by other mechanisms, without vasculitis. For example, some patients with SLE are reported to have premature atherosclerosis [31]; thus, ulcers in these patients may develop due to peripheral arterial disease. Similarly, SLE patients may develop ulcers as a manifestation of secondary antiphospholipid syndrome (16). In other multi-system diseases mentioned above, ulceration is not necessarily associated with vasculitis. Lesions in Behcet's disease may appear without histologic evidence of vasculitis [32].

d. Mixed cryoglobulinemia may be associated with several systemic or infectious diseases such as rheumatoid arthritis, Sjögren's disease, chronic lymphocytic leukemia and hepatitis C.

Table 6.3. Small vessel leukocytoclastic vasculitis[a, b]

Vasculitis induced by an exogenous stimulus:

- Drug-induced vasculitis
- Vasculitis induced by an infectious process
- Serum sickness

As an expression of a connective tissue disease/multi-system diseases:

- Rheumatoid arthritis
- Systemic lupus erythematosus
- Dermatomyositis
- Scleroderma
- Sjögren's disease
- Cryoglubulinemia (mixed, type II & III)
- Polyarteritis nodosa
- Wegener's granulomatosis
- Allergic angiitis and granulomatosis (Churg-Strauss syndrome)
- Behçet's disease

Vasculitis associated with malignancy

a. More detailed discussions regarding vasculitis and its classification can be found in dermatopathology texts. We do wish to make the point, however, that although in most of the conditions listed in the above table the infiltrate is largely neutrophilic, in certain types of vasculitis there is typically a lymphocytic vasculitis (e.g., in collagen diseases such as SLE and some cases of drug-induced vasculitis or arthropod bites [1, 2].
b. Erythema elevatum diutinum also manifests small vessel leukocytoclastic vasculitis [28].

Table 6.4. Cutaneous ulcers in which medium-sized vasculitis or large cell vasculitis may be identified[a, b]

Large-vessel vasculitis

- Temporal arteritis
- Takayasu's disease

Medium-sized vessel vasculitis

- Polyarteritis nodosa
- Kawasaki disease
- Erythema induratum
- Wegener's granulomatosis

a. Wegener's granulomatosis presents as leukocytoclastic vasculitis of small vessels together with vasculitis of large venous vessels [1].
b. Polyarteritis nodosa may present as leukocytoclastic vasculitis of small vessels and as large vessel arterial vasculitis [1].

6.2.4 Other Histologic Patterns

In some cases, a unique histologic pattern may be seen (e.g., a specific type of tumor, or a specific inflammatory process), which provides an accurate diagnosis. Yet, there is a huge range of possible causes of skin ulcers. Hence, many diagnoses may be revealed in a histologic specimen obtained from a cutaneous ulcer. A broad knowledge of dermatopathology is needed to identify all the histologic possibilities.

The classic textbooks of dermatopathology deal with this issue very well
- *Histologic Diagnosis of Inflammatory Skin Diseases: An Algorithmic Method Based on Pattern Analysis (A. B. Ackerman)*
- *Lever's Histopathology of the Skin (Elder, Elenitsas, Jaworsky and Johnson)*

Note that in most cases, the presence of inflammatory cells within the histologic section cannot be used as a diagnostic clue, except where a unique pattern of distribution is identified. Any cutaneous ulcer is subject to inflammatory processes, independent of its primary basic pathology. These inflammatory responses may manifest (but not necessarily) as infiltrations of variable numbers of inflammatory cells within the superficial dermis, usually around blood vessels. Sometimes, the inflammatory infiltrate results from superficial secondary infection and has no etiologic significance. Nevertheless, in some cases, a unique pattern of distribution of inflammatory cells (e.g., numerous plasma cells in syphilis, or a granulomatous pattern) may provide important diagnostic clues. A detailed discussion of inflammatory patterns would entail covering the entire field of dermatopathology, and is beyond the scope of this chapter.

6.2.5 Insufficient Histologic Data

Sometimes the histologic data do not seem to provide even the slightest diagnostic clue. In such a case, it is advisable to thoroughly scan the entire slide and biopsy specimen to see if it shows certain specific histologic characteristics such as fibrin thrombi, vasculitis, a granulomatous pattern (detailed below), or some other specific pattern. If this step does not provide further clues, another biopsy from a different area of the same ulcer should be considered, since there may be considerable variation among different specimens taken from the same ulcer.

When certain conditions are suspected, a biopsy containing deep dermis and subcutaneous tissue should be considered. For example, in polyarteritis nodosa and nodular vasculitis, a superficial biopsy may not reveal the presence of vasculitis. Similarly, as suggested in the section on vasculitis, direct immunofluorescence of a tissue specimen from the ulcer margin may confirm the diagnosis of vasculitis.

Figure 6.7 summarizes the approach to the diagnosis of ulcers when the history and physical examination do not lead to a diagnosis. It includes the main histologic findings and their clinical implications.

6.3 A Non-Healing Ulcer

6.3.1 The Various Histologic Patterns

Biopsy should be considered when dealing with an ulcer that does not heal within 3–4 months of optimal treatment (depending on the clinical set-up). In these cases, additional parameters may influence the decision as to whether the ulcer should be sampled. For example, when the affected area is too close to a bone (i.e., an ulcer located over the anterior tibia), it may be appropriate to postpone the biopsy for a while, giving the ulcer a longer period of time to heal.

Classical examples of non-healing ulcers are those where the clinical features suggest the diagnosis of a 'venous ulcer' or an 'ischemic ulcer' in a patient with peripheral arterial disease. In these cases, it is not the role of the histologic specimen to establish a diagnosis. Diagnoses of such cases are based on physical examination and specific tests such as Doppler flowmetry of leg arteries or Doppler ultrasonography of the lower limb venous system.

In such cases, the main purpose of the biopsy is to confirm that the ulcer, which appears to be benign, is not, in fact, caused by some other underlying process such as malignancy. Occasionally, histologic data may direct the physician towards other conditions such as infectious processes or pyoderma gangrenosum. The histologic possibilities of non-healing ulcers are presented in Fig. 6.8.

6.3.2 Histologic Characteristics of Venous Ulcers

The following may be found in venous ulcers [34]:
- Pericapillary presence of fibrin (fibrin cuffs); this is discussed in detail below
- A variable degree of inflammation
- Presence of hemosiderin
- Extravasation of red blood cells

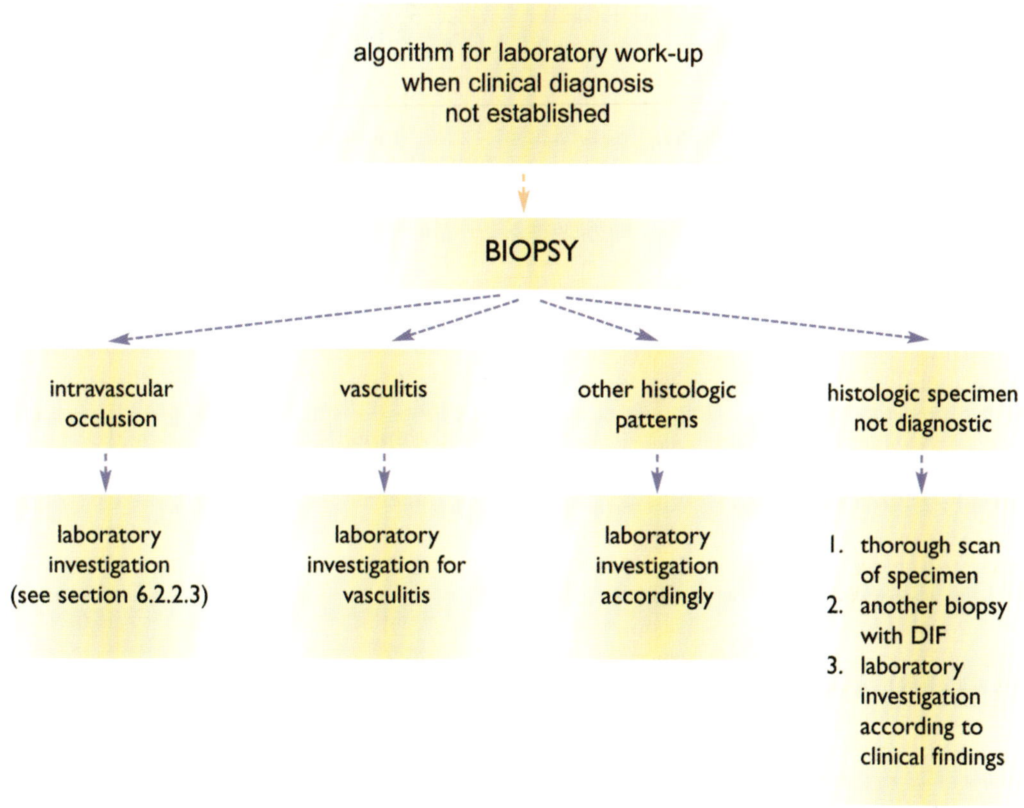

algorithm for laboratory work-up
when clinical diagnosis
not established
BIOPSY
intravascular
occlusion
vasculitis
other histologic
patterns
histologic specimen
not diagnostic
laboratory
investigation
(see section 6.2.2.3)
laboratory
investigation for
vasculitis
laboratory
investigation
accordingly
1. thorough scan
of specimen
2. another biopsy
with DIF
3. laboratory
investigation
according to
clinical findings

Fig. 6.7. Algorithm for laboratory workup when clinical diagnosis has not been established

non-healing ulcer
BIOPSY
correlation with initial
diagnosis (e.g., venous ulcer)
unexpected conditions
not suspected of prior to
biopsy (e.g., BCC)
histologic specimen
not diagnostic

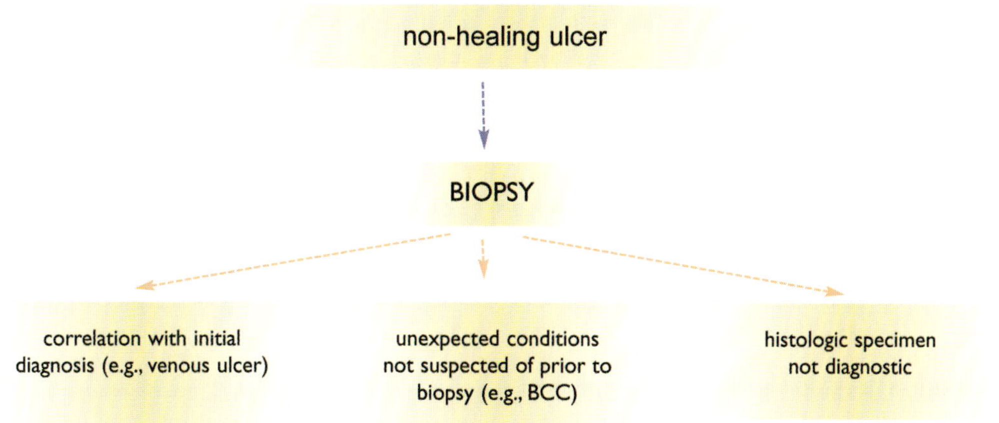

Fig. 6.8. The possible histologic patterns, in the case of a non-healing ulcer

The presence of fibrin cuffs is considered to be a typical histologic finding in venous ulcers. These are organized structures composed of fibrin, laminin, fibronectin, tenascin, collagen, and trapped leukocytes [35]. It is suggested that high venous pressure results in dermal leakage of fibrinogen with subsequent formation of pericapillary fibrin layers [35]. Pericapillary fibrin is positively stained by Martius scarlet blue. Its presence may be also confirmed by direct immunofluorescence [36].

Falanga et al [36] documented the presence of pericapillary fibrin in 14 (93%) of 15 patients with venous ulceration but in only one of 14 patients (7%) who had cutaneous ulcers of other etiologies. Burnard et al. found that pericapillary fibrin can be found in the skin of patients with venous insufficiency, whether the skin is ulcerated or not [37]. However, cuffing can be seen if appropriate staining has been carried out, provided that its structure has not been destroyed by an inflammatory response, which frequently accompanies ulceration.

Note that fibrin cuffs may be seen in diabetic ulcers, including ischemic diabetic ulcers [38] and in pressure ulcers [39]. However, while in venous insufficiency the fibrin is organized in concentric lamellae, in diabetic ulcers the fibrin tends to appear as fragmented and diffuse deposits [38].

6.3.3 The Histologic Characteristics of Ischemic Ulcers

The narrowing or occlusion of blood vessels can be seen in diabetic ulcers and ischemic ulcers as a result of thickening of the blood vessel wall [38]. This process is caused by an abnormal proliferation of endothelial cells or smooth muscle cells [38]. Narrowing or occlusion of blood vessels may also be seen as a result of atherosclerotic disease.

These processes involve only blood vessels of the deep plexus, and these histologic characteristics are not seen within the superficial plexus; therefore, most punch biopsies, which are relatively superficial, will not reveal the above findings [2].

6.3.4 'Unexpected' Histologic Findings in Certain Types of Cutaneous Ulcers

Sometimes, 'unexpected' findings may be encountered while examining cutaneous ulcers histologically. The biopsy may show evidence of malignancy (see below) or various infectious processes (such as the presence of fungi); the histologic findings may direct the physician towards conditions such as pyoderma gangrenosum, or many other situations, which are described in Chaps. 4 and 5. In such cases, the initial clinical diagnosis should be reevaluated. Because of the clinical importance of identifying pyoderma gangrenosum, this will be discussed in a separate section of this chapter.

6.4 Suspected Malignancy

6.4.1 When Should Malignancy Be Suspected?

Tumors and malignant lesions may ulcerate. In most cases, such an ulcer develops within the primary lesion, which will most probably be a plaque or a nodule. A list of these conditions is presented in Table 6.5.

Malignancy may be suspected under the following circumstances:
- When an ulcer arises within a prominent, heavily infiltrated nodule or tumor (e.g., ulceration of melanoma or a cutaneous lesion of lymphoma).
- When granulation tissue extends beyond the ulcer margin: this may occur in basal cell carcinoma (BCC) or squamous cell carcinoma (SCC) [40].
- When specific characteristic features are observed, such as the typical pearly border of a BCC.

Table 6.5. Ulceration in malignancy

Lymphoproliferarive diseases	Tumors of skin appendages
● B-cell Lymphoma ● T-cell lymphoma	● Sebaceous carcinoma
Leukemia	**Sarcomas**
● Acute and chronic leukemia	● Kaposi's sarcoma ● Lymphangiosarcoma
Epithelial tumors	**Other soft tissue tumors**
● Basal cell carcinoma ● Squamous cell carcinoma ● Keratoacanthoma	● Histiocytosis syndromes ● Neural tumors
Other epidermal tumors	**Other tumors (non-cutaneous) that may affect the skin**
● Malignant melanoma ● Merkel cell carcinoma	● By direct invasion into the skin ● Skin metastases (from an internal tumor)

In all these cases, a biopsy is the accepted approach.

However, there are often diagnostic pitfalls when dealing with epitheliomas, especially BCC and SCC; these ulcers may closely resemble other types of ulcers, particularly venous ulcers.

> The combination of a cutaneous ulcer and epithelioma may occur in two different situations:
> - Epithelioma as the primary lesion
> - Epithelioma arising in a long standing cutaneous ulcer

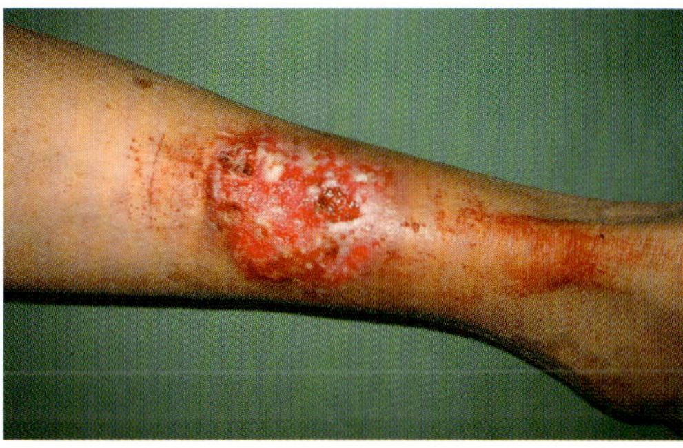

Fig. 6.9. A 2-year-old leg ulcer, labeled as a 'venous' ulcer; a biopsy revealed the presence of SCC

6.4.2 Epithelioma as a Primary Lesion

A BCC or SCC may develop *de novo* on the leg [41], but in some cases it does not present the typical morphologic features. Sometimes the tumor has the appearance of healthy granulation tissue, extending beyond the ulcer margin [40]. Thus, a patient may long be labeled as having a 'venous' ulcer, until the lesion is biopsied (Fig. 6.9). Note that BCC is the most common neoplasm of the lower extremities [42].

6.4.3 Epithelioma Developing in a Long-Standing Cutaneous Ulcer

Epithelioma may develop in long-standing chronic ulcers. This type of malignant transformation is known as a Marjolin ulcer. It often presents as an SCC appearing in burn scars or chronic ulcers [43, 44]. Simmons et al. [44] and Steffen [45] traced the history of the eponym and suggested that Marjolin probably never actually described the pathologic process that currently bears his name. As with SCC, many cases of BCC arising within long-standing venous ulcers have been reported [40–42, 46–48].

6.5 An Ulcerated Nodule or Plaque

6.5.1 Ulcers Developing Within a Nodule or a Plaque

An ulcer that develops within a nodule or a plaque can lead to a wide range of differing etiologic diagnoses. The following possibilities may be considered:

- Ulcerating panniculitis
- Certain connective tissue diseases (e.g., ulcerating rheumatoid nodule of rheumatoid arthritis)
- Ulcers developing in malignant lesions such as lymphoma (and mycosis fungoides), leukemia, skin metastases, or Kaposi's sarcoma
- Deep fungal infections
- Certain bacterial infections such as syphilis, yaws, tuberculosis, atypical mycobacterial infections, and leprosy (ulceration in these diseases is detailed in Chap. 4.)
- Leishmaniasis
- Certain reactions to foreign bodies

Such a lesion requires extensive laboratory investigation, including histologic examination. In many of these cases, a granulomatous pattern may be identified, as described below.

6.5.2 Granulomatous Histologic Pattern

A granuloma is a chronic inflammatory lesion containing groups of epitheloid cells. It may also contain multinuclear giant cells. Certain types of granuloma are surrounded by lymphocytes (e.g., 'tuberculoid granuloma') while in others there is no peripheral lymphocyte infiltrate, or only a sparse infiltrate (e.g., 'sarcoidal granuloma'). The main clinical sign of a granulomatous process is the appearance of nodular lesions.

The main purpose of the histologic examination is to identify the specific type of granuloma, i.e., essentially to decide whether it is a tuberculoid, sarcoidal, palisaded, or suppurative granuloma. This topic is dealt with in the classic dermatopathology texts, and we shall not discuss it further here.

Sometimes a granuloma appears following the penetration of a foreign body into the skin. In some cases, a skin ulcer shown in histology to be a foreign body granuloma, can be the result of deliberate injection of medications, drugs, or other substances into the skin. A discussion of factitious ulcers and their diagnosis appears in Chap. 16.

The biopsy specimen should be appropriately stained, depending on the clinical or laboratory findings and the possible etiology of the lesion:

- Ziehl-Neelsen: for typical or atypical mycobacterial infections
- Giemsa: for leishmaniasis
- PAS or methenamine silver: for deep fungi

In addition, one should consider Warthin-Starry silver stain when syphilis is suspected and Fite stain when leprosy is suspected.

6.5.3 Seeking an Infectious Cause

Particularly when dealing with heavily infiltrated lesions, one should consider an infectious cause, including leishmaniasis, deep mycosis, and mycobacterial or atypical mycobacterial infection. Therefore, in addition to a biopsy, the following tests should be considered:

■ **Smear.** Making a smear of material from the lesion is mandatory in a lesion suspected of being caused by Leishmania. The material should be stained with Wright's or Giemsa stain on a microscope slide.

In mycobacterial infection, a smear stained with Ziehl-Neelsen may confirm the diagnosis – although a smear is much less accurate than a tissue culture diagnosis.

An ulcer suspected of having been infected by fungus should be sampled by a smear. Following treatment with a 10% KOH solution to digest epithelial debris within the sample, microscopic examination may reveal fungal elements and the presence of certain deep mycoses. In most cases of deep mycosis, the fungal particles are situated relatively deep in the skin, and a tissue culture (see below) is required.

■ **Polymerase Chain Reaction (PCR).** PCR may identify Leishmania species, deep mycosis, and mycobacterial or atypical mycobacterial infections [49–64].

■ **Chest X-Ray.** This should be done when mycobacterial infection or systemic involvement with another disease such as deep mycosis is suspected.

■ **Tissue Culture.** The optimal site for taking a tissue culture from an ulcerated nodule is the margin of the lesion. The biopsy may be taken with a punch from deep within the active margin [65, 66]. It is also accepted procedure to take a biopsy from the center of a lesion [66], but the chances of identifying a pathogen from that area is lower, since the center of the lesion is often necrotic and may well not contain any live bacteria (or other infecting organisms).

The tissue specimen should be kept moist with sterile saline until it is processed [66]. Note, however, that when mycobacterial infection is suspected, the collected samples should not be exposed to saline solutions, since certain species of Mycobacterium are sensitive to sodium [67].

The tissue specimen should be finely pulverized and sown onto an appropriate culture medium, depending on the clinical suspicion.

To confirm the diagnosis of mycobacteria or atypical mycobacteria, specimens should be inoculated onto an egg- or agar-based medium, such as Lowenstein-Jensen, and incubated at 37°C.

When *Mycobacterium marinum* is suspected (e.g., a typical lesion appearing on the finger of a patient known to indulge in aquatic activities) the bacteriology laboratory should be informed. In this case the organism should be cultured at a temperature below 25°C (it will not grow at 37°C).

Sabouraud's dextrose agar is an appropriate medium for the identification of fungi. When the clinical features suggest a specific fungal infection based on clinical data, including the endemic area where the patient was, the laboratory should be informed.

■ **Specific Tests.** Specific tests for each organism may be considered, such as the Mantoux test for tuberculosis or specific serologic tests for certain fungal infections. When syphilis is suspected, appropriate serological tests should be performed.

6.6 Pyoderma Gangrenosum

Although pyoderma gangrenosum (PG) is a relatively uncommon cause of skin ulcers, it should be included in the differential diagnosis and will be discussed separately.

The diagnosis of PG is based mainly on clinical findings: clinical appearance of an ulcer surrounded by an undermined violet margin, positive pathergy, and, in many cases, the presence of an underlying disease such as ulcerative colitis, Crohn's disease, or rheumatoid arthritis.

The histologic findings are not pathognomonic in PG, since they are non-specific and variable, depending on the clinical stage when biopsy was performed and its specific site on the cutaneous lesion [68]. Nevertheless, when PG is suspected, histology may be helpful in two ways:
1. The typical histologic finding may further support a presumptive clinical diagnosis
2. Histology may rule out or confirm other possible diagnoses

In a fully developed lesion, there is inflammatory cell infiltration. Dense infiltrate of neutrophils may be seen in the dermis [32, 69]. A heavy infiltration of neutrophils may result in early abscess formation with subsequent ulceration. On the other hand, there may be only a mild infiltration of chronic inflammatory cells, depending on the timing of the biopsy and the site within the lesion from where it was obtained [68].

Vasculitis has been reported to appear in PG lesions, including hemorrhagic necrotizing vasculitis [70, 71], or lymphocytic vasculitis [72]. It is reasonable to assume that the presence of vasculitis, its degree, and the type of cells seen depend on the stage when the biopsy was performed.

Today, the vasculitis seen in PG is considered to be only a secondary process, and not the cause of the pathology [1, 2]. It is presumed that the basic underlying pathology of PG is a process of suppurative folliculitis, which presents clinically as a pustule in which ulceration later develops.

References

1. Ackerman AB, Chongchitnant N, Sanchez Y, Guo Y, Benin B, Reichel M, Randall MB (eds) Proceeding to specific diagnoses. Basic patterns and analysis of them. In: Histologic Diagnosis of Inflammatory Skin Diseases: An Algorithmic Method Based on Pattern Analysis, 2nd edn. Baltimore: Williams & Wilkins. 1997; pp 107–144
2. Barnhill RL, Busam KJ: Vascular diseases. In: Elder D, Elenitsas R, Jaworsky C, Johnson B (eds) Lever's Histopathology of the Skin. 8th edn. Philadelphia: Lippincott-Raven. 1997; pp 185–208
3. Diggs LW, Ching RE: Pathology of sickle cell anemia. South Med J 1934; 27:839–845
4. Lima-Maribona J, Kirsner RS, Kerdel FA: Answers to self-assessment examination of the American Academy of Dermatology. J Am Acad Dermatol 1993; 29: 807
5. Chan YC, Valenti D, Mansfield AO, et al: Warfarin-induced skin necrosis. Br J Surg 2000; 87:266–272
6. Schleicher SM, Fricker MP: Coumarin necrosis. Arch Dermatol 1980; 116:444–445
7. Gold JA, Watters AK, O'Brien E: Coumadin versus heparin necrosis. J Am Acad Dermatol 1987; 16: 148–150
8. Kirsner RS, Eaglstein WH, Katz MH, et al: Stanozolol causes rapid pain relief and healing of cutaneous ulcers caused by cryofibrinogenemia. J Am Acad Dermatol 1993; 28:71–74
9. Beightler E, Diven DG, Sanchez RL, et al: Thrombotic vasculopathy associated with cryofibrinogenemia. J Am Acad Dermatol 1991; 24:342–345
10. Wagner DR, Eckert F, Gresser U, et al: Deposits of paraprotein in small vessels as a cause of skin ulcers in Waldenstrom's macroglobulinemia. Clin Investig 1993; 72:46–49
11. Vanscheidt W, Leder O, Vanscheidt E, et al: Leg ulcers in a patient with spherocytosis: A clinicopathological report. Dermatologica 1990; 181:56–59
12. Rietschel RL, Lewis CW, Simmons RA, et al: Skin lesions in paroxysmal nocturnal hemoglobinuria. Arch Dermatol 1978; 114:560–563
13. Stevanovic DV: Atrophie blanche. A sign of dermal blood occlusion. Arch Dermatol 1974; 109:858–862
14. Shornick JK, Nicholes BK, Bergstresser PR, et al: Idiopathic atrophie blanche. J Am Acad Dermatol 1983; 8:792–798
15. Maessen-Visch MB, Koedam MI, Hamulyak K, et al: Atrophie blanche. Int J Dermatol 1999; 38:161–172
16. Gibson GE, Su WP, Pittelkow MR: Antiphospholipid syndrome and the skin. J Am Acad Dermatol 1997; 36:970–982
17. Gilson RT, Milum E: Calciphylaxis: case report and treatment review. Cutis 1999; 63:149–153
18. Oh DH, Eulau D, Tokugawa DA, et al: Five cases of calciphylaxis and a review of the literature. J Am Acad Dermatol 1999; 40:979–987
19. Essary LR, Wick MR: Cutaneous calciphylaxis: An underrecognized clinicopathologic entity. Am J Clin Pathol 2000; 113:280–287
20. Zaytsev P, Miller K, Pellettiere EV: Cutaneous cholesterol emboli with infarction clinically mimicking heparin necrosis: a case report. Angiology 1986; 37: 471–476
21. Falanga V, Fine MJ, Kapoor WN: The cutaneous manifestations of cholesterol crystal embolization. Arch Dermatol 1986; 122:1194–1198
22. Kalter DC, Rudolph A, McGavran M: Livedo reticularis due to multiple cholesterol emboli. J Am Acad Dermatol 1985; 13:235–242
23. Altmeyer P, Welke S, Renger A, et al: Zur pathogenese der sogenannten Cumarin-Nekrose. Aktuel Dermatol 1976; 2:65–68
24. Slutzki S, Bogokowsky H, Gilboa Y, et al: Coumadin induced skin necrosis. Int J Dermatol 1984; 23: 117–119
25. Deschamps P, Leroy D, Mandard J: Cutaneous crystal cholesterol emboli. Acta Derm Venereol (Stockh) 1980; 60:266–269
26. Rosansky SJ: Multiple cholesterol emboli syndrome. South Med J 1982; 75: 677–680
27. Fauci AS: The vasculitis syndromes. In: Fauci AS, Braunwald E, Isselbacher KJ, Wilson JD, Martin JB, Kasper DL, Hauser SL, Longo DL (eds) Harrison's Principles of Internal Medicine, 14th edn. New York: McGraw-Hill. 1998; pp 1910–1922
28. Fiorentino DF: Cutaneous vasculitis. J Am Acad Dermatol 2003; 48:311–340
29. Jennette JC, Falk RJ, Andrassy K, et al: Nomenclature of systemic vasculitides. Proposal of an international consensus conference. Arthritis Rheum 1994; 37: 187–192

30. Soter NA: Cutaneous necrotizing venulitis. Freedberg IM, Eisen AZ, Wolff K, Austen KF, Goldsmith LA, Katz SI (eds) In: Fitzpatrick's Dermatology in General Medicine, 6th edn. New York: McGraw-Hill. 2003; pp 1727– 1735

31. McDonald J, Stewart J, Urowitz MB, et al: Peripheral vascular disease in patients with systemic lupus erythematosus. Ann Rheum Dis 1992; 51:56–60

32. Magro C, Crowson AN, Mihm M: Cutaneous manifestation of nutritional deficiency states and gastrointestinal disease. In: Lever's Histopathology of the Skin. Elder D, Elenitsas R, Jaworsky C, Johnson B (eds) 8th edn. Philadelphia: Lippincott-Raven. 1997; pp 353–368

33. Grunwald MH, Avinoach I, Amichai B, et al: Leukocytoclastic vasculitis – correlation between different histologic stages and direct immunofluorescence results. Int J Dermatol 1997; 36:349–352

34. Herrick SE, Sloan P, McGurk M, et al: Sequential changes in histologic pattern and extracellular matrix deposition during the healing of chronic venous ulcers. Am J Pathol 1992; 141:1085–1095

35. Burnand KG, Whimster I, Clemenson G, et al: The relationship between the number of capillaries in the skin of the venous ulcer bearing area of the lower leg and the fall in foot vein pressure during exercise. Br J Surg 1981; 68:297–300

36. Falanga V, Moosa HH, Nemeth AJ, et al: Dermal pericapillary fibrin in venous disease and venous ulceration. Arch Dermatol 1987; 123:620–623

37. Burnand KG, Whimster I, Naidoo A, et al: Pericapillary fibrin in the ulcer-bearing skin of the leg: the cause of lipodermatosclerosis and venous ulceration. Br Med J 1982; 285:1071–1072

38. Ferguson MW, Herrick SE, Spencer MJ, et al: The histology of diabetic foot ulcers. Diabetic Med 1996; 13:S30–S33

39. Vande Berg JS, Rudolph R: Pressure (Decubitus) ulcer: Variation in histopathology – A light and electron microscope study. Hum Pathol 1995; 26:195–200

40. Harris B, Eaglstein WH, Falanga V: Basal cell carcinoma arising in venous ulcers and mimicking granulation tissue. J Dermatol Surg Oncol 1993; 19:150–152

41. Phillips TJ, Salman SM, Rogers GS: Nonhealing leg ulcers: a manifestation of basal cell carcinoma. J Am Acad Dermatol 1991; 25:47–49

42. Kofler H, Fritsch P: Ulcers due to tumors. In : Westerhof W (ed) Leg Ulcers: Diagnosis and Treatment, 1st edn. Amsterdam: Elsevier. 1993; pp 183–198

43. Kirkham N: Tumors and cysts of the epidermis. In: Elder D, Elenitsas R, Jaworsky C, Johnson B (eds) Lever's Histopathology of the Skin, 8th edn. Philadelphia: Lippincott-Raven. 1997; pp 685–746

44. Simmons MA, Edwards JM, Nigam A: Marjolin's ulcer presenting in the neck. J Laryngol Otol 2000; 114:980–982

45. Steffen C: Marjolin's ulcer. Report of two cases and evidence that Marjolin did not describe cancer arising in scars of burns. Am J Dermatopathol 1984; 6:187–193

46. Blank AA, Schnyder UW: Squamous cell carcinoma and basal cell carcinoma within the clinical picture of a chronic venous insufficiency in the third stage. Dermatologica 1990; 181:248–250

47. Lanehart WH, Sanusi ID, Misra RP, et al: Metastasizing basal cell carcinoma originating in a stasis ulcer black woman. Arch Dermatol 1983; 119:587–591

48. Black MM, Walkden VM: Basal cell carcinomatous changes on the lower leg: a possible association with chronic stasis. Histopathology 1983; 7:219–227

49. Martin-Sanchez J, Lopez-Lopez MC, Acedo-Sanchez C, et al: Diagnosis of infections with Leishmania infantum using PCR-ELISA. Parasitology 2001; 122:607–615

50. Salotra P, Sreenivas G, Pogue GP, et al: Development of a species-specific PCR assay for detection of Leishmania donovani in clinical samples from patients with kala-azar and post-kala-azar dermal leishmaniasis. J Clin Microbiol 2001; 39:849–854

51. Oliveira-Neto MP, Mattos M, Souza CS, et al: Leishmaniasis recidiva cutis in New World cutaneous leishmaniasis. Int J Dermatol 1998; 37:846–849

52. Uezato H, Hagiwara K, Hosokawa A, et al: Comparative studies of the detection rates of Leishmania parasites from formalin, ethanol-fixed, frozen human skin specimens by polymerase chain reaction and Southern blotting. J Dermatol 1998; 25:623–631

53. Smith HR, Connor MP, Beer TW, et al: The use of polymerase chain reaction in New World cutaneous leishmaniasis. Br J Dermatol 1998; 139:539–540

54. Schubach A, Haddad F, Oliveira- Neto MP et al: Detection of Leishmania DNA by polymerase chain reaction in scars of treated human patients. J Infect Dis 1998; 178:911–914

55. Turin L, Riva F, Galbiati G, et al: Fast, simple and highly sensitive double-rounded polymerase chain reaction assay to detect medically relevant fungi in dermatological specimens. Eur J Clin Invest 2000; 30:511–518

56. Brandt ME, Hutwagner LC, Klug LA, et al: Molecular subtype distribution of Cryptococcus neoformans in four areas of the United States. Cryptococcal Disease Active Surveillance Group. J Clin Microbiol 1996; 34:912–917

57. Van Burik J, Myerson D, Schreckhise RW, et al: Pan-fungal PCR assay for detection of fungal infection in human blood specimens. J Clin Microbiol 1998; 36:1169–1175

58. Mayer J, Kovarik A, Vorlicek J, et al: Efficacy of polymerase chain reaction for detection of deep mycotic infections: confirmation by autopsy. Mycoses 1998; 41:471–475

59. Baek SC, Chae HJ, Houh D, et al: Detection and differentiation of causative fungi of onychomycosis using PCR amplification and restriction enzyme analysis. Int J Dermatol 1998; 37:682–686

60. Mert A, Bilir M, Tabak F, et al: Miliary tuberculosis: Clinical manifestations, diagnosis and outcome in 38 adults. Respirology 2001; 6:217–224

61. Su WJ, Huang CY, Perng RP: Utility of PCR assays for rapid diagnosis of BCG infection in children. Int J Tuberc Lung Dis 2001; 5:380–384

62. Tan SH, Tan HH, Sun YJ et al: Clinical utility of polymerase chain reaction in the detection of Mycobacterium tuberculosis in different types of cutaneous tuberculosis and tuberculids. Ann Acad Med Singapore 2001: 30:3–10

63. Nenoff P, Rytter M, Schubert S, et al: Multilocular inoculation tuberculosis of the skin after stay in Africa: detection of mycobacterial DNA using polymerase chain reaction. Br J Dermatol 2000; 143:226–228

64. Arora SK, Kumar B, Sehgal S: Development of a polymerase chain reaction dot-blotting system for detecting cutaneous tuberculosis. Br J Dermatol 2000; 142:72–76

65. Nolte FS, Metchock B: Mycobacterium. In: Murray PR, Baron EJ, Pfaller MA, Tenover FC, Yolken RH (eds) Manual of Clinical Microbiology, 6th edn. Washington DC: ASM Press. 1995; pp 400–437

66. Kern ME, Blevins KS: Laboratory procedures for fungal culture and isolation. In: Medical Mycology: A Self-Instructional Text. 2nd edn. Philadelphia: F.A. Davis Company. 1997; pp 27–72

67. Tappeiner G, Wolff K: Tuberculosis and other mycobacterial infections. Fitzpatrick TB, EisenAZ, Wolff K, Freedberg IM Austen KF, and (eds) In: Fitzpatrick's Dermatology in General Medicine, 4th edn. New York: McGraw-Hill. 1993; pp 2370–2395

68. Schwaegerle SM, Bergfeld WF, Senitzer D, et al: Pyoderma gangrenosum: A review. J Am Acad Dermatol 1988; 18:559–568

69. Ackerman AB, Chongchitnant N, sanchez Y, Guo Y, Benin B, Reichel M, Randall MB (eds) Pyoderma gangrenosum. In: Histologic Diagnosis of Inflammatory Skin Diseases: An Algorithmic Method Based on Pattern Analysis, 2nd edn. Baltimore: Williams & Wilkins. 1997; pg 674

70. English JS, Fenton DA, Barth J, et al: Pyoderma gangrenosum and leukocytoclastic vasculitis in association with rheumatoid arthritis: a report of two cases. Clin Exp Dermatol 1984; 9:270–276

71. Wong E, Greaves MW: Pyoderma gangrenosum and leukocytoclastic vasculitis. Clin Exp Dermatol 1985; 10:68–72

72. Su WP, Schroeter AL, Perry HO, et al: Histopathologic and immunopathologic study of pyoderma gangrenosum. J Cutan Pathol 1986; 13:323–330

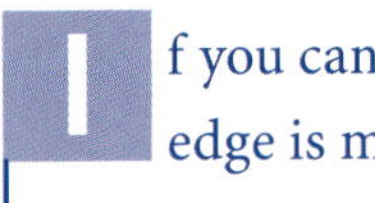

f you cannot measure, your knowledge is meager and unsatisfactory.

(Kelvin's dictum)

provide feedback on the effectiveness of certain treatments.

To begin with, we describe methods used to measure wounds/ulcers. These methods are applicable to acute wounds as well as to chronic ulcers.

Contents

The following basic data are needed at the initial examination and during the course of follow-up to quantify wound/ulcer healing:
- Precise anatomical location
- Assessment of the ulcer area
- Depth
- The presence and extent of undermining
- Parameters of wound/ulcer infection
- Assessment of the appearance of the ulcer surface

Then we detail parameters of assessment in patients suffering from cutaneous ulcers. These parameters are complementary to the etiologic workup (specified in Chaps. 5 and 6). The aim is to determine whether or not there are factors present that may impair the process of normal cutaneous ulcer repair. This assessment should be conducted in the initial evaluation and throughout follow-up.

7.1 Introduction

The clinical follow-up of acute wounds and chronic cutaneous ulcers requires the meticulous recording of several objective parameters. Appropriate recording enables accurate documentation of changes in skin lesions and better assessment of disease progression, and may

The physician should address the following issues:
- Is there evidence of nutritional deficits?
- Does the patient take any medication that could result in ulceration

or may impair the normal healing process?

- In the event of lower limb edema that impairs ulcer healing, a specific workup should be conducted to determine the cause of the edema and appropriate treatment.
- Evaluation and treatment of other conditions that could impair the normal cutaneous ulcer healing process such as hypoxia in general and smoking in particular.

In addition, in the case of a cutaneous ulcer that does not heal within several months, reassessment of ulcer etiology is required and a biopsy from the ulcer margin should be considered.

7.2 Ulcer/Wound Measurements

The measurements detailed below are morphometric. These are the principal measurements required for monitoring and documenting wounds and ulcers. However, there are various non-morphometric tests that can also be carried out, such as measurement of blood flow in the affected limbs and perfusion imaging [1–3], and measurement of transcutaneous oxygen tension [4, 5] or wound pH [6, 7]. Various other biochemical measurements can also be taken from the ulcer area or wound fluid [8–10]. Most of these tests are designed for research or experimental purposes. Here we will limit the scope to measurements that have direct clinical application.

7.2.1 Precise Anatomic Site

A primary and basic requirement for proper recording is the precise determination of the site of the wound or cutaneous ulcer. The site has to be recorded in relation to a clear reference point. It is usually desirable to use a bony or skeletal site that can be clearly identified. Similarly, a natural crease or a specific skin lesion such as a nevus may be used.

Thus, the location can be described, for example, as an ulcer located 2 cm superior to the lateral malleolus, or as an ulcer that is 5.5 cm

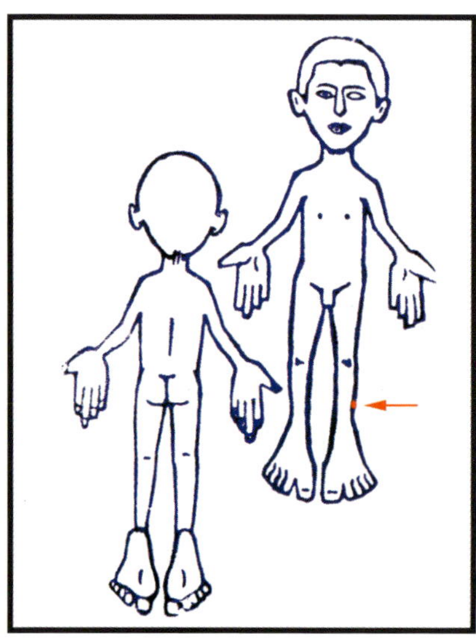
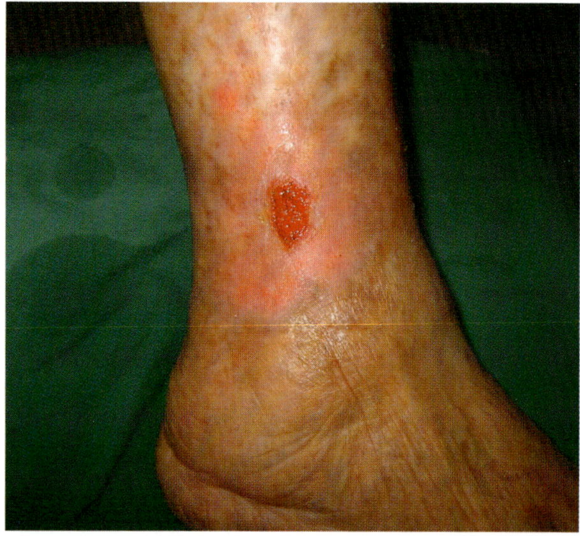

Fig. 7.1. Recording the location of an ulcer on a template drawing (*left*) and its photograph (*right*). The ulcer is located on the right leg, 4 cm above the superior edge of the lateral malleolus

below the inferior border of the patella, on the anterior aspect of the calf.

A precise record of the location of the ulcer is an additional datum that may assist in its etiologic identification. Moreover, any other ulcers that may appear in the future in adjacent areas can be confidently identified. The record should include a tracing or photograph showing the precise location of the ulcer. A stamp or template can be used (Fig. 7.1), designed to facilitate the drawing of various body areas.

7.2.2 Measurement of the Ulcer Area

7.2.2.1 Linear Measurement

The easiest method for assessing the cutaneous ulcer surface area is based on the maximal length and the longest width perpendicular to that length [11, 12]. This method, although less precise than others, enables a degree of objective assessment and can serve as a parameter for therapeutic effectiveness. However, it does not provide a description of the ulcer margins. It does not document the presence of islands of epithelialization within the ulcer area. Repeat measurements can be misleading since different physicians may choose different points of reference.

The measurement is made with a strip of paper or plastic marked in centimeters (Fig. 7.2). To prevent infection, a strip of transparent nylon should be placed on the skin prior to measurement so that the scale does not come into direct contact with the ulcer surface.

7.2.2.2 Tracing the Ulcer Margin

Tracing is a well-accepted, reliable, and practical method [13–15]. It is done on a transparent film (the best type is a transparent film wrap of gauze pads). The film is positioned over the ulcer surface and the ulcer margin is traced. To prevent transmission of infective bacteria, we recommend that a strip of transparent nylon (such as is used for wrapping food) be placed on the skin next to the ulcer, prior to measurement, so that the film does not come into direct contact with the ulcer surface. The tracing should be copied from the transparent film onto a piece of paper appended to the patient's medical chart (Fig. 7.3).

Precise calculation of the surface area is achieved by: (a) counting squares on millimeter paper [11, 15, 16], or (b) scanning of the tracing and planimetric computer analysis in a more precise manner, as done in several studies that have investigated the effectiveness of various therapeutic regimens for cutaneous ulcers [14, 15, 17–23].

When tracing, one should make sure that the transparent film adheres to the ulcer, to avoid measurement errors. Additional characteristics of the ulcer, including areas of clean granulation tissue, islands of epithelialization, and foci of necrosis, can be marked and documented in the tracing.

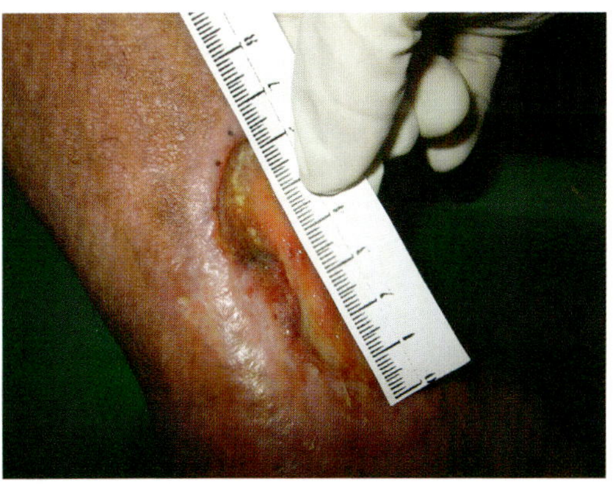

Fig. 7.2. Performance of linear measurement

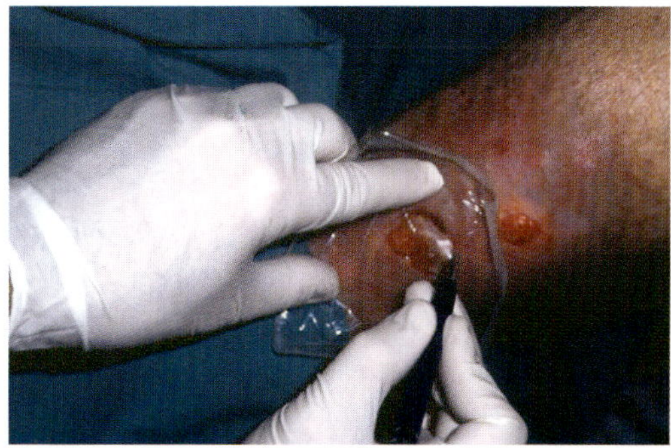

Fig. 7.3. The technique for tracing the ulcer margins

The advantages of tracing are:
- It is more precise than other methods of measurement (e.g. linear measurement).
- It shows the contours of the ulcer.
- Consecutive tracings indicate the progress of the ulcer in terms of its shape and surface area, which can be used to assess the effectiveness of treatment.

Cutler et al. [12] maintained that wound tracing and tracing planimetry were the most sensitive tools for the detection of early wound-size changes.

The few disadvantages, which are minor, include danger of infection if the procedure is not carried out meticulously [20] and discomfort for the patient in cases of particularly sensitive ulcers.

Whenever an ulcer area is recorded or traced, the spread of bacteria to surrounding areas must be prevented by implementing the following safety measures of infection control (see also Chap. 21):
- Use of gloves
- Immediately placing any object that comes into contact with the ulcer (rulers, transparent nylon, etc.) into a disposable trash bag
- In addition to the transparent film upon which the tracing is done, placing a transparent strip of nylon on the ulcer so that the film does not come into direct contact with the surface of the ulcer

7.2.2.3 Photographs

Photos are an effective means of monitoring the surface area and contours of cutaneous ulcers and provide visual documentation of additional indices. Digital photography simplifies the process substantially, since there is no need for photo development.

The following comments on photographic technique are applicable to any skin lesion, not only to cutaneous ulcers:
- A ruler (or a paper strip with millimetric markings) should be placed next to the ulcer/wound margin, so that precise data can be obtained on its area after the photo is scanned into a computer and planimetric analysis is conducted. The name or initials of the patient and the date may be inscribed on the paper on which the millimetric markings appear.
- Follow-up photos should be taken at the same distance as previous ones.
- Regions next to the lesion that are not clinically relevant should be covered with a sheet.
- Appropriate lighting and optimal background should be assured.
- The patient should be positioned in such a way as to prevent discomfort or movement while pictures are being taken.

The advantages of photography over manual tracing are:
- There is no contact or danger of contamination.
- Other information can be obtained, such as the general appearance of the ulcer, its surrounding skin, and the presence of secretions.
- Consecutive photographs provide feedback on the effectiveness of treatment.
- Photographic documentation has medicolegal importance.

The disadvantages are, for one, that failure to place the camera at the identical distance and angle from the ulcer for follow-up photos can

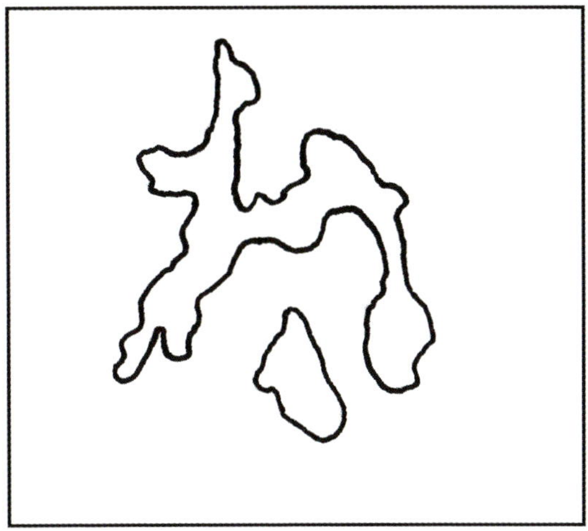 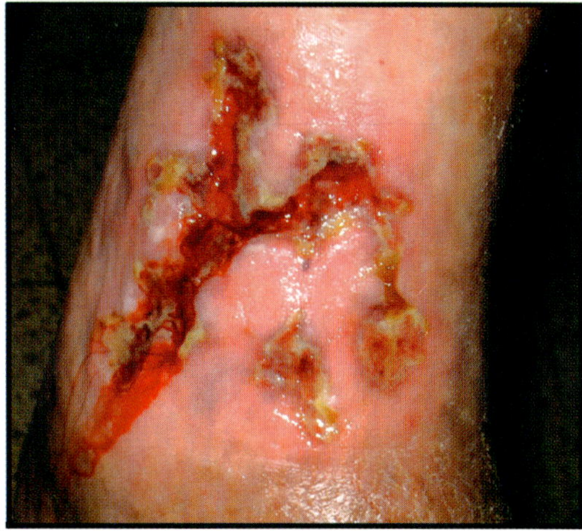

Fig. 7.4. Tracing of an ulcer (*left*) compared with a photograph of the same lesion (*right*)

lead to an erroneous assessment of the dimensions of the ulcer [17, 24]. However, in digital photography, the accuracy of calculating the area is not affected if a ruler is placed next to the ulcer margin and a software for planimetry is used.

Another disadvantage is that, if the ulcer is particularly deep, or if the surface of the ulcer area is curved (e.g., a large, edematous leg), an error in measurement may occur, because the surface area is projected onto a plane. This error, however, is usually negligible and insignificant for clinical monitoring.

If precise measurement is required for research purposes, more exact information can be obtained on the area and volume of the ulcer with stereophotogrammetric or stereophotographic techniques. These techniques are based on photos of the ulcer from different angles that generate a three-dimensional image of the ulcer [15, 25–28]. However, these techniques require relatively expensive equipment that is not needed for routine clinical follow-up of patients with cutaneous ulcers.

Studies have demonstrated a strong correlation between measurement by tracing and measurement by photography (Fig. 7.4) [12, 29, 30]. Cees et al. [17] reported that the combination of transparency tracing with a full-scale photographic technique was practical and highly reliable.

7.2.3 Assessment of Depth

The definitions of staging were originally employed in cases of decubitus ulcers with the objective of fostering better communication among medical personnel. Obviously, these definitions can also be applied to other types of cutaneous ulcers (see Chap. 1, including figures). A commonly accepted system was developed in the United States by The National Advisory Panel (NPUAP) in 1987 [31].

7.2.3.1 Relatively Superficial Ulcers

Relatively superficial ulcers are measured by inserting a sterile swab into the deepest area of the ulcer (Fig. 7.5). The height parallel to the external margin is marked and measured. More sophisticated methods for measuring the depth of relatively superficial ulcers are based on stereophotogrammetry as described above [15, 25–28]. Other methods, not in routine clinical use, include ultrasound imaging [32] and the three-dimensional laser imaging system [33].

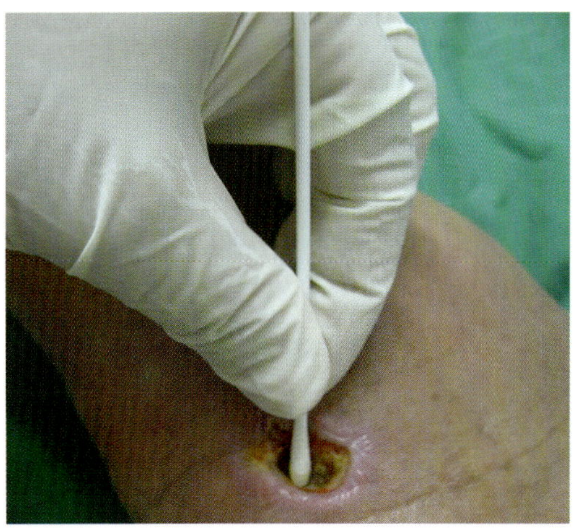

Fig. 7.5. Using a swab to measure the depth of an ulcer

7.2.3.2 Deep Ulcers

Depth measurement is important for deep ulcers as a significant determinant of the ulcer size. A sterile swab can be inserted to the deepest part of the ulcer and then measured. The introduction of saline into the ulcer cavity is also used in the clinic as a means of measuring deeper ulcers. This is done by positioning the patient so that the ulcer is perpendicular to the ground (or, alternatively, by covering the ulcer with a film). The ulcer space is then filled with saline from a syringe. The amount of saline needed to fill the ulcer space to its margins is equivalent to the ulcer volume.

Additional techniques have been developed to calculate the depth of an ulcer and estimate its size [34, 35]. These techniques use high-viscosity materials, usually found in dental laboratories, such as alginate hydrocolloids that solidify quickly after introduction into the ulcer space. The ulcer volume can then be calculated from the mold that forms. However, these techniques are not in routine clinical use.

7.2.4 Undermining

Undermining refers to the spread of the ulcerative process, with its associated destruction of tissue, under apparently normal skin in the region adjacent to the ulcer margins (Fig. 7.6).

The extent of undermining should be assessed with a moist cotton swab or plastic strip with millimetric markings. Either one of the above is inserted into the ulcer under its margin and advanced as gently and precisely as possible. When it is felt that the ulcer's edge has been reached, the depth of insertion is marked. This process should be repeated in several places.

The extent of undermining can be drawn on the skin around the ulcer. These markings are important for assessing the progress of the ulcer and the effectiveness of treatment. Additionally, the type of undermining differs according to the etiology of the ulcer. In ulcers associated with pyoderma gangrenosum the involvement is often symmetrical. In contrast, pressure ulcers have non-symmetrical involvement, with more undermining occurring in the area of maximal pressure.

7.2.5 Measurement in Cases of Infection or Suspected Infection

The presence and color of secretions should be documented. Any change between examinations may provide clinical clues as to the infectious agent. For example, *Staphylococci* tend to cause a purulent creamy yellow discharge, while secretions from *Pseudomonas* spp. are greenish or greenish-blue. Other bacteria, such as anaerobes or *Streptococci*, can cause tissue infection without purulent discharge [36].

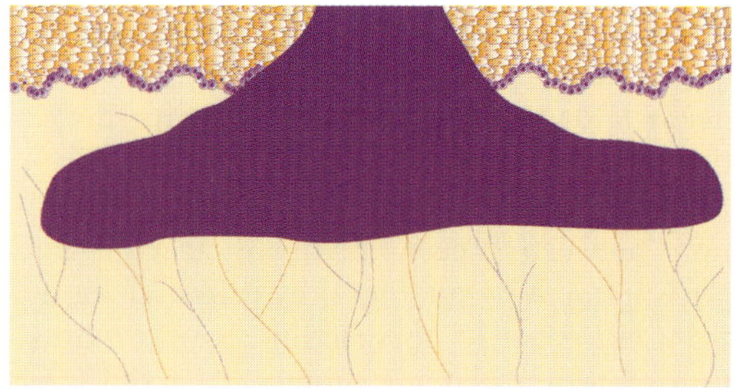

Fig. 7.6. Schematic drawing of an ulcer with undermining in a horizontal section

The following should be documented as indicators either of infection in tissue surrounding the ulcer or of the presence of cellulitis:

- Erythema around the ulcer: Erythema can be documented by the same methods as those described for marking the ulcer margins, i.e., tracing or photography. Documentation should include the shade of erythema, any tendency to pale or darken in color, and any evidence of aggravation.
- The presence of local heat: For practical clinical purposes, this is assessed by touch, noting the presence or absence of increased temperature of the skin adjacent to the ulcer. For more precise measurement of temperature in the ulcer region for research purposes, infrared thermography can be used [6].
- Bacterial swab cultures: Sampling of the deepest point at the ulcer margin, close to healthy skin, is recommended [37]. If there is a sufficient amount of material, it should be drawn from the depth of the ulcer or wound with a sterile needle and syringe [37].

A bacterial swab may also yield some useful data regarding the bacterial antibiotic-susceptibility pattern. The issue of swab sampling compared with biopsy from deep tissue is detailed in the addendum to Chap. 10.

7.2.6 Appearance of the Ulcer Surface and Spectrophotometry

The accepted way to assess the appearance of the surface area of the ulcer is based primarily on the subjective evaluation of its coloration. A clean ulcer in the healing stage contains purple granulation tissue. In contrast, particularly in the presence of peripheral vascular disease, the ulcer might be pinkish. The practical classification of wounds and ulcers according to color was described in the 1980s by Hellgren and Vincent [38], as the 'black-yellow-red' concept. Hence, ulcers can be identified as covered with necrotic tissue that is dark black. Ulcers covered with sloughed necrotic tissue may be grayish white, while infected ulcers may present yellow secretions on the surface. These differences in shading may have implications for identifying the etiology of the ulcer, following the progress of the healing process, and determining the debridement method and topical therapy of choice. As noted above, the presence of infection and its nature may lead to changes in the color of the ulcer surface.

In most reported studies, investigators have used subjective scoring methods to document ulcer surface area. Romanelli [39] suggested an objective method using a skin reflectance analyzer that enables chromatic measurement. It uses a red scale to assess the presence of granulation tissue on the ulcer surface area and a yellow scale for fibrin.

There is no particular value in using spectrophotometric measurements such as this in the routine clinical care of patients with cutaneous ulcers, but it could be of great value in research as an objective and reproducible measuring technique.

7.3 Patient Assessment

7.3.1 General

In addition to the standard, routine patient examination, i.e., history and physical examination, physicians treating patients with cutaneous ulcers should focus on two main aspects: (a) identifying the etiology and (b) identifying factors that might impede ulcer healing. Identification of ulcer etiology is discussed in Chaps. 5 and 6. When a specific etiology has been diagnosed, appropriate treatment should be implemented. In addition, efforts should be made to identify factors that might impede the healing of a cutaneous ulcer such as nutritional deficits, drugs, edema, hypoxia, and smoking.

7.3.2 Nutritional Deficits

Most patients do not present evidence of nutritional deficits on physical examination. At times, anemia can be diagnosed because of obvious pallor. Identification of the cause of anemia (a nutritional deficit such as iron or folate deficiency) and its correction can contribute to the ulcer healing process. On rare occasions it is possible to diagnosis zinc or vitamin C deficiency on the basis of clinical skin findings (as detailed in Chap. 19).

In addition to the routine blood tests conducted for all patients with cutaneous ulcers, i.e., complete blood count and blood chemistry, other tests are advisable: tests for iron (and additonal indicators of iron status, e.g., transferrin iron-binding capacity and ferritin), albumin, and zinc levels. Correction of any such deficiencies is obligatory.

7.3.3 Drugs

A detailed description of drugs that can cause cutaneous ulcers or impede the natural healing process can be found in Chap. 16. Any drug taken by the patient that appears on this list should be discontinued or replaced, if possible.

7.3.4 Edema

Edema of the extremities directly impedes the healing process of a cutaneous ulcer located on the affected skin. It damages the general quality of the skin and its elastic and rheological properties [40]. Impaired lymphatic drainage results in the structural deformity of lymph vessels and subcutaneous tissue. It induces fibroblast proliferation and sclerosis of subcutaneous tissue with subsequent interference in the metabolic processes and gas exchange of the affected tissues, decreased cellular function, and impaired wound healing capacity. Lymph vessels and their valves are subjected to fibrotic changes with further impairment of lymphatic drainage, leading to a vicious cycle of edema [41, 42]. In view of the cumulative damage to tissue integrity, edema may exacerbate ulceration, especially when other factors that induce alteration are already present, such as diabetes or peripheral artery disease. If an ulcer already exists, its chances of healing are significantly reduced in the presence of edema.

The presence of edema necessitates the following steps:
- Measurement of extremity dimensions
- Evaluation of the cause of edema
- Treatment of the edema

Extremity dimensions should be measured with a disposable measuring tape (Fig. 7.7). Both extremities should be measured at a corresponding site. The precise site of measurement should be recorded in relation to a permanent reference point (e.g., 10 cm below the lower edge of the patella) to guarantee that repeat measurements will be reliable. The measurement must be conducted with the patient in the same position each time. The measuring tape should be placed firmly on the skin, but without applying excessive pressure that would reduce the precision of the measurement.

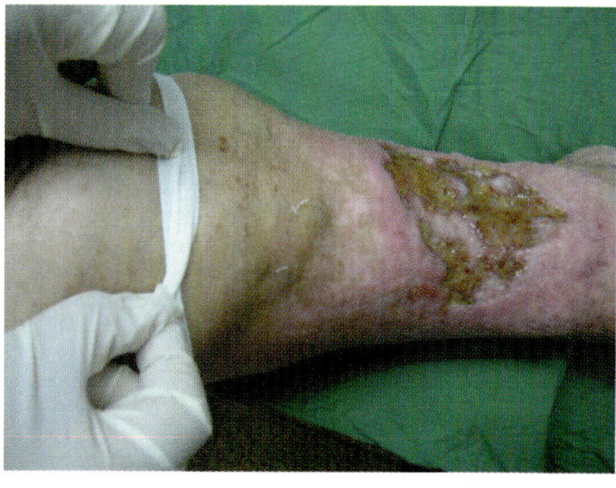

Fig. 7.7. Measurement of the extremity circumference

Using the same tape measure for all patients may increase the spreading of pathogenic bacteria. Instead of using a standard tape measure with millimetric markings, it would be better to use a disposable tape and to mark it by hand prior to each use (and to be thrown away after each use).

Generalized edema and localized edema should be distinguished.

■ **Generalized Edema.** The most common causes of generalized edema are congestive heart failure and pericardial disease, hypoalbuminemia (caused by various factors, including the nephrotic syndrome), and liver disease. Other causes include acute nephritic syndrome, idiopathic edema, myxedema, and trichinosis [43–45].

In generalized edema, when the patient is in a dependent posture, fluids accumulate in the lower extremities. In most cases, but not all, bilateral leg edema is a manifestation of generalized edema. However, bilateral leg edema may also occur in conditions such as bilateral venous insufficiency. The history and physical examination of a patient with generalized edema should focus on the conditions listed above.

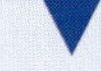

Routine tests indicated in patients with generalized edema include [43–45]:
- Complete blood count
- Urinalysis
- Blood chemistry (including liver function tests), serum albumin, and creatinine
- Chest X-ray
- Electrocardiogram

■ **Localized Edema.** Localized edema is caused by regional obstruction to venous, lymphatic, or venous and lymphatic limb drainage. Possible etiologies may be classified into primary and secondary causes. Primary lymphedema is defined as lymphedema of unknown cause. It may be congenital, caused by processes such as agenesis, hypoplasia, or obstruction of lymphatic vessels. Other forms of primary lymphedema may manifest later in life. Most cases are familial, with a genetic predisposition [46, 47].

The most common form of primary lymphedema, **lymphedema praecox**, constitutes almost 70% of primary lymphedema cases. It begins at puberty, in most cases affecting girls near menarche. Another relatively common form of lymphedema (10–20% of all primary lymphedema cases) is **lymphedema tarda**, which is clinically similar to lymphedema praecox but appears in patients over the age of 35 years.

Secondary lymphedema includes acquired conditions in which previously normal lymphatic vessels do not function properly as a result of a pathological process that causes incomplete or complete obstruction.

Causes of secondary lymphedema are:
- Infectious:
    - Bacterial (e.g., recurrent episodes of bacterial lymphangitis)
    - Fungal
    - Parasitic (e.g., filariasis)
- Vascular:
    - Venous insufficiency
    - Thrombophlebitis
- Traumatic
- Malignant tumors
    - Tumors of the pelvis or abdomen (such as prostate carcinoma or ovarian mass)
    - Propagation of metastases within lymphatic vessels
    - Angiosarcoma (Stewart-Treves syndrome)
- Following medical procedures due to malignancy:
    - Resection of lymph nodes
    - Radiation therapy
- Other causes: e.g., popliteal cyst (Baker's cyst)

Whatever the cause of lymphedema, its course is in most cases progressive and usually causes disability.

In the conditions presented above, venous insufficiency is the most common cause of lymphedema [48–50]. The pathologic process induced by venous insufficiency damages the surrounding tissues, including lymphatic vessels located adjacent to the affected veins [48–50].

Ciocom et al. [51] studied 245 patients with leg edema. The most common causes were venous insufficiency (63.2%), heart failure (15.1%) and drug-induced edema (13.8%). Less common conditions included post-phlebitis syndrome, cirrhosis, lymphedema, lipedema, and prostatic carcinoma.

Evaluation of a patient with localized edema requires a thorough physical examination in order to identify an obstructing tumor (e.g., lymphoma or prostate cancer). Enlarged lymph nodes in the groin area and abdominal masses should be sought. In view of the above, rectal examination is mandatory. The workup should also include abdominal and pelvic ultrasound or computerized tomography. When needed, lymphoscintigraphy or lymphangiography may be considered in order to distinguish between primary and secondary edema. In primary lymphedema the lymphatic vessels are absent, hypoplastic, or ectatic. In contrast, they tend to be dilated in secondary lymphedema [46].

■ **Treatment of Edema.** Once the cause of edema has been identified, treatment should be initiated accordingly. In addition, certain steps should be considered that are detailed in Chap. 21.

7.3.5 Other Factors to Be Considered

The physician should seek and identify other factors and conditions that may result in impaired healing (such as hypoxia caused by congestive heart failure or chronic lung disease) and treat them accordingly. If the patient smokes, explain to him/her the clinical implications of smoking on wound healing (as well as the detrimental effects of smoking in general).

7.3.5.1 Hypoxia

In the initial stages of healing, hypoxia may, in fact, serve as a stimulus for the secretion of growth factors and proliferation of granulation tissue. Later, however, the process of healing is impeded under conditions of hypoxia [52]. Local tissue hypoxia contributes to the formation of cutaneous ulcers of many etiologies, including venous ulcers, ulcers of peripheral arterial disease, diabetic ulcers, and pressure ulcers. In conditions such as congestive heart failure or chronic lung disease there is generalized hypoxia involving all tissues in the body. In patients with cutaneous ulcers, these conditions may further impair wound healing, since peripheral organs are especially affected.

In an animal model, exposure to reduced oxygen levels was shown to reduce wound tensile strength [53].

7.3.5.2 Anemia

Similar to the correction of hypoxia states, correction of anemia is important in order to improve the oxygen-carrying capacity of the blood.

7.3.5.3 Hydration

For nursing-home residents – a population that is prone to developing pressure ulcers – maintaining adequate hydration status becomes a significant clinical issue. Inadequate hydration results in impaired perfusion and reduced tissue oxygenation, with a subsequent detrimental effect on the healing process. In these patients, signs of dehydration such as decreased blood pressure, tachycardia, and decreased urine output should be monitored regularly [54].

It has been suggested that inadequate hydration may have a certain effect on the healing of pressure ulcers in a number of nursing home residents in whom mild states of dehydration may go unnoticed [54]. Some patients do not present with clear clinical signs of dehydration; yet, following the administration of intravenous

Table 7.1. Tests to be performed on a patient with a cutaneous ulcer, at first visit

Blood tests:

- Complete blood count
- Blood chemistry (including hepatic and renal function tests)
- Serum iron (and additonal indicators for iron status e.g., transferrin iron-binding capacity and ferritin), zinc, albumin

Measurements:

- Obtain precise anatomical location
- Note the presence of erythema, record the nature and color of granulation tissue as well as the presence and color of secretions
- Make a tracing of the ulcer margin (or take a photograph)
- Note the depth of the ulcer
- Record the presence and extent of undermining
- Swab for bacterial culture

Identification of factors that may impair healing:

- General factors such as nutritional deficit, anemia, hypoxia, smoking
- Drugs to be avoided, where relevant (see chapter 16)
- Leg edema (and measurement of leg circumference in that case)

Documentation of past treatments: This information may affect decisions regarding optional treatments (avoid treatments shown to be ineffective in the past)

Work-up for determination of ulcer etiology in accordance with the clinical data (see Chaps. 5 and 6).

---

fluids, tissue oxygenation improves. In this respect, Chang et al [55] coined the term "subclinical hypovolemia", suggesting that even 'subclinical' inadequate hydration may hinder the normal course of wound repair. The issue of 'subclinical hypovolemia' and its practical implications, e.g., the administration of supplemental fluid, have to be clarified by further research.

7.3.5.4 Smoking

Patients with cutaneous ulcers should be instructed to refrain froom smoking. Smoking may impair wound healing via several mechanisms. The damage to blood vessels due to smoking, already widely described [56], causes decreased perfusion to an ulcer or wound area. Other effects of smoking on wound healing are decreased production of collagen [57] and impaired migration of keratinocytes [58]. Cigar-

Table 7.2. Follow-up

1. Trace the ulcer margin or photograph it every 2–3 weeks, depending on the general impression of the rate of change occurring in the ulcer. Islands of epithelialization on the ulcer bed or peripheral epithelialization should be documented.

2. Record ulcer depth.

3. Document features related to infection:

   Presence of secretion and its color

   Erythema or local heat of the surrounding skin

   Repeated bacterial cultures

4. Measure leg circumference in the case of leg edema

5. Depending on the clinical situation, consider repeating the blood tests listed in Summary Table 7.1; try to identify factors that impair healing.

Table 7.3. Tests to be considered in the case of any ulcer that does not heal within 3–4 months[a]

1. Biopsy to establish etiology or rule out certain conditions

2. X-ray and bone scan to rule out osteomyelitis

3. Nutritional follow-up including hemoglobin level, albumin, and iron

4. Doppler flowmetry of leg arteries or Doppler ultrasonography of the lower-limb venous system

[a] If necessary, the above tests should be performed earlier, depending on the clinical circumstances

ette smoking also impairs wound healing following surgical procedures [59–62].

7.3.5.5 Physical Activity

The beneficial effects of physical activity in cases of leg edema are described in Chap. 21. Its beneficial effects on the cardiovascular system are well documented [63–65]. Physical activity, if possible, is recommended for every patient suffering from a leg ulcer. (Note: For patients with ulcers of the foot, physical activity such as walking may result in undesirable effects of intermittent pressure and shearing forces. In such cases, the type of physical activity should be adjusted to the nature and location of the ulcer.)

7.4 Summary Tables

Tables 7.1–7.3 summarize the initial workup of patients with cutaneous ulcers, the follow-up of such patients, and tests to be done for non-healing ulcers.

References

1. He C, Cherry GW: Measurement of blood flow in patients with leg ulcers. In: Mani R, Falanga V, Shearman CP, Sandman D (eds): Chronic Wound Healing. Clinical Measurement and Basic Science, 1st edn. London: WB Saunders. 1999; pp 50–67

2. Mayrovitz HN, Larsen PB: Periwound skin microcirculation of venous leg ulcers. Microvasc Res 1994; 48:114–123

3. Svedman C, Cherry GW, Ryan TJ: The veno-arteriolar reflex in venous leg ulcer patients studied by laser Doppler imaging. Acta Derm Venereol 1998; 78:258–261

4. Romanelli M, Falanga V: Measurement of transcutaneous oxygen tension in chronic wounds. In: Mani R, Falanga V, Shearman CP, Sandman D (eds): Chronic Wound Healing. Clinical Measurement and Basic Science, 1st edn. London: WB Saunders. 1999; pp 68–80

5. Mani R, Gorman FW, White JE: Transcutaneous measurements of oxygen tension at edges of leg ulcers: preliminary communication. J R Soc Med 1986; 79:650–654

6. Romanelli M, Gaggio G, Piaggesi, A et al: Technological advances in wound bed measurements. Wounds 2002; 14:58–66

7. Wilson IA, Henry M, Quill RD, et al: The pH of varicose ulcer surfaces and its relationship to healing. Vasa 1979; 8:339–342

8. Stacey MC, Trengove NJ: Biochemical measurements of tissue and wound fluids. In: Mani R, Falanga V, Shearman CP, Sandman D (eds): Chronic wound healing. Clinical measurement and basic science, 1st edn. London: WB Saunders. 1999; pp 99–123

9. James TJ, Hughes MA, Cherry GW, et al: Simple biochemical markers to assess chronic wounds. Wound Rep Reg 2000; 8:264–269

10. Trengove NJ, Langton SR, Stacey MC: Biochemical analysis of wound fluid from nonhealing and healing chronic leg ulcers. Wound Rep Reg 1996; 4:234–239

11. Langemo DK, Melland H, Hanson D, et al: Two-dimensional wound measurement: comparison of 4 techniques. Adv Wound Care 1998; 11:337–343

12. Cutler NR, George R, Seifert RD, et al: Comparison of quantitative methodologies to define chronic pressure ulcer measurements. Decubitus 1993; 6:22–30

13. Sussman C: Wound measurement. In: Sussman C, Bates-Jensen BM (eds): Wound Care: A Collaborative Practice Manual for Physical Therapists and Nurses, 1st edn. Gaithersburg, MD: Aspen Publishers 1999; pp 83–102

14. Mani R, Ross JN: Morphometry and other measurements. In: Mani R, Falanga V, Shearman CP, Sandman D (eds): Chronic Wound Healing. Clinical Measurement and Basic Science, 1st edn. London: WB Saunders. 1999; pp 81–98

15. Wysocki AB: Wound measurement. Int J Dermatol 1996; 35:82–91

16. Majeske C: Reliability of wound surface area measurements. Phys Ther 1992; 72:138–141

17. Lucas C, Classen J, Harrison D, et al: Pressure ulcer surface area measurement using instant full- scale photography and transparency tracings. Adv Skin Wound Care 2002; 15:17–23

18. Etris MB, Pribble J, LaBrecque J: Evaluation of two wound measurement methods in a multi-center, controlled study. Ostomy Wound Manage 1994; 40:44–48

19. Brown-Etris M: Measuring healing in wounds. Adv Wound Care 1995; 8:53–58

20. Fuller FW, Mansour EH, Engler PE, et al: The use of planimetry for calculating the surface area of a burn wound. J Burn Care Rehabil 1985; 6:47–49

21. Brown GL, Nanney LB, Griffen J, et al: Enhancement of wound healing by topical treatment with epidermal growth factor. N Engl J Med 1989; 321:76–79

22. Wieman TJ, Smiell JM, Su Y: Efficacy and safety of a topical gel formulation of recombinant human platelet-derived growth factor-BB (becaplermin) in patients with chronic neuropathic diabetic ulcers. Diabetes Care 1998; 21:822–827

23. Robson MC, Phillips TJ, Falanga V, et al: Randomized trial of topically applied repifermin (recombinant human keratinocyte growth factor-2) to accelerate wound healing in venous ulcers. Wound Rep Reg 2001; 9:347–352

24. Xakellis GC Jr, Frantz RA: Pressure ulcer healing. What is it? What influences it? How is it measured? Adv Wound Care 1997; 10:20–26

25. Eriksson G, Eklund AE, Torlegard K, et al: Evaluation of leg ulcer treatment with stereophotogrammetry: A pilot study. Br J Dermatol 1979; 101:123–131

26. Bulstrode CJ, Goode AW, Scott PJ: Stereophotogrammetry for measuring rates of cutaneous healing: a comparison with conventional techniques. Clin Sci 1986; 71:437–443

27. Bulstrode CJ, Goode AW, Scott PJ: Measurement and prediction of progress in delayed wound healing. J R Soc Med 1987; 80:210–212

28. Frantz RA, Johnson DA: Stereophotography and computerized image analysis: a three-dimensional method of measuring wound healing. Wounds 1992; 4:58–64

29. Harding KG: Methods for assessing change in ulcer status. Adv Wound Care 1995; 8:37–42

30. Griffin JW, Tolley EA, Tooms RE, et al: A comparison of photographic and transparency based methods for measuring wound surface area. Phys Ther 1993; 73:117–122

31. The National Pressure Ulcer Advisory Panel. Pressure ulcers prevalence, cost and risk assessment: consensus development conference statement. Decubitus 1989; 2:24–28

32. Whiston RJ, Melhuish J, Harding KG: High resolution ultrasound imaging in wound healing. Wounds 1993; 5:116–121

33. Smith RB, Rogers B, Tolstykh GP, et al: Three-dimensional laser imaging system for measuring wound geometry. Lasers Surg Med 1998; 23:87–93

34. Covington JS, Griffin JW, Mendius RK, et al: Measurement of pressure ulcer volume using dental impression materials: suggestion from the field. Phys Ther 1989; 69:690–694

35. McCulloch JM: Evaluation of patints with open wounds. In: McCulloch JM, Kloth LC, Feedar JA (eds) Wound Healing: Alternative in Management, 2nd edn. Philadelphia: FA Davis. 1995; pp 111–134

36. Harkess N: Bacteriology. In: McCulloch JM, Kloth LC, Feedar JA (eds): Wound Healing: Alternative in Management, 2nd edn. Philadelphia: FA Davis. 1995; pp 60–86

37. Niedner R, Schopf E: Wound infections and antibacterial therapy. In: Westerhof W (ed) Leg ulcers – Diagnosis and treatment, 1st edn. Amsterdam: Elsevier Science Publishers. 1993; pp 293–303

38. Hellgren L, Vincent J: Debridement: an essential step in wound healing. In: Westerhof W (ed) Leg ulcers – Diagnosis and treatment, 1st edn. Amsterdam: Elsevier. 1993; pp 305–312

39. Romanelli M: Objective measurement of venous ulcer debridement and granulation with a skin color reflectance analyzer. Wounds 1997; 9:122–126

40. Pierard-Franchimont C, Letawe C, Fumal I, et al: Gravitational syndrome and tensile properties of skin in the elderly. Dermatology 1998; 197:317–320

41. Olszewski W: Pathophysiology and clinical observations of obstructive lymphedema of the limbs. In: Clodius L (ed) Lymphedema. Stuttgart: Georg Thieme Verlag. 1977; pp 79–102

42. Casley-Smith JR, Casley-Smith JR: Pathology of oedema – Effect of oedema. In: Casley-Smith JR, Casley-Smith JR (eds.) Modern Treatment for Lymphoedema, 5th revised edn. Adelaide: The Lymphoedema Association of Australia. 1997; pp 60–73

43. Friedman HH: Edema. In: Friedman HH (ed) Problem-Oriented Medical Diagnosis, 7th edn. Boston: Little, Brown 2001; pp 1–3

44. Ciocon JO, Fernandez BB, Ciocon DG: Leg edema: Clinical clues to the differential diagnosis. Geriatrics 1993; 48:34–40, 45

45. Braunwald E: Edema. In: Braunwald E, Fauci AS, Kasper DL, Hauser SL, Longo DL, Jameson JL (eds) Harrison's Principles of Internal Medicine, 15th edn. New York: McGraw-Hill. 2001; pp 217–222

46. Creager MA, Dzau VJ: Vascular disease of the extremities. In: Braunwald E, Fauci AS, Kasper DL, Hauser SL, Longo DL, Jameson JL (eds) Harrison's Principles of Internal Medicine, 15th edn. New York: McGraw-Hill. 2001; pp 1434–1442

47. Casley-Smith JR, Casley-Smith JR: The etiology of lymphoedema. In: Casley-Smith JR, Casley-Smith JR (eds) Modern Treatment for Lymphoedema, 5th revised edn. Adelaide: The Lymphoedema Association of Australia. 1997; pp 74–78

48. Bull RH, Gane JN, Evans JE, et al: Abnormal lymph drainage in patients with chronic venous leg ulcers. J Am Acad Dermatol 1993; 28:585–590

49. Prasad A, Ali-Khan A, Mortimer PS: Leg ulcers and oedema: a study exploring the prevalence, aetiology, and posssible significance of oedema in venous ulcers. Phlebology 1990; 5:181–187

50. Partsch H: Investigations on the pathogenesis of venous leg ulcers. Acta Chir Scand 1988; [Suppl] 544: 25–29
51. Ciocon JO, Galindo Ciocon D, Galindo DJ: Raised leg exercises for leg edema in the elderly. Angiology 1995; 46:19–25
52. Stadelmann WK, Digenis AG, Tobin GR: Impediments to wound healing. Am J Surg 1998; 176 [Suppl]: 39S–47S
53. Niinikoski J: Effect of oxygen supply on wound healing and formation of experimental granulation tissue. Acta Physiol Scand 1969; 334:1–72
54. Stotts NA, Hopf HW: The link between tissue oxygen and hydration in nursing home residents with pressure ulcers: preliminary data. J Wound Ostomy Continence Nurs 2003; 30:184–190
55. Chang N, Goodson WH III, Gottrup F, et al: Direct measurement of wound and tissue oxygen tension in postoperative patients. Ann Surg 1983; 197: 470–478
56. Burns DM: Nicotine addiction. In: Braunwald E, Fauci AS, Kasper DL, Hauser SL, Longo DL, Jameson JL (eds) Harrison's Principles of Internal Medicine, 15th edn. New York: McGraw-Hill 2001; pp 2574–2577
57. Jorgensen LN, Kallehave F, Christensen E et al: Less collagen production in smokers. Surgery 1998; 123: 450–455
58. Zia S, Ndoye A, Lee TX et al: Receptor-mediated inhibition of keratinocyte migration by nicotine involves modulations of calcium influx and intracellular concentration. J Pharmacol Exp Ther 2000; 293: 973–981
59. Nolan J, Jenkins RA, Kurihara K et al: The acute effects of cigarette smoke exposure on experimental skin flaps. Plast Reconstr Surg 1985; 75:544–551
60. Chang LD, Buncke G, Slezak S et al: Cigarette smoking, plastic surgery, and microsurgery. J Reconstr Microsurg 1996; 12:467–474
61. Reus WF, Colen LB, Straker DJ: Tobbaco smoking and complications in elective microsurgery. Plast Reconstr Surg 1992; 89:490–494
62. Gu YD, Zhang GM, Zhang LY et al: Clinical and experimental studies of cigarette smoking in microvascular tissue transfers. Microsurgery 1993; 14: 391–397
63. Maiorana A, O'Driscoll G, Cheetham, C et al: The effect of combined aerobic and resistance exercise training on vascular function in type 2 diabetes. J Am Coll Cardiol 2001; 38: 860–866
64. Leng GC, Fowler GC, Ernst E: Exercise for intermittent claudication (Cochrane Review). The Cochrane Library. Issue 4, 2001. Oxford: Update Software
65. Jolliffe JA, Rees K, Taylor RS et al. Exercise-based rehabilitation for coronary heart disease. (Cochrane Review). The Cochrane Library. Issue 1, 2003. Oxford: Update Software

Dressing Materials

8

Contents

8.1 Overview

Many dressings have been introduced during the past decade. The dressing modalities available at present demand that the physician gain a better understanding of the wound healing process, to distinguish between the various types of dressing materials, and to identify the conditions for which each class of dressing should be used.

The four main classes of dressings, as suggested by the Food and Drug Administration (FDA) on November 4, 1999, are:
- Non-resorbable gauze/sponge
- Hydrophylic/absorptive
- Occlusive
- Hydrogel

Other types may be classified as follows:
- Dressings that combine two of the above groups
- Interactive dressings
- Dressings with unique features
- Biological dressings (discussed in Chap. 13)

8.2 Traditional Dressings: Non-Resorbable Gauze/ Sponge Dressings

Non-resorbable gauze/sponge dressings are made of woven or non-woven cotton-mesh cellulose or cellulose derivatives and can be manufactured in the form of pads or strips.

> These are the basic dressings that fulfill the classic roles expected from any kind of dressing, including advanced-type dressings, which should:
> - Protect the wound from external infection and prevent bacteria in the wound from contaminating the surroundings
> - Protect the wound and its surrounding from mechanical trauma
> - Absorb secretions, if needed
> - Improve patient comfort

Gauze/sponge dressings are used mainly to cover a wound surface area following application of topical preparations (e.g., antibacterial creams or advanced spreadable preparations).

8.3 Development of Advanced Dressing Modalities

The accepted and traditional approach to wound healing 40–50 years ago was that, in optimal treatment, wounds or cutaneous ulcers should be left to dry out, preferably exposed to the air. In 1962, Winter et al. [1] presented a domestic pig model indicating that a moist environment was ideal for healing a wound or a cutaneous ulcer. These results were confirmed in human subjects in 1963 by Hinman and Maibach, who demonstrated the beneficial effect of a moist environment on wounds (vs. air-exposed wounds) in human volunteers [2].

A suitable degree of moisture within an ulcer's environment creates a desirable biological medium that provides optimal conditions for the complex processes of wound healing. It enables a more efficient metabolic activity of each cell and the whole tissue, cellular interaction, and growth-factor activities that cannot occur within dry tissues.

> Occlusive dressings, representing the next generation of dressing materials, were developed in the 1960s and 1970s, but it was not until the 1980s that other types of advanced dressings were introduced, each for a specific purpose:
> - Hydrogel dressings: used to maintain a moist environment and to induce autolytic debridement of necrotic debris within the ulcer area
> - Hydrophilic dressings: used to absorb secretions
> - Hydrocolloid dressings: used to maintain a moist environment (see below)

All these advanced dressing materials can fulfill the classical roles of dressings (as described above) much better than the traditional gauze dressings. In most cases they offer better protection from mechanical trauma and/or external contamination. Newer dressing materials are usually easy and convenient to apply; they are flexible and conform to various body parts. Today, when absorption of secretions is needed, it can be achieved more efficiently with certain types of modern dressings.

8.4 Features of Dressings

In each class of the advanced dressings discussed below, various subtypes have been introduced, according to certain physical features.

8.4.1 Transparency

A transparent dressing enables visual monitoring of the ulcer surface area. An ulcer covered by a non-transparent dressing may gradually become infected, without this being noticed. When non-transparent dressings are used, frequent removal and changing of the dressings is mandatory.

8.4.2 Adhesiveness

Adhesives lead to the attachment of the dressing to the wound surface. Removal of the dressing may then strip away newly forming epithelium [3]. On the other hand, the probability of epithelial injury with the use of hydrogel or hydrocolloid dressings is relatively low, due to the formation of a gelatinous substance that intervenes between the dressing material and the wound surface.

The clinical appearance of the ulcer's surrounding should be taken into account.

Adhesive dressings should not be used in the following cases:
- When the area surrounding the wound is macerated
- When the surrounding skin is affected by dermatitis [3, 4]
- In easily injured/atrophic skin – as in patients on steroid treatment – that may be damaged on removal of the dressing. One should avoid dressings which are excessively adhesive, since these may damage healthy skin around the treated ulcer. By the same token, avoid using adhesives (plasters) to fix a dressing onto a wound.

Note that damage to newly forming epithelium and to healing granulation tissue with removal of a dressing may occur with non-adhesive dressings as well: A dressing may adhere to the wound surface due to the presence of exudate and its gradual desiccation.

8.4.3 Form of Dressing

Current dressing materials appear in a variety of forms, the main ones being sheet forms and spreadable forms (such as gels or pastes). Other forms of dressings do exist, for example, alginate dressings marketed in a rope form. A sheet-form dressing should be placed 2–3 cm beyond the ulcer margin. When using a spreadable form of advanced dressing modality, a secondary dressing is needed to affix it and to ensure that it is well attached to the ulcer bed.

8.4.4 Absorptive Capacity

The absorptive capacity of each dressing type varies greatly, according to the type of dressing and manufacturer.

8.4.5 Permeability/Occlusiveness

The level of permeability to fluids, gases, vapor, and bacteria varies according to the type of dressing and manufacturer. As the level of secretion increases, more permeable dressings should be used.

Thomas et al. [5] compared the beneficial effect of a polyurethane foam, highly permeable to moisture vapor, with that of hydrocolloid dressings on 100 patients with leg ulcers and 99 patients with pressure sores. No statistically significant difference was demonstrated regarding the healing rates of the two groups. However, the foam dressing was found to better control dressing leakage and odor formation. One may assume that these results were not related to the class of dressing (hydrocolloid vs. foam), but rather to the different degrees of permeability according to the specific manufacturing of each dressing.

Occlusive dressings, in general, are used mainly to maintain a moist environment within the ulcer area. The significance of a moist environment for all the complex processes of wound healing was noted earlier in this chapter. This approach was confirmed by a variety of research studies, demonstrating the beneficial effect of occlusive dressings on surgical wounds [6–9] and chronic cutaneous ulcers [10–12]. In most of these studies, a more efficient healing was manifested by improved granulation tissue formation as well as enhanced epithelialization. However, one should avoid 'over-moisturizing' cutaneous ulcers, since this may lead to maceration, skin breakdown, and infection.

Note that some degree of autolytic debridement (described in Chap. 9) may be achieved by using occlusive dressings, as a result of the moist environment they produce.

8.4.6 Antimicrobial Effect

The issue of an antimicrobial effect in respect to dressing materials is discussed below. This applies to products such as cadexomer-iodine (Iodosorb®) and dressings that combine activated charcoal with silver (Actisorb®). A certain antimicrobial effect may also be achieved by other means, for instance, by absorbing exudate with hydrophilic dressings, thereby creating an environment unsuitable for multiplication of bacteria.

Studies that compare dressing materials of various types should be regarded with a certain degree of scientific criticism. In some articles, the authors give only a general definition of the examined ulcer type (e.g., venous ulcers or pressure ulcer), while significant data (such as the presence of slough, its color, the presence of discharge within the ulcer bed) are not provided.

8.5 Advanced Dressing Modalities

8.5.1 Occlusive Dressings: Films, Hydrocolloids, Foams

An occlusive or moisture-retentive dressing is one that maintains an appropriate moisture vapor transmission rate within the ulcer's environment, thus providing ideal conditions for wound healing [13].

Sub-types of occlusive dressings according to the FDA classification are:
- Thin films
- Hydrocolloid dressings
- Foam dressings

In its basic form, an occlusive dressing is composed of a synthetic polymer, such as polyethylene or polyurethane, with or without adhesive backing. Films were the first occlusive dressings to be developed, followed by more complex products such as hydrocolloid dressings and foam dressings. As discussed above, occlusive dressings are used to maintain a moist environment within the ulcer area.

The 'classical' FDA classification, as presented above, is becoming less and less relevant. The boundaries between various groups of dressing materials are becoming continuously blurred. Not all foams, for example, are occlusive. Similarly, certain hydrogel sheet dressings, which do not belong to the occlusive group according to the FDA classification are, in fact, occlusive.

8.5.1.1 Thin Films

Films are composed of a thin sheet of polyurethane, permeable to moisture vapor and gases (to different degrees, according to type and manufacturer), but impermeable to fluid and bacteria [3, 13]. They maintain a moist wound environment, but since they are non-absorbent, they should not be used on secreting ulcers.

The first commercial film dressing (Opsite®) was intended to be used for a wide range of lesions, including burn wounds, donor sites, cutaneous ulcers, and surgical wounds [14]. According to textbooks, films may be used for numerous types of ulcers and wounds [13]; the fact that films are impermeable to bacteria and fluids makes them ideal for a clean, sutured surgical wound (Fig. 8.1). Currently, physicians tend to use film dressings less frequently for chronic cutaneous ulcers, preferring the more advanced modern dressings.

Most films are adhesive, so they may also be used as a secondary dressing applied over other topical preparations [14]. Certain dressings are manufactured as a combination of polyurethane films and other dressing materials (e.g., alginates or hydrogels).

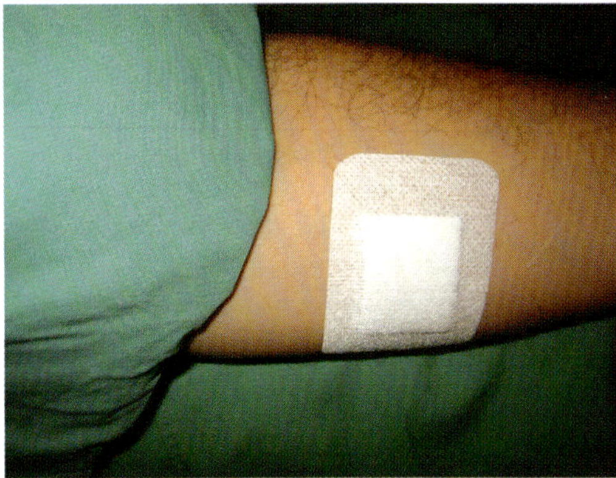

Fig. 8.1. A film dressing covers a clean sutured surgical wound

Examples of film dressing:
- Bioclusive transparent dressing® – Johnson & Johnson
- Blisterfilm transparent dressing® – Kendall
- Carrafilm transparent film dressing® – Carrington Laboratories
- Cutifilm – Beiersdorf-Jobst
- Dermafilm intelligent film dressing® – Derma Sciences
- Epiview® – Convatec
- Mefilm® – Mölnlycke Health Care
- Opsite® – Smith & Nephew
- Orifilm transparent film dressing® – Orion Medical Products
- Polyskin® – Kendall
- 3M Tegaderm transparent dressing® – 3M Health Care

8.5.1.2 Hydrocolloid Dressings

Hydrocolloid dressings contain hydrocolloidal hydrophilic particles (mainly sodium carboxy methyl cellulose) that are gel-forming. Other substances may be included such as gelatin or pectin. The composition and amount of each ingredient varies according to the manufacturer.

Hydrocolloid materials are available in a spreadable form or as sheets. The sheet form is composed of an inner hydrocolloid lining and an external hydrophobic coating (usually polyurethane) that is impermeable to gases, water, and bacteria [15, 16]. The sheet dressings are adhesive.

When hydrocolloids dressings are applied onto an ulcer surface (Fig. 8.2), there is interaction between the hydrocolloid substance and the ulcer's fluid, resulting in a characteristic gelatinous yellow mass over the ulcer. This gelatinous mass contributes to the formation of a moist environment, facilitating autolytic debridement, granulation tissue formation, and epithelialization.

The hydrocolloid substance absorbs necrotic material and fluids from the ulcer's environment, as well as wound fluid. There is accumulating evidence that ingredients in the fluids of chronic, long-standing ulcers (unlike acute wound fluid) may diminish the proliferative capacity of keratinocytes [17, 18].

The gelatinous mass is located between the dressing and the ulcer bed. Thus, when the dressing is removed or changed there is no damage to superficial tissues within the ulcer bed, namely, the granulation tissue and the new regenerative epithelium (Fig. 8.3).

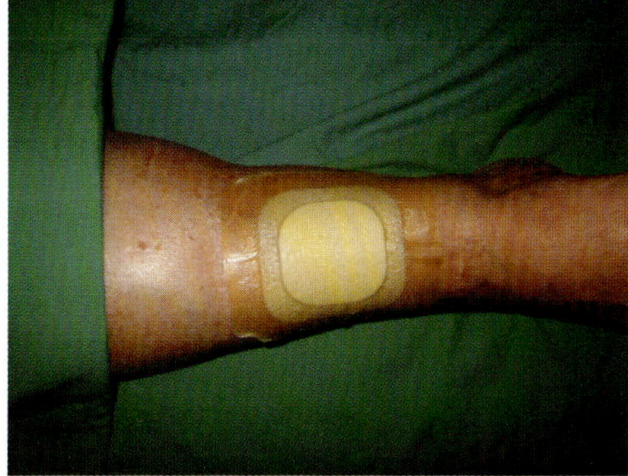

Fig. 8.2. A hydrocolloid dressing is placed onto a cutaneous ulcer

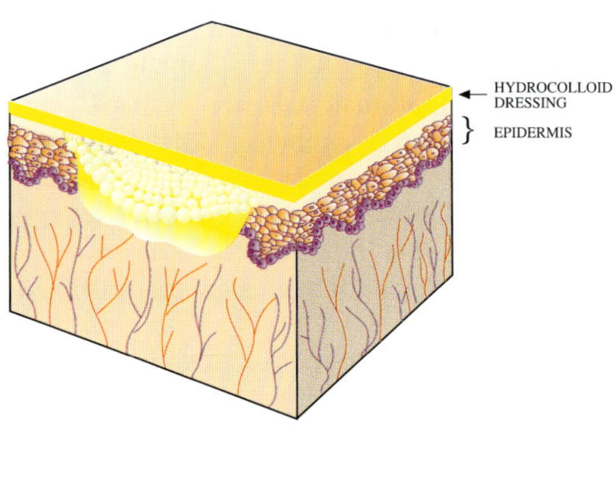

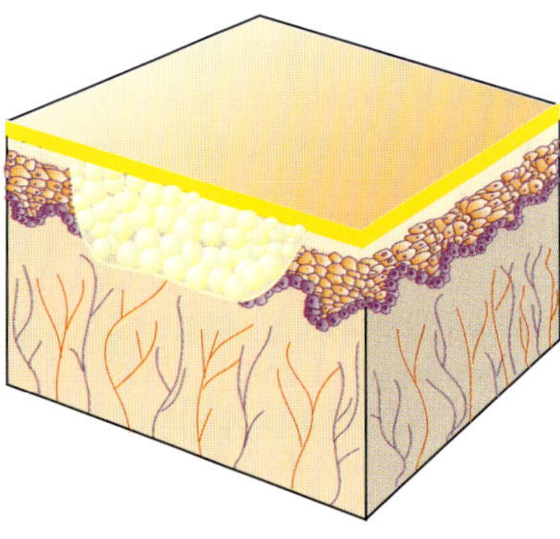

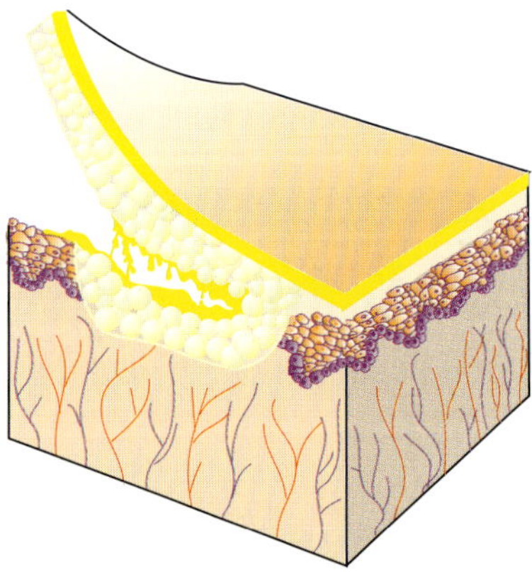

Fig. 8.3. The mode of action of a hydrocolloid dressing. A hydrocolloid dressing on a cutaneous ulcer (*top*). Hydrocolloid particles absorb secretions and increase in size (*center*). While the dressing is being changed, a protective gelatinous layer remains on the surface, which can be removed by gentle rinsing (*bottom*)

Further possible advantages of hydrocolloid dressings have been documented:

- The hypoxic environment induced by hydrocolloid dressings is said to stimulate proliferation of fibroblasts and angiogenesis, presumably by the formation of growth factors [19, 20]. However, this information should not be taken for granted, especially regarding chronic cutaneous ulcers that usually appear in elderly populations. In 1972, Hunt et al. [21] stated that wound healing processes may be delayed and impeded by relative hypoxia. It is currently accepted that apart from the very initial stages of healing, hypoxia is not essential to the overall healing process. In most cases, when dealing with chronic ulcers, it impedes healing. Xia et al. [22] recently reported that keratinocytes derived from an elderly donor showed a delay in migratory activity under hypoxic conditions, while young keratinocytes showed enhanced migratory activity.
- The acidic microenvironment induced by hydrocolloids may be active against bacteria, including strains of *Pseudomonas aeruginosa* [23].

The accepted indications for hydrocolloid dressings are mild-to-moderate exudating ulcers, burn wounds, and donor sites [3, 24–26]. This recommendation is based on clinical observations indicating that chronic cutaneous ulcers treated by occlusive hydrocolloid dressings have been shown to improve, even though the presence of bacteria on the ulcer bed was confirmed by swab cultures [23, 27]. The use of hydrocolloid dressings on infected or necrotic wounds is definitely contraindicated [28]. The presence of pus on an ulcer bed is a clear marker of infection and under such cirumstances, hydrocolloid dressing should not be used [29–32].

The question as to the level of turbidity of discharge and the cut-off point above which it would be reasonable to avoid the use of occlusive dressings remains under debate and subject to the clinical judgement of the treating physician. It has been suggested that the presence of seropurulent/turbid discharge on a non-healing ulcer may indeed reflect local infection [33]. This being the case, placing such an ulcer under occlusive conditions may aggravate the infection. Based on our experience, the application of hydrocolloid dressings should be limited only to relatively clean ulcers and ulcers with minimal serous (clear) secretion.

■ **Mode of Use.** After application of sheet-form hydrocolloid dressings (as well as other sorts of occlusive dressings in sheet form) onto the ulcer, creases in the dressing should be smoothed out. This should be followed by light pressure for about 20 seconds with the objective of allowing the dressing to conform to the ulcer bed. These recommendations may vary according to the dressing's type and manufacturer's instructions.

■ Changing Dressings. It is common practice to leave hydrocolloid dressings in place for 5–7 days before changing. However, this is debatable. The main argument for leaving the dressings on for this period of time is to avoid damaging the surrounding skin when stripping off the adhesive. In addition, it has been suggested that frequent changing and cleansing can inflict a certain amount of trauma on the granulation tissue and newly forming epithelium.

The main argument for changing the dressing more frequently, on the other hand, is to enable appropriate visual monitoring. Even transparent dressings do not allow a thorough enough examination of the ulcer. We have, in fact, encountered several ulcers that have worsened under prolonged occlusive conditions. In any case, the frequency of changing dressings depends on the appearance of the ulcer. If an ulcer is not clean, frequent monitoring is required. In such cases, the dressing should be changed every 48 h, and in some cases even every 24 h.

Note that when hydrocolloid dressings are used, a gelatinous mass of characteristic appearance is formed on the ulcer surface. It is not purulent material. Nevertheless, having been made aware of this fact by medical staff, some patients remain oblivious to the increased amounts of discharge within the ulcer and can, at their next visit, present with a severely infected ulcer.

> Examples of hydrocolloid dressings:
> - Comfeel® – Coloplast
> - Cutinova® – Beiersdorf-Jobst
> - Dermacol® – Derma Sciences
> - Dermatell® – Gentell
> - Duoderm® – Convatec
> - Exuderm® – Medline Industries
> - Granuflex® – Convatec
> - Hydrocol® – Bertek Pharmaceuticals
> - Hydrocoll® – Hartmann
> - Nu-derm (hydrocolloid)® – Johnson & Johnson
> - Oriderm® – Orion Medical Products
> - Replicare® – Smith & Nephew
> - Restore® – Hollister Incorporated
> - Tegasorb® – 3M Health Care
> - Ultec® – Kendall

Being manufactured by many different companies, hydrocolloid dressings are not uniform in their quality and features. There is wide variation between the properties of different dressings [34]. Further research studies are required to determine the exact type of ulcer or wound for which each type of dressing is ideally intended.

8.5.1.3 Foam Dressings

Foam dressings are composed of polymeric material such as polyurethane, that is manufactured to contain air bubbles. The spaces embedded within the dressing material are capable of absorbing fluids. These dressings are generally occlusive or semi-occlusive, and are permeable to gases and water vapor [13, 35].

The absorptive capacity is dependent on the thickness of the dressing as well as on the substances impregnated in it and varies with type and manufacturer. Foam dressings are usually opaque and non-adherent.

Foam dressings are available in sheet form or as spreadable foams. In sheet form, they have a hydrophilic side that is in contact with the wound surface and absorbs secretions. The external hydrophobic side contributes to a moist environment. Spreadable foams are used for cavities. In this case, a secondary dressing is needed to affix the preparation to the ulcer bed.

Since most of the foam dressings are occlusive, the indication, in principle, is similar to that for hydrocolloids. In view of their absorptive capacity, their use may be considered when dealing with secreting ulcers. However, above a certain level of turbidity, other modalities are advocated.

Examples of foam dressings:
- Allevyn® – Smith & Nephew
- Biatain® – Coloplast
- Carrasmart foam® – Carrington Lab
- Curafoam plus® – Kendall
- Cutinova foam® – Beiersdorf-Jobst
- Flexzan® – Bertek Pharmaceuticals
- Hydrasorb® – Convatec
- Lyofoam® – Convatec
- Mepilex® – Mölnlycke Health Care
- 3M Foam® – 3M Health Care
- Orifoam® – Orion Medical Products
- Sof-foam® – Johnson & Johnson
- Reston foam® – 3M Health Care
- Tielle® – Johnson & Johnson
- Vigifoam® – Bard Med. DivisioN

8.5.2 Hydrogels

Hydrogels are made up of a three-dimensional matrix of hydrophylic polymers, such as carboxy-methylcellulose (Intrasite gel®) or polyethylene oxide (Vigilon®), combined with a high (usually more than 90%) water content.

Hydrogel preparations may also contain glycerin and pectin. As in the case of other dressings, they are available in sheet form or as a spreadable viscous gel.

Hydrogel dressings are semipermeable to gases and water vapor. Note that certain hydrogel dressings may contain polyurethane and thus, to a certain extent, have occlusive properties. However, the unique feature of hydrogels (as distinguished from other occlusive dressings) is due to the presence of hydrophylic polymers in their content: The amorphous gel formed by hydrogel dressings maintains a moist and hydrated environment within the ulcer.

This makes hydrogel dressings suitable in two main situations:
- Since hydrogel dressings maintain a moist wound environment, they may be used for clean, red ulcers.
- The hydrated moist conditions within the ulcer area enable the separation of necrotic tissue and induce processes of autolytic debridement. Therefore, hydrogel dressings may be applied to ulcers that present white or yellowish slough on their surface. Autogenous enzymes released by dead or damaged tissue disintegrate the sloughy material and enable its detachment from the ulcer's surface area [36–39]. That being the case, amorphous gels are indicated, and not the sheets.

Hydrogel dressings may also be considered for softening black, dry necrotic material, due to their water-donating properties. However, a beneficial effect (if any) is expected to occur relatively slowly. Other forms of debridement, such as surgical debridement, should be considered when dealing with dry, black necrotic material on an ulcer bed (see Chap. 20). Due to the water-donating properties of hydrogels, care must be taken that the ulcer and the healthy tissue around it do not become macerated [36].

Among research studies performed with hydrogel dressings, Bale et al. [36] demonstrated beneficial effects of hydrogel dressings on 50 pressure ulcers, with effective debridement of necrotic tissue within the ulcer bed. Flanagan [40] documented a research study containing 47 patients, each with one cutaneous ulcer in which non-viable tissue covered more than 30% of the ulcer's surface area. The cutaneous ulcers included in the study were leg ulcers and pressure ulcers, as well as other sorts of lesions such as traumatic wounds. Efficient removal of necrotic material from the ulcer bed was observed. After 21 days of treatment, 10 ulcers (21%) were completely clean. In 20 other ulcers, 50% or more of non-viable material was removed. Other randomized controlled studies have shown the beneficial effect of hydrogels on diabetic foot ulcers as compared with standard care [41].

Examples of hydrogel dressings:
- Aquaflo® – Kendall
- Aquasorb® – Deroyal
- Carrasyn gel wound dressing® – Carrington Laboratories
- Curafil® – Kendall
- Cutinova gel® – Beiersdorf-Jobst
- Dermagran hydrogel zinc-saline wound dressing® – Derma Sciences
- Duoderm hydroactive gel® – Convatec
- Granugel® – Convatec
- Hydrosorb® – Hartmann
- Hyfil wound gel® – B. Braun Medical
- Hypergel® – Molnlycke Health Care
- Iamin hydrating gel® – CR Bard
- Intrasite gel® – Smith & Nephew
- Macropro gel® – Brennen Medical
- MPM Excel gel® – MPM Medical
- Purilon gel® – Coloplast
- Sterigel® – Seton Scholl
- Vigilon® – Bard Med. Division

8.5.3 Hydrophilic/ Absorptive Dressings

Hydrophilic dressings are intended to absorb exudate. Although cotton dressings and cotton

derivates are capable of this, currently used advanced dressings have been shown to do this better. The main representatives of this group are discussed below.

8.5.3.1 Alginate Dressings

Alginate dressings are made of polysaccharide fiber, containing alginic acids, derived from various species of seaweed. The fibers absorb the ulcer exudate with the formation of a highly absorbent hydrophilic gel. This interaction results in a moist wound environment that may provide appropriate conditions for autolytic debridement. Alginate fibers are biodegradable [42].

Alginate dressings are indicated for moderate-to-heavy exudating cutaneous ulcers [43]. In view of this fact, they should be changed at least once daily.

Alginate dressings are available in sheet form (Fig. 8.4). In addition, rope forms or gel forms are intended for cavity ulcers (Fig. 8.5).

Sayag et al. [44] documented the beneficial effects of alginate dressings on full-thickness pressure ulcers. A minimal 40% reduction in ulcer area was demonstrated in 74% of patients treated with alginate dressings, compared with 42% of patients treated with dextranomer paste.

The question as to whether alginates have certain pharmacologic qualities that contribute to wound healing (beyond absorbing exudate

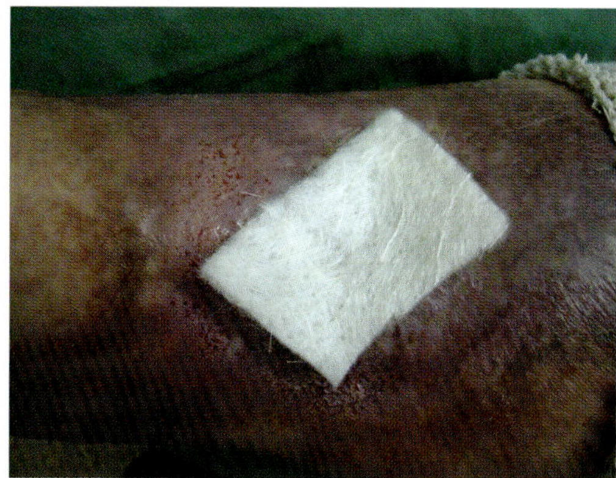

Fig. 8.4. Alginate dressing – sheet form

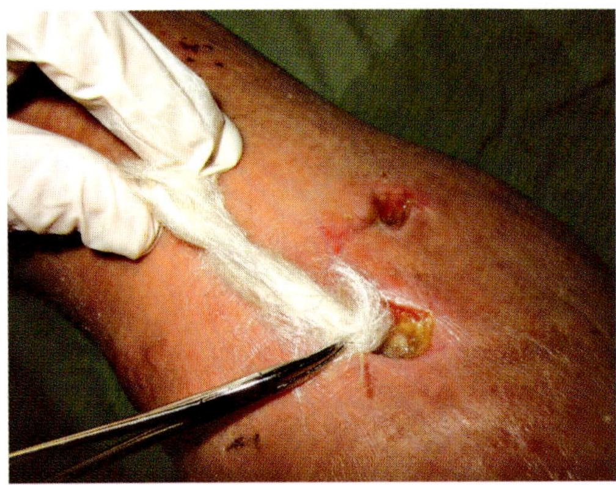

Fig. 8.5. Rope-form alginate dressing on an ulcer

and induction of a better wound environment) requires further investigation. Bowler et al. [45] documented *in vitro* the effect of calcium alginate dressings against pathogenic bacteria.

Examples of alginate dressings:
- Algiderm® – Bard Med. Division
- Algisite® – Smith & Nephew
- Carrasorb® – Carrington Lab
- Curasorb® – Kendall
- Cutinova alginate® – Beiersdorf-Jobst
- Fybron® – B. Braun Medical
- Hyperion® – Hyperion Medical
- Kalginate® – Deroyal
- Kaltostat® – Convatec
- Maxorb® – Medline Industries
- Melgisorb® – Molnlycke Health Care
- Nu-derm® – (alginate) – Johnson & Johnson
- Nutrastat® – Derma Sciences
- Orisorb® – Orion Medical Products
- Restore Calcicare® – Hollister
- Seasorb® – Coloplast
- Sorbalgon® – Hartmann
- Sorbsan® – Bertek Pharmaceuticals
- Tegagen alginate dressing® – 3M Health Care

8.5.3.2 Dextranomer Hydrophilic Granules

Dextranomer hydrophilic preparations contain microspheres, i.e., granules with a diameter of 0.1–0.3 mm in dry form, composed of the dextranomer hydrophilic polysaccharide. When the granules come into contact with fluid, they absorb water and swell until saturated. When placed on a secreting ulcer, the granules absorb exudate with subsequent swelling and formation of a gel-like mass [46]. Only water and small molecules (with molecular weights of less than 1000) are absorbed into the granules. Particles of molecular weight between 1000 and 5000 have limited penetration, while larger particles, such as bacteria or tiny pieces of necrotic tissue (molecular weight of more than 5000), remain in the interspaces between the granules (Fig. 8.6). The osmotic flow carries the larger particles and bacteria from the ulcer's surface into the layer of granules. When the ulcer surface is rinsed, the larger particles and bacteria tend to be swept away from the ulcer bed, between the swelling granules.

Sawyer et al. [47] conducted a randomized trial, using dextranomer granules for cutaneous ulcers of various etiologies. After three weeks of treatment, a 53.6% increase in epithelialized area was observed in 25 ulcers treated with dextranomer preparation, compared with a 19.8% increase in 25 ulcers treated with conventional therapy. In addition, a reduction of pus and debris in the ulcer beds in 21 of the 25 ulcers treated with dextranomer was reported, compared with only eight of the 25 ulcers in the control group.

Dextranomer hydrophilic granules have been found to be an efficient method of reducing exudate and removing debris from cutaneous ulcers [46–48] and thus can be regarded as another option for treating heavily secreting ulcers. A modification of the above method is based on similar hydrophilic microspheres containing active iodine in a concentration of 0.9% (Cadexomer-iodine). In addition to absorptive qualities similar to those of conventional dextranomer granules, the preparation is said to release iodine into the ulcer's environment and to provide some antiseptic effect. In most of the studies conducted, the use of cadex-

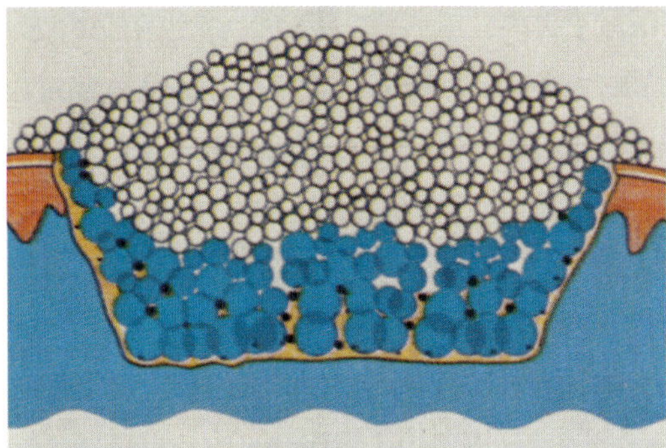

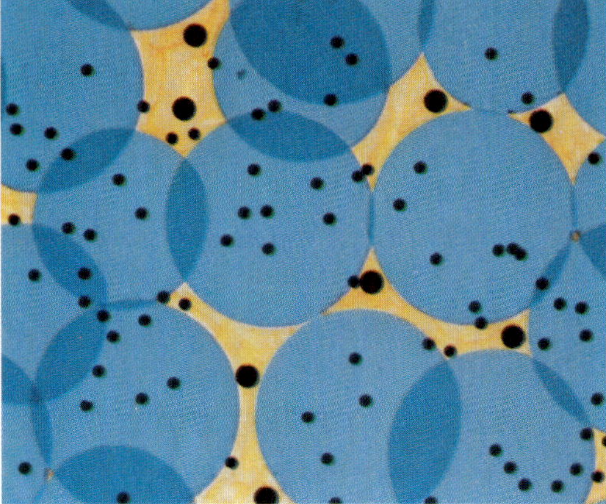

Fig. 8.6 a, b. Mode of action of dextranomer granules. **a.** Wound exudate is absorbed into dextranomer granules (*top*). **b.** (Magnification of Figure **a.**) Small molecules are absorbed into the granules; larger particles remain in the interspaces between the granules (*bottom*)

omer-iodine was associated with enhanced healing and efficient cleansing of the ulcers treated [49–52]. The current view considers advanced forms of iodine compounds such as Cadexomer-iodine as being effective in the treatment of chronic cutaneous ulcers [53].

Preparations containing hydrophilic granules are:
- Dextranomer granules: Debrisan® – Pharmacia & Upjohn
- Cadexomer-iodine granules: Iodosorb® – Smith & Nephew

8.5.3.3 Activated Charcoal Dressings

In these dressings, activated charcoal is bound to a semi-permeable membrane. These dressings protect the ulcer from external infection and trauma. The semi-permeable dressing is said to encourage the formation of a moist environment, optimal for enhanced wound healing.

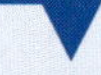

The two main unique features of activated charcoal are:
- It absorbs exudate and bacteria from the ulcer bed onto the dressing material. Thus, it may be regarded as a form of mechanical debridement. The absorptive effect of the activated charcoal has been proven by *in vitro* studies [54].
- Activated charcoal acts as a barrier that absorbs and filters the malodorous chemicals which evaporate and are released from the ulcer (similar to the way in which activated charcoal acts in air filters and gas masks). It has been used for several years in the management of suppurating malodorous ulcers and has been shown to reduce exudate and malodor from cutaneous ulcers [55–57].

Recently, dressings that combine activated charcoal and silver (0.15%) have been developed, i.e., silver-impregnated activated charcoal dressings (Fig. 8.7). The rationale behind this combination is to obtain, in addition to the absorptive effect, some degree of antibacterial effect. Silver has been shown to have some antibacterial effect [58–60] (see Chap. 11). These dressings have a beneficial effect on cutaneous ulcers infected by both gram-positive and -negative strains, including *Pseudomonas* and methicillin-resistant *Staphylococcus aureus* [61].

Wunderlich and Orfanos [62] conducted a controlled randomized study of 40 patients with venous leg ulcers. Silver-impregnated acti-

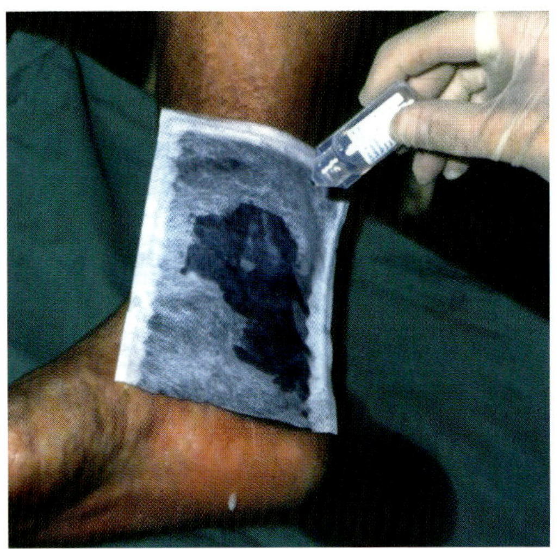

Fig. 8.7. A silver-impregnated activated-charcoal dressing

vated charcoal dressings were compared with various conventional therapies such as granulating ointments or zinc paste and were found to be superior to conventional therapy. Six of 19 patients (31.6%) treated with silver-impregnated activated charcoal dressings healed completely compared with only two of 19 (10.5%) treated with conventional therapy. While examining other parameters, such as the increase of epithelialization and the reduction of ulcer size, better results were obtained by using silver-charcoal dressings compared with other topical therapies.

In our clinical experience, silver-impregnated activated-charcoal dressings may definitely be considered as a therapeutic option. They should be used especially in ulcers from which resistant strains of bacteria are cultivated, such as *Pseudomonas* strains and methicillin-resistant *Staphylococcus aureus*.

Examples of dressings containing activated charcoal:
- Carboflex® – Convatec
- Carbonet® – Smith & Nephew
- Clinisorb® – Clinimed Ltd.
- Kaltocarb® – Convatec

Silver-impregnated activated charcoal dressings:
- Actisorb Plus® – Johnson & Johnson
- Actisorb Silver 220® – Johnson & Johnson

8.5.3.4 Other Absorptive/ Osmotic Methods

Other topical methods may be based, at least in part, on absorptive/osmotic activity. These include preparations such as sugars [63, 64] and honey [65–68]. Treatment with honey is described in Chap. 17.

8.6 Other Types of Dressings

8.6.1 Dressings Combining Two of the Above Groups

Certain dressings combine two or more of the above dressing materials in the manufacturing process, i.e., hydrogels with alginates, or hydrogels with hydrocolloids.

Examples of 'combined' products:
- Nu-gel® – (hydrogel and alginate) – Johnson & Johnson
- Granugel® – (hydrocolloid and hydrogel) – Convatec
- Carboflex odor control dressing® – (alginate, hydrocolloid, and charcoal) – Convatec

8.6.2 Interactive Dressings

The FDA defines interactive dressings as dressings that contain topical medications, such as antimicrobial preparations, growth factors, or other biological compounds. These medications may be integrated within highly permeable dressings. For the time being, the FDA has deferred classification of this group.

The issue of an antimicrobial effect in respect to dressing materials, regarding products such as cadexomer-iodine (Iodosorb®) and dressings that combine activated charcoal with silver (Actisorb®), has been discussed above. Other interactive dressings that contain silver are detailed in Chap. 11.

Other advanced dressing materials intended to enhance healing are described in Chap. 13.

8.6.3 Dressings with Unique Features

Several types of dressing materials have unique features that impart to these dressings a unique mode of action for certain types of cutaneous ulcers. For example, there is a multi-layered polyacrylate dressing with Ringer's lactate solution (Tenderwet®): The main component of a multi-layered dressing is polyacrylate, which functions as an absorbent core. The polyacrylate is enveloped within a layer of polypropylene-knitted fabric. The structure of the dressing enables frequent rinsing with Ringer's lactate solution every 12–24 h. The amount of Ringer's lactate used is dependent on the size of the ulcer, the dressing, and the quantity of secretions within the ulcer bed.

The polyacrylate absorbs secretions. It is also capable of retaining bacteria. Thus, wound exudate is replaced by Ringer's lactate solution [69]. The presence of Ringer's solution results in a moist environment that is essential for the wound repair process. In addition, a debriding effect can be achieved in that it softens and loosens sloughy material, leading to its detachment from the ulcer bed [70].

The absorbent core has a greater affinity for the protein compounds of wound exudate than for Ringer's lactate solution. Therefore, there is a continuous exchange of Ringer's solution (instead of ulcer secretions) onto the ulcer bed. This type of dressing may be recommended for ulcers with necrotic sloughy material on their surface.

There are also dressings that apply topical negative pressure. This mode of treatment may be regarded as a special type of dressing with unique features. However, since the active component here is a mechanical device, and not the foam, it is described in the addendum section of Chap. 20.

8.6.4 Biological Dressings

Biological dressings are those derived from living tissues or those containing ingredients originating from living tissues. These are discussed in Chap. 13.

8.7 Summary

A large variety of dressing materials are currently available (Fig. 8.8). Each type of cutaneous ulcer should be treated with the most appropriate dressing material. The ulcer's clinical appearance is the main parameter in determining the most suitable dressing.

Two main questions should be asked regarding any dressing material that is introduced to the market: (a) To which class of dressing does this product belong? and (b) For which types of cutaneous ulcers is the product intended? Knowing the answers for each type of dressing to be used is mandatory for better patient care.

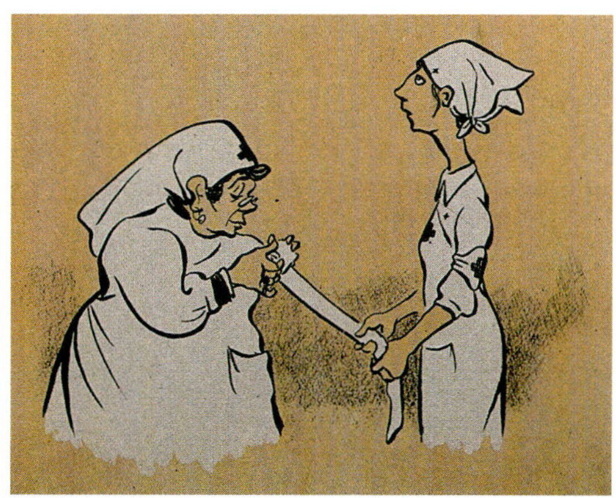

Fig. 8.8. Two nurses roll a bandage. (Taken from comical hospital scenes; color lithograph after L. Ibels, 1916, The Wellcome Library, London)

References

1. Winter GD: Formation of the scab and the rate of epithelization of superficial wounds in the skin of the young domestic pig. Nature 1962; 193:293–294
2. Hinman D, Maibach H: Effect of air exposure and occlusion on experimental human skin wounds. Nature 1963; 200:377–378
3. Phillips TJ, Dover JS: Leg Ulcers. J Am Acad Dermatol 1991; 25:965–987
4. Falanga V: Occlusive wound dressings: Why, when, which? Arch Dermatol 1988; 124:872–877
5. Thomas S, Banks V, Bale S, et al: A comparison of two dressings in the management of chronic wounds. J Wound Care 1997; 6:383–386
6. Rovee DT, Kurowsky CA, Labun J, et al: Effect of local wound environment on epidermal healing . In Maibach H, Rovee DT (eds) Epidermal Wound Healing. Chicago: Year Book Medical Publishers. 1972; pp 159–181
7. Barnett A, Berkowitz RL, Mills R, et al: Comparison of synthetic adhesive moisture vapor permeable and fine mesh gauze dressings for split-thickness skin graft donor sites. Am J Surg 1983; 145:379–381
8. Pickworth JJ, De Sousa N: Angiogenesis and macrophage response under the influence of Duoderm. In: Fibrinolysis and Angiogenesis in Wound Healing. Amsterdam: Excerpta Medica. 1988; pp 45–48
9. Madden MR, Finkelstein JL, Hefton JM, et al: Optimal healing of donor site wounds with hydrocolloid dressings. In: Ryan TJ (ed) An Environment for Healing: The Role of Occlusion. London: Royal Society of Medicine. 1985; pp 133–137
10. Cherry GW, Cherry CA, Jones RL, et al: Clinical experience with DuoDERM in various ulcers and clot resolution in experimental full thickness wounds. In: Cederholm-Williams SA, Ryan TJ, Lydon MJ (eds) Fibrinolysis and Angiogenisis in Wound Healing. Princeton: Excerpta Medica. 1988; pp 19–23
11. Cherry GW, Ryan T, McGibbon D: Trial of a new dressing in venous leg ulcers. Practitioner 1984; 228:1175–1178
12. Mumford JW, Mumford SP: Occlusive hydrocolloid dressings applied to chronic neuropathic ulcers. A study of efficacy in patients at a rural South Indian Hospital. Int J Dermatol 1988; 27:190–192
13. Choucair M, Phillips TJ: Wound dressings. In: Freedberg IM, Eisen AZ, Wolff K, Austen KF, Goldsmith LA, Katz SI, Fitzpatrick TB (eds) Fitzpatrick's Dermatology in General Medicine, 5th edn. New York: McGraw-Hill. 1999; pp 2954–2958
14. Thomas S, Banks V, Fear M, et al: A study to compare two film dressings used as secondary dressings. J Wound Care 1997; 6:333–336
15. Field CK, Kerstein MD: Overview of wound healing in a moist environment. Am J Surg 1994; 167 [Suppl]: 2S–6S
16. Lawrence JC, Lilly HA: Are hydrocolloid dressings bacteria proof? Pharmaceutical J 1987; 239:184
17. Mendez MV, Raffetto JD, Phillips T, et al: The proliferative capacity of neonatal skin fibroblasts is reduced after exposure to venous ulcer wound fluid: A potential mechanism for senescence in venous ulcers. J Vasc Surg 1999; 30:734–743
18. Bucalo B, Eaglstein WH, Falanga V: Inhibition of cellular proliferation by chronic wound fluid. Wound Rep Reg 1993; 1:181–186
19. O'Toole EA, Marinkovich MP, Peavey CL, et al: Hypoxia increases human keratinocyte motility on connective tissue. J Clin Invest 1997; 100:2881–2891
20. Varghese MC, Balin AK, Carter DM, et al: Local environment of chronic wounds under synthetic dressings. Arch Dermatol 1986; 122:52–57
21. Hunt TK, Pai MP: The effect of varying ambient oxygen tensions on wound metabolism and collagen synthesis. Surg Gynecol Obstet 1972; 135:561–567
22. Xia YP, Zhao Y, Tyrone JW, et al: Differential activation of migration by hypoxia in keratinocytes isolated from donors of increasing age: Implication for chronic wounds in the elderly. J Invest Dermatol 2001; 116:50–56
23. Gilchrist B, Reed C: The bacteriology of chronic venous ulcers treated with occlusive hydrocolloid dressings. Br J Dermatol 1989; 121:337–344
24. Findlay D: Modern dressings: what to use. Austral Fam Physician 1994; 23:824–839
25. Hermans MH, Hermans RP: Duoderm, an alternative dressing for smaller burns. Burns Incl Therm Inj 1986; 12:214–219
26. Turner TD: The development of wound management products. In: Krasner DL, Rodeheaver GT, Sibbald RG (eds) Chronic Wound Care, 3rd edn. Wayne PA: HMP Communications. 2001; pp 293–310
27. Friedman SJ, Su WP: Management of leg ulcers with hydrocolloid occlusive dressing. Arch Dermatol 1984; 120:1329–1336
28. Browne A, Dow G, Sibbald G: Infected wounds: definitions and controversies. In: Falanga V (ed) Cutaneous Wound Healing. London: Martin Dunitz. 2001; pp 203–219
29. Parish LC, Witkowski JA: The infected decubitus ulcer. Int J Dermatol 1989; 28:643–647
30. Niedner R, Schopf E: Wound infections and antibacterial therapy. In: Westerhof W (ed) Leg Ulcers: Diagnosis and Treatment. Amsterdam: Elsevier. 1993; pp 293–303
31. Lipsky BA, Berendt AR: Principles and practice of antibiotic therapy of diabetic foot infections. Diabet Metab Res Rev 2000; 16 [Suppl 1]: S42–S46
32. Robson MC: Wound Infection: a failure of wound healing caused by an imbalance of bacteria. Surg Clin North Am 1997; 77:637–650
33. Cutting KF, Harding KG: Criteria to identify wound infection. J Wound Care 1994; 3:198–201
34. Limova M, Troyer-Caudle J: Controlled, randomized clinical trial of two hydrocolloid dressings in the management of venous insufficiency ulcers. J Vasc Nurs 2002; 20:22–34

35. Ovington LG: Wound dressings: their evolution and use. In: Falanga V (ed) Cutaneous Wound Healing,1st edn. London: Martin Dunitz. 2001; pp 221–232

36. Bale S, Banks V, Haglestein S, et al: A comparison of two amorphous hydrogels in the debridement of pressure sores. J Wound Care 1998; 7:65–68

37. Williams C: The role of Sterigel hydrogel wound dressing in wound debridement. Br J Nurs 1997; 6:494–496

38. Bale S, Harding KG: Using modern dressings to effect debridement. Prof Nurse 1990; 5:244–245

39. Williams C: Intrasite Gel: a hydrogel dressing. Br J Nurs 1994; 3:843–846

40. Flanagan M: The efficacy of a hydrogel in the treatment of wounds with non-viable tissue. A report of a multicentre clinical trial that assessed the efficacy of a hydrogel in wound debridement. J Wound Care 1995; 4:264–267

41. Smith J: Debridement of diabetic foot ulcers (Cochrane Review). In: The Cochrane Library, Issue 1, 2003. Oxford: Update Software

42. Gilchrist T, Martin AM: Wound treatment with Sorbsan – an alginate fibre dressing. Biomaterials 1983; 4:317–320

43. Motta GJ: Calcium alginate topical wound dressings: a new dimension in the cost-effective treatment for exudating dermal wounds and pressure sores. Ostomy Wound Manage 1989; 25:52–56

44. Sayag J, Meaume S, Bohbot S: Healing properties of calcium alginate dressings. J Wound Care 1996; 5:357–362

45. Bowler PG, Jones SA, Davies BJ, et al: Infection control properties of some wound dressings. J Wound Care 1999; 8:499–502

46. Jacobsson S, Rothman U, Arturson G, et al: A new principle for the cleansing of infected wounds. Scand J Plast Reconstr Surg 1976; 10:65–72

47. Sawyer PN, Dowbak G, Sophie Z, et al: A preliminary report of the efficacy of Debrisan (dextranomer) in the debridement of cutaneous ulcers. Surgery 1979; 85:201–204

48. Ljungberg S: Comparison of dextranomer paste and saline dressings for management of decubital ulcers. Clin Ther 1998; 20:737–743

49. Skog E, Arnesjo B, Troeng T, et al: A randomized trial comparing cadexomer iodine and standard treatment in the out-patient management of chronic venous ulcers. Br J Dermatol 1983; 109:77–83

50. Hansson C: The effects of cadexomer iodine paste in the treatment of venous leg ulcers compared with hydrocolloid dressing and paraffin gauze dressing. Cadexomer Iodine Study Group. Int J Dermatol 1998; 37:390–396

51. Danielsen L, Cherry GW, Harding K, et al: Cadexomer iodine in ulcers colonised by Pseudomonas aeruginosa. J Wound Care 1997; 6:169–172

52. Hillstrom L: Iodosorb compared to standard treatment in chronic venous leg ulcers – a multicenter study. Acta Chir Scand Suppl 1988; 544:53–56

53. Kirsner RS, Martin LK, Drosou A: Wound microbiology and the use of antibacterial agents. In: Rovee DT, Maibach HI (eds) The Epidermis in Wound Healing. Boca Raton: CRC Press. 2004; pp 155–182

54. Frost MR, Jackson SW, Stevens PJ: Adsorption of bacteria onto activated charcoal cloth: an effect of potential importance in the treatment of infected wounds Microbios Letts 1980; 13:135–140

55. Butcher G, Butcher JA, Maggs FA: The treatment of malodorous wounds. Nurs Mirror Midwives 1976; 142:64

56. Beckett R, Coombs TJ, Frost MR, et al: Charcoal cloth and malodorous wounds. Lancet 1980; 2:594

57. Mulligan CM, Bragg AJ, O'Toole OB: A controlled comparative trial of Actisorb activated charcoal cloth dressings in the community. Br J Clin Pract 1986; 40:145–148

58. Deitch EA, Marino AA, Gillespie TE, et al: Silver nylon: a new antimicrobial agent. Antimicrob Agents Chemother 1983; 23:356–359

59. Tsai WC, Chu CC, Chiu SS, et al: *In vitro* quantitative study of newly made antibacterial braided nylon sutures. Surg Gynecol Obstet 1987; 165:207–211

60. Falcone AE, Spadaro JA: Inhibitory effects of electrically activated silver material on cutaneous wound bacteria. Plast Reconstr Surg 1986; 77:455–459

61. Furr JR, Russell AD, Turner TD, et al: Antibacterial activity of Actisorb Plus, Actisorb and silver nitrate. J Hosp Infect 1994; 27:201–208

62. Wunderlich U, Orfanos CE: Treatment of venous ulcera cruris with dry wound dressings. Phase overlapping use of silver impregnated activated charcoal xerodressing. Hautarzt 1991; 42:446–450

63. Thomlinson RH: Kitchen remedy for necrotic malignant breast ulcers. Lancet 1980; 2:707

64. Chirife J, Scarmato G, Herszage L: Scientific basis for the use of granulated sugar in treatment of infected wounds. Lancet 1982; 1:560–561

65. Cooper RA, Molan PC, Harding KG: Antibacterial activity of honey against strains of Staphylococcus aureus from infected wounds. J R Soc Med 1999; 92:283–285

66. Efem SE: Clinical observations on the wound healing properties of honey. Br J Surg 1988; 75:679–681

67. Zumla A, Lulat A: Honey – a remedy rediscovered. J R Soc Med 1989; 82:384–385

68. Molan PC: Potential of honey in the treatment of wounds and burns. Am J Clin Dermatol 2001; 2:13–19

69. Mahr R: The mode of action of a superabsorbent polymer wound dressing (Tenderwet). Ostomy Wound Manage 2003; 49:8–9

70. Paustian C: Debridement rates with activated polyacrylate dressings (Tenderwet). Ostomy Wound Manage 2003; 49:13–14

Debridement

9

From the stump of the arm,

the amputated hand,

I undo the clotted lint, remove the

slough, wash the matter and blood,

Back on his pillow the soldier

bends with curv'd neck and side

failing head,

His eyes are closed, his face is pale,

he dares not look on the bloody

stump,

And has not yet look'd on it.

(The Wound Dresser, Leaves of Grass,
Walt Whitman)

Contents

9.1 Definition of Debridement

The term 'debridement' was first coined by Desault (1744–1795), in Paris, referring to the surgical removal of necrotic material from open wounds [1]. Since then, this term has taken on a much broader meaning, and other forms of debridement have been developed, as presented below.

Debridement is defined in *Dorland's Medical Dictionary* as "the removal of foreign material and devitalized or contaminated tissue from or adjacent to a traumatized or infected lesion, until surrounding [and underlying, in the case of a cutaneous ulcer] healthy tissue is exposed." Choosing the appropriate method of debridement and employing it correctly may have a significant effect on the healing process.

Debridement can be a lengthy process. Occasionally, one must change the method of debridement during the treatment of an ulcer. This chapter reviews the various types of devitalized tissues and current methods of debridement.

9.2 Appearance of Necrotic Material on an Ulcer's surface

Necrotic material on the surface of an ulcer usually appears in one of two major forms: slough, and eschar or crust. Slough may be yellow, green, or gray/white (Fig. 9.1). It is usually soft, ranging from a liquefied mass to semi-solid or relatively solid material; it is composed of necrotic proteins, devitalized collagen, and fibrin.

Necrotic material may dry, desiccate, and harden to form **eschar**, which is brown or black (Fig. 9.2). The term 'eschar' was originally used

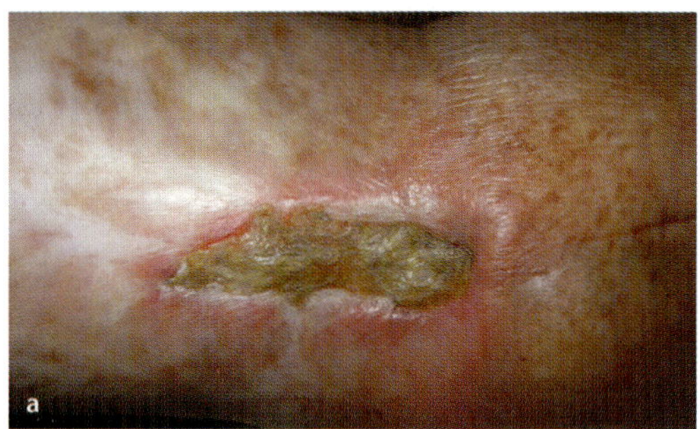

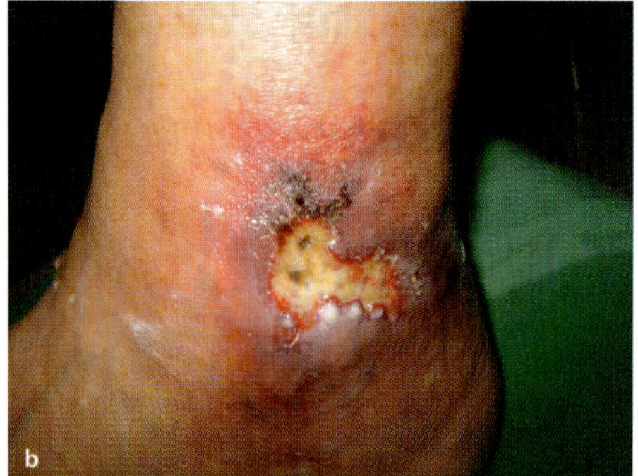

Fig. 9.1a, b. Sloughy ulcers

In this chapter we discuss the various techniques for removing eschar and slough. Treatment of secretions is detailed in Chap. 20. The discussion on absorptive dressings (which are actually a form of mechanical debridement) intended for secreting ulcers can be found in Chap. 8.

Sometimes, the surface of a cutaneous ulcer may present a combination of two or more of the above forms of necrotic material, and the appropriate debridement measures should be considered accordingly.

9.3 Why Should Ulcers Be Debrided?

The observation that wounds and chronic cutaneous ulcers improve following appropriate debridement therapy has been made for centu-

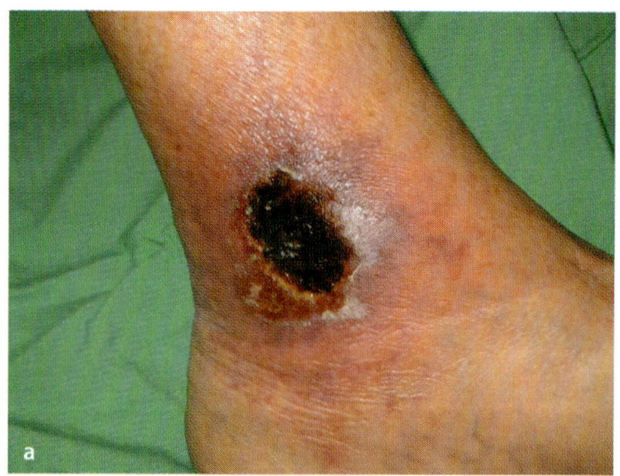

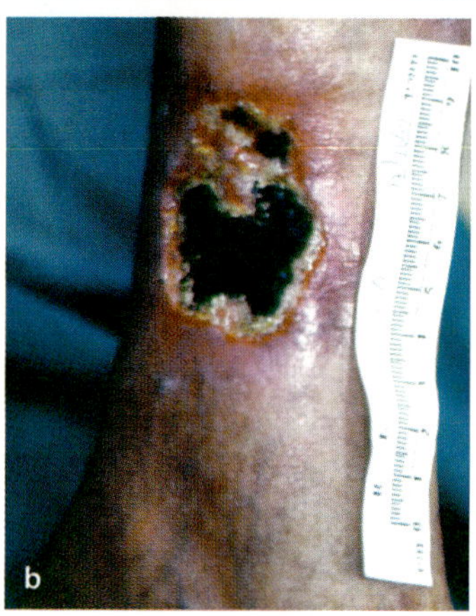

Fig. 9.2a, b. Ulcers covered by black eschar

to describe the devitalized tissue that appears in burns [2]. Eschar consists of devitalized proteins and collagen from burnt tissue, with cellular debris and solidified secretions. This term has since been applied to the field of cutaneous ulcers, indicating the presence of dry necrotic tissue within an ulcer bed.

Secretions that have dried out on an ulcer bed may form a crust. Although it does not contain dead tissue, a **crust** that is thick and black may resemble eschar, and it may require similar techniques of debridement for its removal.

Purulent or seropurulent discharge is composed of the debris of dead cells and liquefied tissue (Fig. 9.3). It may indicate the presence of infective bacteria within the ulcer bed. Therefore, according to the dictionary definition of debridement, its removal may be regarded as a form of a debriding procedure. However, the currently accepted concept of debridement relates to the removal of slough and eschar only.

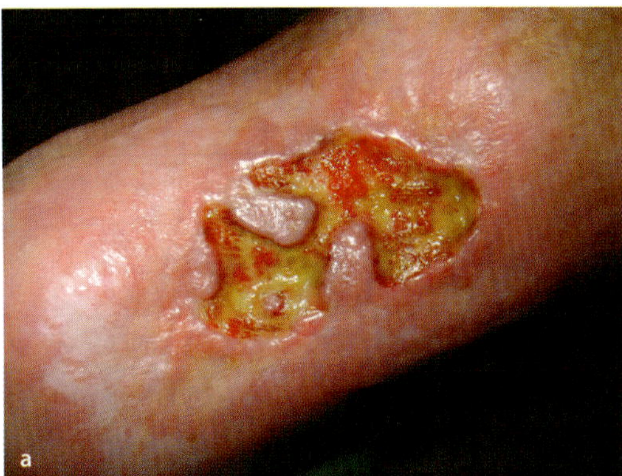

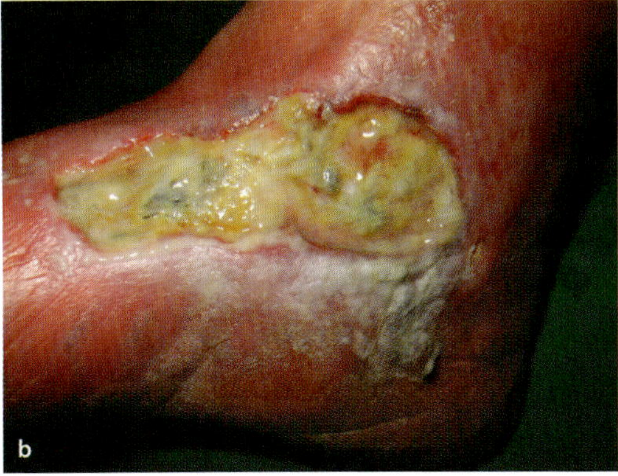

Fig. 9.3a, b. Ulcers with purulent discharge

ries. Nevertheless, it is worth clarifying here how debridement contributes to improved wound repair.

The presence of necrotic material on an ulcer bed enhances bacterial colonization and may lead to infection [3, 4, 5]. Necrotic material may induce activation of the alternative pathway of the complement system [6]. This may result in ongoing inflammation, destruction of surrounding healthy tissue, and delay of the wound healing process.

Foreign matter within a cutaneous ulcer, acting as a physical barrier, prevents the normal course of wound contraction and interferes with epithelialization [3, 5]. The presence of a dry crust or eschar on an ulcer bed results in slower epithelialization, compared with a faster healing rate within a moist wound environment [7].

In addition, a specific type of surgical debriding procedure is recommended prior to skin grafting and several advanced healing modalities, such as keratinocyte transplantation, grafting 'living' skin substitutes or topical application of growth factors [8–12]. This kind of debridement should extend (very superficially) to viable healthy tissue until a minor degree of bleeding (pinpoint bleeding) is achieved, and vital granulating tissue is exposed. This can be done by shaving the superficial upper (healthy) layer of an ulcer bed.

This procedure should be done with the following objectives:

- Removal of a fibrin layer: A layer of fibrin (which may be thin and, in some cases, almost invisible) may coat the ulcer bed, acting as a physical barrier that impedes penetration of growth factors and prevents the attachment of a skin graft or transplanted keratinocytes. Removal of this layer by shaving results in a cleaner surface area.
- Achieving a better vascular bed: Shaving results in an ulcer bed which is more vascular, thus producing a better substrate for advanced treatment modalities.
- Removal of senescent cells: Senescent cells, whose ability to produce cytokines and to proliferate is reduced, are present in chronic cutaneous ulcers [13–15]. Removal of senescent cells from the ulcer's margin and its surface may improve wound repair [8].

9.4 Methods of Debridement

Debridement can be achieved by several methods, as summarized in Table 9.1: Surgical debridement, several types of mechanical debridement (or variants of mechanical debridement), chemical/enzymatic debridement, and autolytic debridement. Maggot debridement therapy can also be considered under certain conditions, as described below.

Table 9.1. Methods of debridement

Type of debridement	Purpose	Comments
Surgical	For solid or semi-solid necrotic material that can be handled effectively with a scalpel or forceps	Contraindicated when bleeding disorders are suspected. Contraindicated in pyoderma gangrenosum
Mechanical		
Hydrodebridement and 'wet to moist' dressing	To soften slough or dry necrotic tissue	Avoid prolonged soaking
Repeated saline irrigation (enabling the ulcer to dry out)	To remove purulent or seropurulent secretions with liquefying slough	Irrigation should be done gently
'Wet-to-dry' dressing	Necrotic tissue with exudate	Healthy tissues may be damaged
Scrubbing	To remove necrotic tissue	Should be avoided
Absorptive		
Dextranomer granules	Secreting ulcers	
Activated charcoal	Secreting ulcers	Beneficial effect against *Pseudomonas* strains and methicillin resistant *Staph. aureus*
Chemical		
Enzymatic	Ulcers with slough	
Mild acidic preparations	Ulcers with slough	
Autolytic	Ulcers with slough	Hydrogel dressings are used to induce autolytic debridement
Maggot therapy	Ulcers with slough (with/without purulent secretions)	

9.4.1 Surgical Debridement

Surgical instruments such as a scalpel or scissors are used to cut away and remove necrotic tissue. Forceps should be used to grasp necrotic tissue while it is being cut and to remove it from the ulcer.

Surgical debridement is usually done to remove firm, black necrotic material. Note that it may be possible to use this procedure on yellow/gray slough, provided the slough is relatively solid. Soft, liquefying material cannot be handled efficiently by a surgical knife or forceps. Moreover, when liquefying material covers the ulcer bed it becomes difficult to distin-

guish between necrotic and vital tissues. When a definite demarcation between viable and necrotic tissue cannot be identified clearly, other debridement methods should be used. Sometimes a piece of tissue that seems to be pale and slough-like may recover following appropriate treatment (such as topical growth factors or antibiotic treatment). In this case, hasty surgical procedures may result in the unnecessary loss of potentially healthy and vital tissue.

Some make a distinction between two methods of surgical debridement [16]: 'Surgical debridement' refers to a major procedure that requires an operating room and is done under general or regional anesthesia. 'Sharp debridement' is usually regarded as a minor form of surgical debridement, which can be handled in a clinic, and for which topical anesthesia suffices (see below). These definitions are not always accepted in the literature, and the term 'surgical debridement' may refer to either of the above. Here, we shall refer to 'surgical debridement' as any type of debriding procedure where surgical instruments are used to cut away and remove devitalized tissue.

9.4.1.1 Guidelines to Follow Regarding Surgical Debridement

■ **Avoid Spreading Infection.** Adhere strictly to sterile conditions before, during, and after the procedure. It is of the utmost importance to prevent the spread of bacteria to the surroundings, thereby exposing other patients to infection. Thorough cleansing is required: The ulcer should be rinsed with antiseptics (e.g., povidone-iodine solution) and then with saline solution before and following the procedure.

■ **Provide Optimal Conditions.** To ensure optimal conditions for the procedure, the patient should be lying down, while the physician is seated nearby as comfortably as possible. Good lighting is essential.

■ **Debridement in the Operating Room.** It is generally accepted that in the following cases surgical debridement should be done in an operating room [2]:

> – For patients suffering from extremely painful ulcers
> – When bone needs to be removed
> – In cases where the necrotic tissue is adjacent to a vital organ
> – In cases where it is difficult to assess the extent of the required procedure

■ **Topical Anesthetics.** A more superficial procedure that does not require an operating room is better tolerated if the ulcer is treated previously with topical anesthetics such as a mixture of lidocaine and prilocaine (EMLA®) [17, 18].

■ **Contraindications to Surgical Debridement.** Surgical debridement should be avoided in cases where (a) patients are taking anticoagulants; (b) patients have thrombocytopenia; and (c) pyoderma gangrenosum or other conditions associated with pathergy are present.

The term 'pathergy', in the context of debridement of cutaneous ulcers, refers to the formation of a new lesion or aggravation of existing lesions following minor and trivial trauma. In some patients with pathergy, venepuncture may be followed by pustulation. The classical condition known to be aggravated following surgical debridement is pyoderma gangrenosum (PG) [19–22]. Therefore, debridement of a lesion suspected of being PG is contraindicated. Other diseases associated with pathergy are Behçet's disease, Sweet's syndrome, and Wegener's granulomatosis [23–26]. If pathergy is suspected, avoid surgical debridement.

Note: Identification of pathergy, apart from the clinical impression of the worsening of ulcers following debridement, is made by the 'pathergy test'. This is performed by pricking the skin with a sterile needle, or by injecting 0.1 ml of saline into the skin. A positive test is indicated by the appearance of a pustule within 24 h [27].

■ **Avoid Damaging Healthy Tissue.** While debriding wounds, be cautious and ensure that only necrotic tissue is removed. When nearing vital tissue, the procedure should be discontinued and further debridement may be accomplished by using an alternative method. Exposed nerves, tendons, and blood vessels should be identified and left intact. Obviously, any damage to newly forming epithelium appearing on the ulcer bed must be avoided.

> In spite of precautions taken, vital, healthy tissues may be injured in the course of surgical debridement. Injury to healthy tissues may result in:

— Bacteremia: Transient bacteremia with leukocytosis and fever may occur. It has been shown that in 50% of patients with pressure ulcers, surgical debridement was followed by bacteremia [28].

— Injured nerves: If the patient complains of pain during the procedure, it is an indication that healthy tissue is involved and one should discontinue debridement in that area.

— Injured blood vessels: While surgically debriding a cutaneous ulcer containing necrotic and foreign material, injury to blood vessels should be avoided as much as possible. Bleeding may indicate that vital tissue is being damaged. In addition, penetration of infective material into injured blood vessels may induce bacteremia. If surgical debridement cannot be carried out without bleeding, alternative methods of debridement should be used.

■ **Debridement and Bleeding.** As mentioned in Sect. 9.3, when dealing with relatively clean cutaneous ulcers, debridement should be carried out as a preparatory stage, prior to advanced therapeutic modalities such as keratinocyte transplantation, skin grafting, or the application of growth factors. The purpose is not just to remove devitalized material, but also to create an optimal vascular substrate for advanced treatment modalities [8, 10–12]. Therefore, debridement should extend (very superficially) to viable healthy tissue until a minor degree of bleeding (pinpoint bleeding) is achieved. Particular care must be taken not to damage or remove newly forming epithelium. This may occur especially when debridement is performed inappropriately following keratinocyte grafting or the application of growth factors.

9.4.1.2 Research Studies of Surgical Debridement

In a multicenter, randomized, double-blind study, Steed et al. [8] showed that topical recombinant human platelet-derived growth factor (rhPDGF) was superior to placebo in the management of 118 patients with diabetic foot ulcers. However, a significant observation of this study was associated with the frequency of debridement procedures in these patients: Improved healing was associated with a higher frequency of debridement, independent of treatment group. The highest degree of healing occurred in patients where the use of topical growth factors was combined with frequent debridement.

Schmeller et al. [29] used surgical debridement in the form of shave therapy in 80 patients with 105 chronic leg ulcers. A Schink dermatome was used to remove the ulcer surface and the surrounding lipodermatosclerosis in successive horizontal flat layers, until a pulsating bleeding pattern was achieved, indicating the presence of tissue with better microcirculation. This procedure was followed by covering the wounds with meshed split-skin grafts. Schmeller et al. documented short-term healing rates (3 months follow-up) of 79% for 59 patients with 76 ulcers. For 18 patients with 26 ulcers, for whom the follow-up was longer (more than 20 months), a healing rate of 88% was reported.

9.4.1.3 The Appropriate Technique of Surgical Debridement Prior to Advanced Modalities

Shaving the superficial upper layer of the ulcer bed may be performed with a scalpel, or with a fine curette (Figs. 9.4, 9.5). The shape of a curette makes it suitable for accurate outlining of the ulcer margin, so it is used to remove layers near the margin. Debridement of the ulcer margin is extremely important, since marginal, peripheral epithelialization can be stimulated by this procedure. As mentioned above, particular care should be taken not to damage or remove newly forming epithelium.

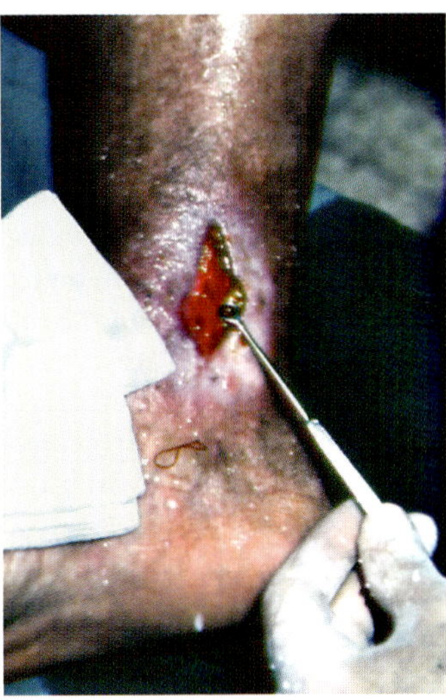

Fig. 9.4. Shaving the superficial layer of a cutaneous ulcer with a fine curette prior to application of a preparation containing growth factors

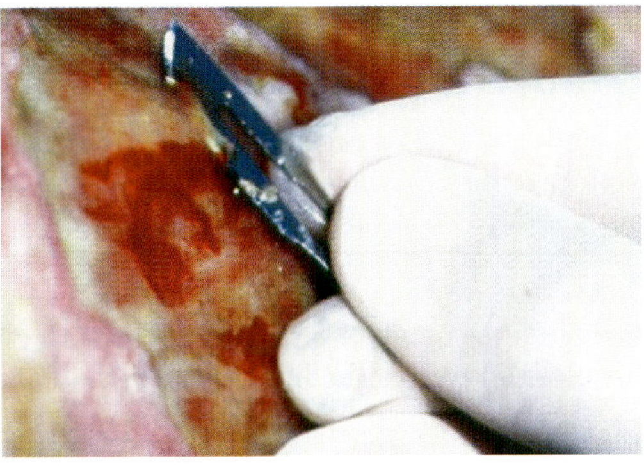

Fig. 9.5. Debridement performed with a scalpel

9.4.2 Mechanical Debridement

Subtypes of mechanical debridement are: hydrodebridement, 'wet-to-moist' dressings, 'wet-to-dry' dressings, irrigation with saline, and mechanical scrubbing.

9.4.2.1 Hydrodebridement

Soaking the ulcer in a bath of water may soften and loosen slough or dry necrotic tissue, there-

by easing its separation from the ulcer bed. In addition, bacteria and residues of topical preparations are washed away [3, 30].

> The procedure may be combined with:
> — Topical preparations such as Burow's solution, or diluted solutions of potassium permanganate or chlorine [31], which achieve a certain antibacterial effect (see Chap. 11).
> — Whirlpool for removal of loose necrotic debris [16].

> While using hydrodebridement avoid:
> — Prolonged soaking, which may result in maceration and damage to healthy tissue. The duration of this procedure should not exceed 15 min each time.
> — Aggressive whirlpooling: Overly aggressive water agitation may mechanically damage granulation tissue and the newly forming epithelium.
> — Spreading infection: The equipment used should be thoroughly cleansed with an antiseptic preparation.

9.4.2.2 'Wet-to-Moist' Technique

An effect similar to that of soaking may be obtained by covering the ulcer with layers of cloth or gauze saturated with fluid (e.g., saline), with repeated wetting. In the 'wet-to-moist' dressing technique, the ulcer is *not* supposed to dry out.

The 'wet-to-moist' technique is aimed at keeping ulcers moist. Similar to the hydrodebridement method, the water may soften and loosen slough or dry necrotic tissue. The efficacy of this technique as a debridement method depends on the frequency of wetting and the amount of fluid used.

'Wet-to-moist' dressings may be used on leg ulcers, when one prefers to avoid soaking of certain body regions, such as the foot. Unnecessary immersion of the feet may lead to maceration, which is not desirable, especially for diabetic patients.

A special form of dressing consisting of a multilayered polyacrylate dressing with Ringer's lactate solution may be regarded as a modification of the 'wet-to-moist' technique. The presence of Ringer's lactate creates a moist environment, with softening and loosening of slough. This type of dressing is discussed in detail in Chap. 8.

There is a clear distinction between soaking the ulcer region in water, as described above, and repeated washing or the repeated placing of a single-layered damp cloth on the ulcer, enabling the ulcer to dry out. Soaking or covering the ulcer with saturated cloth, preventing the ulcer from drying out, results in a debriding effect, as described above. It is intended to soften and loosen slough or dry necrotic tissue.

In contrast to soaking, repeated wetting achieves the opposite effect, as described below. When the added water (either by washing or repeatedly applying a damp cloth or a damp gauze) evaporates, the treated area gradually dries out. This is intended for secreting ulcers. Repeated wetting is *not* considered to be a debridement technique – it is just a cleansing method that can also be used for drying out any other types of inflamed, secreting areas of the skin. This mode of treatment is also discussed in Chap. 20.

A modification of the latter method is repeated wetting when the gauze is left to dry, so as to adhere to the ulcer bed, as in the 'wet-to-dry' technique described below.

9.4.2.3 'Wet-to-Dry' Technique

The 'wet-to-dry' technique is a modification of the 'repeated wetting' technique, in which the gauze dressing is left to adhere to the ulcer surface. It is a useful method in cases where necrotic tissue is accompanied by relatively moderate amounts of exudate. In this procedure, a gauze dressing is applied to the ulcer, onto the

necrotic material. It is moistened with saline and left to dry. After a few hours, when the gauze is dry and adherent to the ulcer bed, it is pulled firmly, with the necrotic tissue attached to the gauze. This procedure may be repeated several times a day. The main disadvantage of this debridement method is that, being non-selective, newly regenerated epithelium and healthy granulation tissue are removed from the ulcer bed together with necrotic material. In view of this, a 'wet-to-dry' dressing is generally not favored as a debridement procedure.

9.4.2.4 Irrigation with Saline

Frequent irrigation with saline is an excellent method for removing seropurulent or purulent secretions and liquefied slough. Nevertheless, it will not remove relatively solid slough or black necrotic eschar firmly attached to the ulcer bed. Note that forceful, high-pressure irrigation may damage healthy tissue. Therefore, wound irrigation should be done as gently as possible. The procedure can be performed once or twice daily, while the wound dressing is being changed, with the aim of removing remnants of topical preparations previously used on the ulcer.

A basin, or nylon sheets, should be placed under the area to be treated, to collect the irrigating fluid and avoid spreading bacteria from the ulcer to the surrounding environment.

9.4.2.5 Mechanical Scrubbing

Removal of necrotic tissue by scrubbing has an adverse effect similar to that of the 'wet-to-dry' technique and may cause damage to regenerating epithelium and granulation tissue. It should therefore be avoided.

9.4.3 A Variant of Mechanical Debridement: Absorptive Debridement

The mechanical effect of absorption may be regarded as an additional method of debridement. Such procedures use the absorptive qualities of hydrophilic dextranomer granules or activated charcoal for removal of tiny pieces of necrotic material and bacteria from the ulcer bed. These preparations, intended for secreting ulcers, are described in Chap. 8.

Other topical methods of debridement may be based, at least in part, on absorptive/osmotic activity. These include preparations such as sugars [32, 33], honey [34–37], and alginates. Treatment with honey is described in Chap. 19. Alginates are discussed in Chap. 8.

9.4.4 Chemical Debridement

Chemical debridement mainly involves the use of lytic enzymes, whose purpose it is to dissolve the necrotic material. In addition, cutaneous ulcers can to some extent also be debrided by using mild acidic preparations.

9.4.4.1 Enzymatic Debridement

There are commercial enzymatic preparations directed specifically towards certain substances contained in necrotic tissue such as fibrin, collagen, or various other proteins. In order not to damage healthy tissue, enzymatic debridement is used for an ulcer whose entire surface is covered by necrotic material. In addition, there is a basic assumption with this approach (requiring further investigation) that vital cells are capable of producing inhibitors against these enzymatic preparations and remain intact, while necrotic tissue is being dissolved.

Enzymes for chemical debridement are classified as proteolytics, fibrinolytics, or collagenases.

The approach recommended in several articles [16, 38–42] is to vary the type of enzyme being used, depending on the appearance of the necrotic tissue seen on the ulcer surface:
- Thin superficial necrotic tissue is probably composed mainly of fibrin and necrotic proteins which tend to be located more superficially than devitalized collagen [16, 38]. If chemical debridement is chosen, fibrinolytics and proteolytic enzymes should be used. Hence, ulcers with fibrinous exudates may be effectively treated with fibrinolytic enzymes.
- Thick necrotic tissue is probably composed mainly of devitalized, necrotic collagen. This layer of collagen adherent to the base of the ulcer may appear as black eschar or may be yellowish in its moistened state. In both cases, the upper layer contains fibrin and necrotic proteins. In this situation, some suggest the initial use of fibrinolytic and proteolytic enzymes. Collagenases may be used following the dissolution and removal of the upper layer [16, 40, 41].
- Purulent discharge is thought to contain large amounts of DNA/RNA degradation products [42]. Another group of debriding enzymes worthy of mention includes DNA/RNA-dissolving agents. Preparations such as bovine pancreatic deoxyribonuclease or streptodornase are able to degrade DNA and RNA, thereby reducing the viscosity of purulent secretions and making them easier to remove from the ulcer bed [43, 44].

However, the distinction presented above is not clear-cut. There are no definite data in the literature regarding the preferred enzymatic preparation for any particular type of necrotic material. Moreover, for the time being, there is insufficient evidence to recommend the use of enzymatic preparations for debriding ulcers, and their use is still controversial. More randomized controlled studies are required regarding specific preparations. In many of these studies, basic information regarding the appearance of the ulcer bed prior to enzymatic therapy is not provided. In other studies, as indicated previously [45], the effectiveness of certain enzymatic preparations was assessed by using inappropriate parameters (i.e., achieving complete healing), instead of merely measuring their debriding effect. One may expect that in the coming years more selective and more efficient preparations will be developed.

9.4.4.1.1
Guidelines for Using Enzymatic Preparations

Eschar-like, hard, necrotic tissue has to be cross-hatched or incised prior to the chemical/enzymatic treatment [38, 46]. Intact skin around the ulcer should be protected by the application of substances such as zinc-oxide paste. To minimize chemical irritation and damage to healthy granulation tissue, enzymatic debridement should not be used in cases where necrotic material covers only part of the ulcer surface, with some of the surface clean and red.

9.4.4.1.2
Enzymatic Preparations Documented in the Literature

Collagenase is derived from *Clostridium histolyticum* [46, 47]. However, collagenases may be produced from other sources such as the hepatopancreas of the king crab (*Paralithodes camtschatica*) [48]. Collagenases degrade both denatured and undenatured collagen. They are also thought to dissolve strands of undenatured collagen that have been shown to anchor necrotic debris to the base of the ulcer, resulting in a more efficient debridement [3, 40, 41].

Fibrinolysin is derived from bovine plasmin. In commercial preparations it is combined with bovine pancreatic deoxyribonuclease. Fibrinolysin is thought to break down fibrin in necrotic material, while deoxyribonuclease is thought to degrade DNA residues of necrotic cells [49, 50]. The effectiveness of an ointment consisting of fibrinolysin and deoxyribonuclease (Elase®) was evaluated in a double-blind randomized study, published in 1998 [50]. No long-term clinical benefit was demonstrated in reducing purulent exudates or necrotic tissue.

A streptokinase/streptodornase preparation, produced from Streptococcus A is another type of enzymatic product [43].

Sutilains are derived from *Bacillus subtilis*. Their use is documented in the management of amputation-stump wounds and in burns, but their use in chronic cutaneous ulcers has not been documented [51–53].

Papain is derived from the fruit *Carica papaya*. A commonly used formulation is the papain-urea combination [54–56]. Papain is used to break down cysteine residues, while urea, by affecting the three-dimensional structure of proteins, enhances papain's proteolytic effect. This combination was found to be much more efficacious than papain alone [57]. The addition of chlorophyllin to this combination is thought to prevent agglutination of erythrocytes, thereby reducing the inflammatory response and pain sensation frequently observed with the use of papain-urea preparations [45]. In an open randomized clinical trial, a papain-urea preparation was found to be more effective than collagenase in reducing the amount of necrotic tissue of cutaneous ulcers. However, the possibility that papain-urea preparations may damage viable components of the ulcer bed still has to be examined [45].

Trypsin is derived from an extract of ox pancreas [44, 58]. It is nonspecific and hydrolyzes various proteins. The mode of activity of chymotrypsin is similar to that of trypsin [59].

Krill enzymes are derived from the digestive system of a small shrimp (Antarctic krill – *Euphausia superba*) [60–62].

Examples of enzymatic preparations:
- Santyl®, Iruxol®, Novoxol® (collagenase) – Abbott Lab (distributed by Smith & Nephew)
- Elase® (fibrinolysin-desoxyribonuclease solution) – Fujisawa, Inc.
- Fibrolan® (fibrinolysin-desoxyribonuclease solution) – Pfizer AG
- Varidase® (streptokinase/streptodornase) – Wyeth Lederle Lab.

- Accuzyme® (papain-urea combination) – Healthpoint
- Panafil® (papain-urea combination with chlorophyllin) – Healthpoint
- Gladase® – (papain-urea combination) Smith & Nephew
- Granulex spray® (trypsin) – Bertek Pharmaceuticals

9.4.4.2 Debridement with Mildly Acidic Preparations

Certain topical preparations contain a mixture of relatively mild acids, which are thought to dissolve necrotic material on ulcer surfaces [63]. Such preparations are manufactured as creams. They may be combined with silver-sulfadiazine, either mixed together or used alternately, to obtain both an antibacterial and a debriding effect. Aserbine®, which contains benzoic acid, malic acid and salicylic acid, is used for this purpose.

9.4.5 Autolytic Debridement

Autolytic debridement is a natural process that occurs normally in cutaneous ulcers, whereby endogenous enzymes digest and break down devitalized tissues. This process is much more efficient in well-hydrated ulcers. To some extent, every time occlusive or semi-occlusive dressings or preparations are used, there is some degree of autolytic debridement, because these dressings prevent water from evaporating, thus enabling tissue fluids to accumulate within the ulcer's environment. These fluids contain macrophages, neutrophils, lytic enzymes, and growth factors that may contribute to the healing process.

Therefore, occlusive dressings such as films, polyurethane foams, or hydrocolloid dressings may result in better environmental conditions for autolysis. This may explain the relative effectiveness of these dressing materials in the treatment of surgical wounds and chronic skin ulcers [64–67].

However, the use of hydrogels achieves a more effective autolytic debridement [68–71]. Colin et al. [68] compared the beneficial effects of an amorphous hydrogel (Intrasite®) and a dextranomer paste (Debrizan®). This study included 120 patients with sloughing pressure ulcers. After 21 days, the median reduction in ulcer area was 35% in ulcers treated with hydrogels as compared with 7% in those treated with dextranomer. Mulder et al. [72] demonstrated that using hypertonic gel dressings was more beneficial than the old procedure of 'wet-to-dry' dressings for debriding dry necrotic tissue in chronic cutaneous ulcers.

While autolytic debridement is being used, the ulcer should be cleansed once daily to ensure that the moist environment does not turn the ulcer into a breeding-ground for bacterial growth with subsequent infection [71].

By the same token, one may conclude that using a fatty preparation (i.e., ointment) may have a similar effect. An occlusive layer above dry necrotic material prevents water evaporation, thereby increasing the water content in the treated area. This may, to a certain extent, also facilitate the autolytic process.

9.4.6 Maggot Therapy

A type of debridement which may also be considered a variant of mechanical debridement is maggot therapy. The procedure is also termed 'biological debridement', 'biotherapy', or 'biosurgery'.

This debridement method is based on the finding that certain strains of maggots are nourished only by dead tissue and do not damage healthy living tissues. The type of larvae that are commonly used for this procedure, being safe and therapeutically efficient, are *Lucilia sericata* (green bottle blowfly) [73].

Using maggots for wound cleansing is an old method. Ambroise Paré [74] documented the beneficial effect of maggots a few centuries ago. Observations during Napoleon's battles and during the American Civil War indicated that the wounded soldiers whose wounds were infested by maggots had a better prognosis than those without maggots [74, 75]. Modern use of maggot therapy was documented in the 1930s and the 1940s. Hewitt [76] published research studies on maggot therapy that took place at Johns Hopkins University in Baltimore, Maryland.

This mode of treatment was abandoned in the 1940s, when antibiotic therapy was introduced. However, additional research studies in the past 20 years have confirmed their beneficial effect [73, 77, 78].

In their life cycle maggots reach maturity within a few days. During that period, as they eat, they grow to 8–10 mm. At that stage maggots are transformed into **puparium** – their next stage of development.

Maggots exert their debriding and healing activity via several mechanisms:
- Removal of necrotic debris by eating it. Because of their small size they are able to penetrate all areas of the ulcer.
- Secretion of proteases that degrade, liquefy, and dissolve necrotic material [73, 79]
- Secretion of substances such as antibacterial compounds [80] and compounds that may enhance healing (e.g., allantoin) [81]. Allantoin is said to be a 'soothing' substance; however, for the time being, there is no scientific substantiation of its effect on wound healing. It has been suggested that larvae secrete substances that are similar to growth factors and may affect proliferation of fibroblasts [82].
- Several investigators suggest that the motion of maggots within the wound may result in mechanical stimulation that enhances granulation tissue formation.

In this form of debridement, maggots are collected from a sterile container and placed onto the ulcer's surface, on a saline-moistened gauze. This is covered with a gauze and an external dressing.

The dressing is changed every 1–3 days, when the maggots discontinue eating and debriding necrotic debris. The ulcer is then rinsed thoroughly and the procedure is repeated until the ulcer is entirely debrided [73] (see Figs. 9.6–9.8).

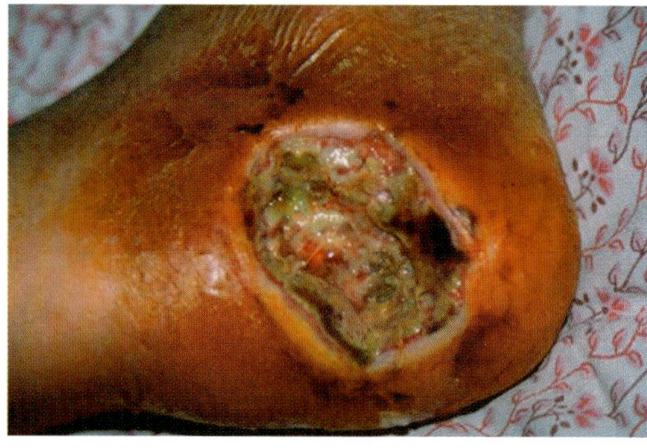

Fig. 9.6. An ulcer prior to maggot therapy

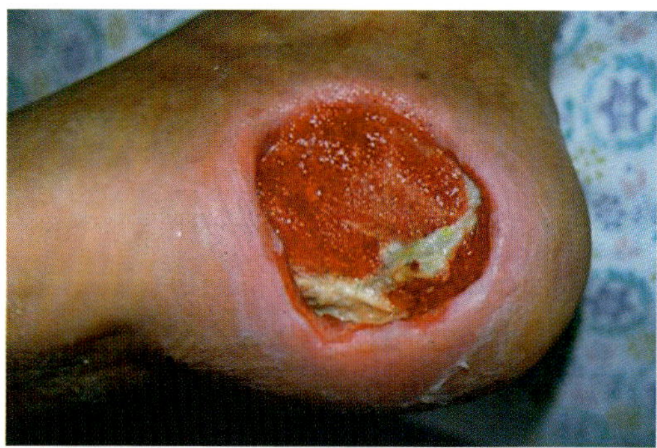

Fig. 9.7. The same ulcer as in Fig. 9.6, following maggot therapy

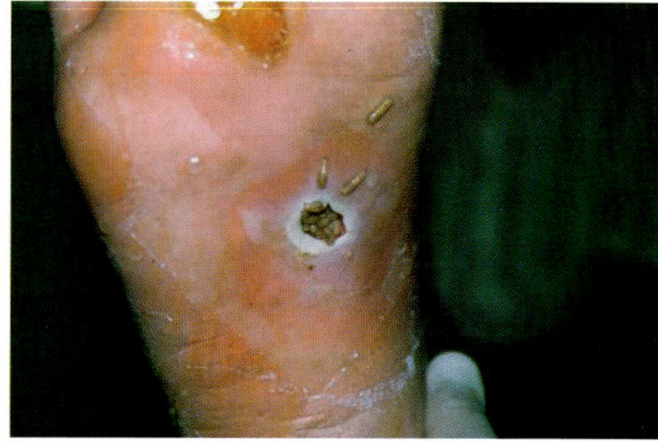

Fig. 9.8. Maggots on a cutaneous ulcer

An external dressing should be applied onto the gauze containing the maggots. The dressing is expected to [77]:
- Prevent the maggots from leaving the ulcer area and wandering around freely in the medical facility
- Enable transfer of oxygen
- Enable adequate drainage from the ulcer
- Allow inspection of the ulcer surface

Maggot therapy is currently considered to be a highly selective, efficient, and relatively fast debridement method [73,77,78]. The main indication for using maggots nowadays is for ulcers containing sloughing necrotic debris that was not effectively debrided by other methods.

The main contraindications to maggot therapy are (a) an ulcer adjacent to a body cavity, internal organ, or a relatively large vessel, and (b) a patient who is or may become psychologically disturbed by the procedure.

Sterile maggots are produced in laboratories in the UK, Germany, USA and several other countries. The 'International Biotherapy Society' was established in 1996. Details about maggot therapy and the society can be found on the Internet at: http://www.homestead.com/biotherapy.

9.5 Disadvantages of and Contraindications to Debridement: Final Comments

When debridement therapy is carried out correctly, adverse effects are rare but may occur. For example, sensitivity to a component of a debriding topical preparation may result in contact dermatitis.

However, most adverse effects that may be seen in debridement are usually attributed to its improper use.

This may occur in the following circumstances:
- When an inadequate mode of debridement is used: This generally involves using a method that is not appropriate for the ulcer surface, i.e., absorptive agents for dry necrotic material or enzymatic debriding agents for an ulcer whose surface is mostly red and clean.
- When certain older debridement methods such as scrubbing or 'wet-to-dry' dressings are used, that actually damage newly forming epithelium and healthy granulation tissue
- When a contraindicated debridement method is used

Contraindications to maggot therapy and to surgical debridement are detailed earlier in this chapter. In conditions associated with pathergy, such as pyoderma gangrenosum, it is advisable to avoid not only surgical debridement, but any type of physical or chemical manipulation (such as enzymatic debriding agents) that may cause irritation to ulcer tissue.

9.6 Summary

A variety of debridement methods exist for the removal of necrotic material from the surface of a cutaneous ulcer. A physician should adopt the preferred debridement method in accordance with the type and appearance of the necrotic material, as presented below in Table 9.2. A detailed flow-chart displaying all possibilities and recommended therapeutic approaches in accordance with the ulcer's appearance is presented in Chap. 20.

Black eschar or a thick crust may be removed by surgical debridement. A fatty topical preparation or hydrogel preparation may be applied to the surface to increase moisture level within the ulcer, thereby enabling its spontaneous removal, or as a preparatory stage before surgical debridement. Before application of

Table 9.2. Suggested approach according to appearance of necrotic material

Slough	Black crust or eschar	Purulent or sero-purulent discharge
Autolytic or chemical debridement	Hydrogel preparations may be used to produce autolysis	Discussed in Chap. 20
Polyacrylate dressings with Ringer's lactate solution may be considered	Consider softening the dry material with ointment	
Hydrodebridement may be used	Hydrodebridement may be used (before appliction of hydrogels or ointments)	
Consider maggot therapy	Surgical debridement	
Topical negative pressure		

these preparations, the treated area may be soaked in water for approximately 15 min to hydrate dry necrotic debris.

For sloughly ulcers, surgical debridement is used when slough is relatively solid and when a clear demarcation line can be identified between necrotic material and vital tissues. Autolytic or enzymatic debridement may be considered. Maggot therapy may also be ideal due to its high selectivity. Other methods of treatment such as the use of certain topical preparations may be combined with debridement.

Certain types of dressings may provide a debriding effect as well. The use of hydrophilic dextranomer granules or activated charcoal is intended for absorption of secretions. In addition, polyacrylate dressings with Ringer's lactate solution may be considered for removal of slough. Dressings applying topical negative pressure absorb fluid and debris from the ulcer bed. These are reviewed in Chap. 8. A detailed discussion with a flow chart regarding the appearance of a cutaneous ulcer and the appropriate treatment is presented in Chap. 20.

Note that after an ulcer has been debrided, and it looks clean and red with healthy granulation tissue, the optional therapeutic modalities change. For a clean red ulcer following debridement one should consider using skin substitutes containing living cells, keratinocyte transplantation, or the application of preparations containing growth factors.

References

1. Brown RF: The management of traumatic tissue loss in the lower limb, especially when complicated by skeletal injury. Br J Plast Surg 1965; 18:26–50
2. Monafo WW, Freedman B: Topical therapy for burns. Surg Clin North Am 1987; 67:133–145
3. Witkowski JA, Parish LC: Debridement of cutaneous ulcers: Medical and surgical aspects. Int J Dermatol 1992; 9:585–591
4. Reed BR, Clark RA: Cutaneous tissue repair: Practical implications of current knowledge. J Am Acad Dermatol 1985; 13:919–941
5. Bates-Jansen BM: Management of necrotic tissue. In: Sussman C, Bates-Jensen BM (eds): Wound Care, 1st edn. Gaithersburg: Aspen Publishers. 1998; pp 139–158
6. Clark RA: Cutaneous tissue repair: Basic biologic considerations. J Am Acad Dermatol 1985; 13:701–725
7. Winter GD: Formation of the scab and the rate of epithelization of superficial wounds in the skin of the young domestic pig. Nature 1962; 193:293–294
8. Steed DL, Donohoe D, Webster MW et al: Effect of extensive debridement and treatment on the healing of diabetic foot ulcers. J Am Coll Surg 1996; 183:61–64
9. Fisher JC: Skin grafting. In: Georgiades GS, Riefkohl R, Levin LS (eds): Plastic, Maxillofacial and Reconstructive Surgery, 3rd edn. Baltimore: Williams & Wilkins 1996; pp 13–18
10. Marcusson JA, Lindgren C, Berghard A, et al: Allgeneic cultured keratinocytes in the treatment of leg ulcers: A pilot study. Acta Derm Venereol (Stockh) 1992; 72:61–64
11. Teepe RG, Roseeuw DI, Hermans J, et al: Randomized trial comparing cryopreserved cultured epidermal allgrafts with hydrocolloid dressings in healing chronic venous ulcers. J Am Acad Dermatol 1993; 29:982–988

12. Pham HT, Rosenblum BI, Lyons TE, et al: Evaluation of a human skin equivalent for the treatment of diabetic foot ulcers in a prospective, ramdomized, clinical trial. Wounds 1999; 11:79–86

13. Raffetto JD, Mendez MV, Phillips TJ, et al: The effect of passage number on fibroblast cellular senescence in patients with chronic venous insufficiency with and without ulcer. Am J Surg 1999; 178:107–112

14. Mendez MV, Stanley A, Park HY, et al: Fibroblasts cultured from venous ulcers display cellular characteristics of senescence. J Vasc Surg 1998; 28:876–883

15. Agren MS, Steenfos HH, Dabelsteen S, et al: Proliferation and mitogenis response to PDGF-BB of fibroblasts isolated from chronic venous leg ulcers is ulcer-age dependent. J Invest Dermatol 1999; 112:463–469

16. Feedar JA: Clinical management of chronic wounds. In: McCulloch JM, Kloth LC, Feedar JA (eds): Wound Healing: Alternatives in Management, 2nd edn. Philadelphia. F.A. Davis Company: 1995; pp 137–185

17. Holm J, Andren B, Grafford K: Pain control in the surgical debridement of leg ulcers by the use of a topical lidocaine-prilocaine cream, Emla. Acta Derm Venereol 1990; 70:132–136

18. Vanscheidt W, Sadjadi Z, Lillieborg S: EMLA anaesthetic cream for sharp leg ulcer debridement: a review of the clinical evidence for analgesic efficacy and tolerability. Eur J Dermatol 2001; 11:90–96

19. Wolff K, Stingl G: Pyoderma gangrenosum. In: Freedberg IM, Eisen AZ, Wolff K, Austen KF, Goldsmith LA, Katz SI and Fitzpatrick TB (eds) Fitzpatrick's Dermatology in General Medicine, 5th edn. New York: McGraw-Hill. 1999; pp 1140–1148

20. Schwaegerle SM, Bergfeld WF, Senitzer D, et al: Pyoderma gangrenosum: A review. J Am Acad Dermatol 1988; 18:559–568

21. Hopfl R, Hefel L, Fritsch P: Pyoderma gangraenosum: differential diagnosis in ulcus cruris and postoperative exacerbating processes. Wien Med Wochenschr 1994; 144:279–280

22. McCalmont CS, Leshin B, White WL, et al: Vulvar pyoderma gangraenosum. Int J Gynaecol Obstet 1991; 35:175–178

23. Ergun T, Gurbuz O, Harvell J et al: The histopathology of pathergy: a chronologic study of skin hyperreactivity in Behçet's disease. Int J Dermatol 1998; 37:929–933

24. Gul A, Esin S, Dilsen N, et al: Immunohistology of skin pathergy reaction in Behcet's disease. Br J Dermatol 1995; 132:901–907

25. Gonzales AZ, Gonzales E: Pyoderma gangrenosum: self assessment. J Am Acad Dermatol 1990;23:545–548

26. Odom BO, James WD, Berger TG (eds): Erythema and urticaria. In: Andrews' Diseases of the Skin: Clinical Dermatology, 9th edn. Philadelphia: W.B. Saunders. 2000; pp 146–171

27. Odom BO, James WD, Berger TG (eds): Disorders of mucous membranes. In: Andrews' Diseases of the Skin: Clinical Dermatology, 9th edn. Philadelphia: W.B. Saunders. 2000; pp 991–1010

28. Glenchur H, Patel BS, Pathmarajah C: Transient bacteremia associated with debridement of decubitus ulcers. Mil Med 1981; 146:432–433

29. Schmeller W, Gaber Y, Gehl HB: Shave therapy is a simple, effective treatment of persistent venous leg ulcers. J Am Acad Dermatol 1998; 39:232–238

30. Marquez RR: Wound debridement and hydrotherapy. In: Gogia PP (ed): Clinical Wound Management, 1st edn. New Jersey: Slack Incorporated. 1995; pp 115–130

31. Steve L, Goodhart P, Alexander J: Hydrotherapy burn treatment: Use of chloramine T against resistant microorganisms. Arch Phys Med Rehabil 1979; 60:301–303

32. Thomlinson RH: Kitchen remedy for necrotic malignant breast ulcers. Lancet 1980; 2:707

33. Chirife J, Scarmato G, Herszage L: Scientific basis for the use of granulated sugar in treatment of infected wounds. Lancet 1982; 1:560–561

34. Cooper RA, Molan PC, Harding KG: Antibacterial activity of honey against strains of Staphylococcus aureus from infected wounds. J R Soc Med 1999; 92:283–285

35. Efem SE: Clinical observations on the wound healing properties of honey. Br J Surg 1988; 75:679–681

36. Zumla A, Lulat A: Honey – a remedy rediscovered. J R Soc Med 1989; 82:384–385

37. Molan PC: Potential of honey in the treatment of wounds and burns. Am J Clin Dermatol 2001; 2:13–19

38. Sieggreen MY, Maklebust J: Debridement: Choices and challenges. Adv Wound Care 1997; 10:32–37

39. Rodeheaver GT, Baharestani M, Brabec ME, et al: Wound healing and wound management: Focus on debridement. Adv Wound Care 1994; 7:22–36

40. Howes EL, Mandl I, Zaffuto S, et al: The use of Clostridium histolyticum enzymes in the treatment of experimental third degree burns. Surg Gynecol Obstet 1959; 109:177–188

41. Boxer AM, Gottesman N, Bernstein H, et al: Debridement of dermal ulcers and decubiti with collagenase. Geriatrics 1969; 24:75–86

42. Poulsen J, Kristensen VN, Brygger HE, et al: Treatment of infected surgical wounds with varidase. Acta Chir Scand 1983; 149:245–248

43. Hellgren L, Vincent J: Degradation and liquefaction effect of streptokinase-streptodornase and stabilized trypsin on necroses, crusts of fibrinoid, purulent exudate and clotted blood from leg ulcers. J Int Med Res 1977; 5:334–337

44. Hellgren L: Cleansing properties of stabilized trypsin and streptokinase-streptodornase in necrotic leg ulcers. Eur J Clin Pharmacol 1983; 24:623–628

45. Falanga V: Wound bed preparation and the role of enzymes: A case for multiple actions of therapeutic agents. Wounds 2002; 14:47–57

46. Varma AO, Bugatch E, German FM: Debridement of dermal ulcers with collagenase. Surg Gynecol Obstet 1973; 136:281–282

47. Barrett D Jr, Klibanski A: Collagenase debridement. Am J Nurs 1973; 73:849–851

48. Glyantsev SP, Adamyan AA, Sakharov Y: Crab collagenase in wound debridement. J Wound Care 1997; 6: 13–16

49. Westerhof W, Jansen FC, De Wit FS, et al: Controlled double-blind trial of fibrinolysin-desoxyribonuclease (Elase) solution in patients with chronic leg ulcers who are treated before autologuos skin grafting. J Am Acad Dermatol 1987; 17: 32–39

50. Falabella AF, Carson P, Eaglstein WH, et al: The safety and efficacy of a proteolytic ointment in the treatment of chronic ulcers of the lower extremity. J Am Acad Dermatol 1998; 39: 737–740

51. Singh GB, Snelling CFT, Hogg GR, et al: Debridement of the burn wound with sutilains ointment. Burns 1979; 7: 41–48

52. Makepeace AR: Enzymatic debridement of burns: a review. Burns Incl Therm Inj 1983; 9: 153–157

53. Dimick AR: Experience with the use of proteolytic enzyme (Travase) in burn patients. J Trauma 1977; 17: 948–955

54. Berger MM: Enzymatic debriding preparations. Ostomy Wound Manage 1993; 39: 61–66

55. Rodeheaver G, Marsh D, Edgerton MT, et al: Proteolytic enzymes as adjuncts to antimicrobial prophylaxis in contaminated wounds. Am J Surg 1975; 129: 537–544

56. Alvarez OM, Fernandez-Obregon A, Roisin S, et al: A prospective, randomized, comparative study of collagenase and papain-urea for pressure ulcer debridement. Wounds 2000; 14: 293–301

57. Silverstein P, Ruzicka FJ, Helmkamp GM, et al: In-vitro evaluation of enzymatic debridement of burn eschar. Surgery 1973; 73: 15–22

58. Suomalainen O: Evaluation of two enzyme preparations: Trypure and Varidase in traumatic ulcers. Ann Chir Gynaecol 1983; 72: 62–65

59. Nduwimana J, Guenet L, Dorval I, et al: Proteases. Ann Biol Clin 1995; 53: 251–264

60. Westerhof W, Van Ginkel CJ, Cohen EB, et al: Prospective randomized study comparing the debriding effect of Krill enzymes and a non-enzymatic treatment in venous leg ulcers. Dermatologica 1990; 181: 293–297

61. Hellgren L, Karlstam B, Mohr V, et al. Krill enzymes. A new concept for efficient debridement of necrotic ulcers. Int J Dermatol 1991; 30: 102–103

62. Hellgren L, Vincent J: Debriding properties of krill enzymes in necrotic leg ulcers. Arch Dermatol 1989; 125: 1006

63. Kathleen Parfitt (ed) Aserbine. In: Martindale – The Complete Drug Reference, 32nd edn. London: The Pharmaceutical Press. 1999; pp 1678

64. Madden MR, Finkelstein JL, Hefton JM, et al: Optimal healing of donor site wounds with hydrocolloid dressing. In: Ryan TJ (ed) An Environment for Healing: The Role of Occlusion. London: Royal Society of Medicine. 1985; pp 133–137

65. Barnett A, Berkowitz, RL, Mills R, et al: Comparison of synthetic adhesive moisture vapor permeable and fine mesh gauze dressings for split-thickness skin graft donor sites. Am J Surg 1983; 145: 379–381

66. Mumford JW, Mumford SP: Occlusive hydrocolloid dressings applied to chronic neuropathic ulcers. Int J Dermatol 1988; 27: 190–192

67. Choucair M, Phillips T: Wound dressing. In: Freedberg IM, Eisen AZ, Wolff K, Austen KF, Goldsmith LA, Katz SI, Fitzpatrick TB (eds): Fitzpatrick's Dermatology in General Medicine, 5th edn. New York: McGraw-Hill. 1999; pp 2954–2958

68. Colin D, Kurring PA, Yvon C, et al: Managing sloughy pressure sores. J Wound Care 1996; 5: 444–446

69. Flanagan M: The efficacy of a hydrogel in the treatment of wounds with non-viable tissue. J Wound Care 1995; 4: 264–267

70. Bale S, Banks V, Haglestein S, et al: A comparison of two amorphous in the debridement of pressure sores. J Wound Care 1998; 7: 65–68

71. Rodeheaver GT: Pressure ulcer debridement and cleansing: A review of current literature. Ostomy Wound Management 1999; 45 [Suppl 1A]: 80S–85S

72. Mulder GD: Cost-effective managed care: gel versus wet-to-dry for debridement. Ostomy Wound Manage 1995; 41: 68–76

73. Mumcuoglu KY: Clinical applications for maggots in wound care. Am J Clin Dermatol 2001; 2: 219–227

74. Bear WS: The treatment of chronic osteomyelitis with the maggot (larva of the blow fly). J Bone Joint Surg 1931; 13: 438–475

75. Chernin E: Surgical maggots. South Med J 1986; 79: 1143–1145

76. Hewitt F: Osteomyelitis: Development of the use of maggots in treatment. Am J Nurs 1932; 32: 31–38

77. Sherman RA: A new dressing design for use with maggot therapy. Plast Reconstr Surg 1997; 100: 451–456

78. Mumcuoglu KY, Ingber A, Gilead L, et al: Maggot therapy for the treatment of intractable wounds. Int J Dermatol 1999; 38: 623–627

79. Ziffren SE, Heist HE, May SC, et al: The secretion of collagenase by maggots and its implication. Ann Surg 1953; 138: 932–934

80. Robinson W, Norwood VH: Destruction of pyogenic bacteria in the alimentary tract of surgical maggots implanted in infected wounds. J Lab Clin Med 1934; 19: 586–581

81. Robinson W: Stimulation of healing in non-healing wounds by allantoin occurring in maggot secretions and of wide biological distribution. J Bone Joint Surg 1935; 17: 267–271

82. Prete PE: Growth effects of Phaenicia sericata larval extracts on fibroblasts: mechanisms of wound healing by maggot therapy. Life Sci 1997; 60: 505–510

Antibiotics, Antiseptics, and Cutaneous Ulcers   10

> orten Kiil: Let me see, what was the story? Some kind of beast that had got into the water-pipes, wasn't it?
>
> Dr. Stockmann: Infusoria – yes.
>
> Morten Kiil: And a lot of these beasts had got it, according to Petra – a tremendous lot.
>
> Dr. Stockmann: Certainly; hundreds of thousands of them, probably.
>
> Morten Kiil: But no one can see them – isn't that so?
>
> Dr. Stockmann: Yes; you can't see them.
>
> (*An Enemy of The People,*
> Henrik Ibsen)

Contents

10.1 Overview: Detrimental Effects of Bacteria on Wound Healing

Cutaneous ulcers constitute exposed tissue devoid of a layer of intact skin, and are contaminated by bacteria, some of which may be pathogenic [1–3]. The traditional rationale for using antibiotics and antiseptics in the management of cutaneous ulcers is based on the reasonable assumption that the presence of bacteria on an ulcer may lead to active infection, with subsequent interference to the process of wound healing [4–9].

Note that there is often a confusing lack of uniformity in the way the terms 'contamination', 'colonization', and 'infection' are presented in the literature. According to the currently accepted approach, the term 'contamination' simply refers to the presence of microorganisms in living tissue. The term 'colonization' describes the multiplication of microorganisms without causing a specific immune response or a disruption of normal bodily function [10, 11]. Bacteria require specific mechanisms of adherence in order to colonize; hence, they cannot be washed away from the affected tissue [12].

In contrast, 'infection' implies that the presence of microorganisms on tissue is accompanied by a host reaction and, in most cases, actual damage to the affected tissue. Note that it is not just the presence of organisms which leads to infection. 'Infection' is defined quantitatively as virulence multiplied by bacterial load, divided by host resistance. The final outcome of this equation determines whether a wound is merely colonized or advances towards clinical infection. Clinical signs of infection in cutaneous ulcers are described below.

The traditional definition suggests that the presence of more than 10^5 bacteria per gram of tissue should be considered as an infection, assuming that this number of bacteria indeed represents a significant biological burden [4, 13]. The issue of tissue biopsy and culture has since been questioned by others. Detailed discussion on methods of collection and identification of pathogenic bacteria appears in Addendum A to this chapter.

The detrimental effect of bacteria on wound healing results from several mechanisms. Bacteria release a variety of endotoxins and exotoxins that may reduce the proliferative capacity of fibroblasts and epithelial cells. Moreover, bacteria may affect cell function even to the extent of cellular destruction. Secreted toxins may cause lysis of collagen and fibrin [5, 14–17], as well as the degradation of growth factors [5]. In addition, consumption of nutrients and oxygen by the invading bacteria at the expense of the newly forming tissue leads to tissue anoxia, with further delay in the healing process [6, 14].

Stephens et al. [18] demonstrated that lower concentrations of supernatants of *Peptostreptococcus spp.* isolated from venous ulcers exerted a profound *in vitro* inhibiting effect on keratinocyte wound repopulation and endothelial tubule formation. Further research, however, is required in order to determine the ramifications of *in vitro* findings for *in vivo* conditions.

Impaired healing is not only attributed directly to the offending bacteria but is also caused by the host response to bacterial invasion and subsequent prolonged inflammatory response. The release of proteases and free-oxygen radicals by activated leukocytes may affect infecting organisms but may damage host tissue as well [5, 6]. This should be taken into account when the therapeutic approach is being planned.

The issue of antibiotics, antiseptics, and cutaneous ulcers is a complex one. This chapter does not aim to dictate rigid rules regarding the use of antibiotics and antiseptics on cutaneous ulcers. We shall limit ourselves to examining certain aspects of this issue.

10.2 Antibiotics and Antiseptics: Definitions and Properties

In this chapter, we make a distinction between antibiotic and antiseptic preparations. The dictionary definition of antibiotics is "… substances that destroy or suppress the growth or reproduction of microorganisms and are produced by various species of microorganisms …". However, in current usage, the term 'antibiotics' is extended to include synthetic antibacterial products such as sulfonamides and quinolones [19].

Other antimicrobial agents such as antiseptics are usually defined as substances that kill or inhibit the growth and development of microorganisms. In this category are included substances such as iodine or hydrogen peroxide.

The practical reason for differentiating between antibiotics and antiseptics relates to their differing modes of action. Antibiotics exert their effect against bacteria by using a specific mechanism that is unique to each class of antibiotic. However, in most cases, this specific mode of action limits the antibiotic effect against bacteria, since bacteria may develop defense mechanisms against specific modes of action of antibiotic compounds and acquire resistance to these antibiotics.

By way of contrast, antiseptics act via nonselective toxicity, directed against any living tissue: The damage is not only to the pathogenic microorganisms but to the host's cells as well [20].

Following is a list of antibiotics that may be used topically under certain conditions [21]:
- Bacitracin
- Chloramphenicol
- Fusidic acid
- Garamycin
- Mupirocin
- Neomycin
- Polymyxin B

Antiseptic preparations that may be considered for use on cutaneous ulcers are shown in Table 10.1.

10.3 Infected Ulcers, Clean Ulcers, and Non-Healing 'Unclean' Ulcers

In the following discussion we shall distinguish between infected cutaneous ulcers, clean ulcers, and an intermediate group, referred to as non-healing 'unclean' ulcers.

Table 10.1. Antiseptic preparations[a]

Oxidizing agents

- Hydrogen peroxide
- Potassium permanganate

Iodine compounds

- Povidone iodine
- Cadexomer iodine

Chlorine compounds

- Eusol
- Dakin's solution
- Milton's solution

Silver compounds

- Silver nitrate
- Silver sulfadiazine[b]

Other antiseptics

- Burow's solution

a. A detailed discussion on antiseptic preparations appears in chap. 11
b. Silver sulfadiazine cannot be considered a pure antiseptic agent, since it contains an antibiotic component – sulfadiazine.

10.3.1 Infected Ulcers

In the currently accepted practical approach, ulcers defined as 'infected' are those accompanied by cellulitis or erysipelas. Cellulitis and erysipelas are manifested mainly by classical signs of infection in the skin around the ulcer, and by systemic signs. According to an article by Cavanagh et el. [22], the presence of two or more local signs such as erythema, warmth, pain, or local tenderness can be regarded as evidence of infection. It is also accepted that the presence of purulent secretions on an ulcer bed should be regarded as evidence of infection [10, 23–26] (Fig. 10.1).

Cellulitis or erysipelas may be identified by systemic signs such as elevated temperature or an elevated white blood-cell count. In elderly patients, this may result in alterations in the conscious state, such as confusion. Obviously,

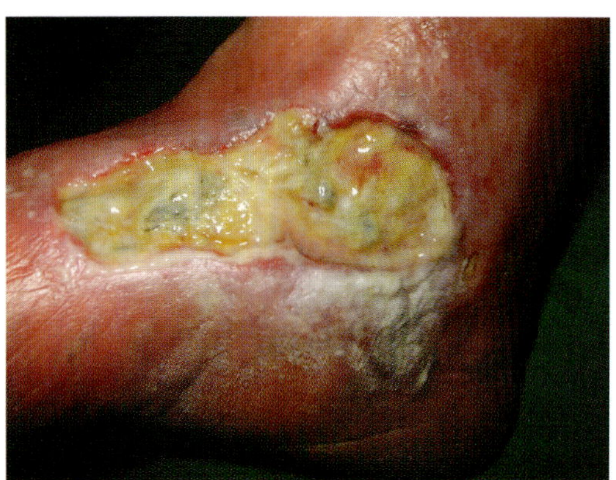

Fig. 10.1. An infected ulcer secreting a purulent discharge. The marked redness in its surrounding is a manifestation of cellulitis

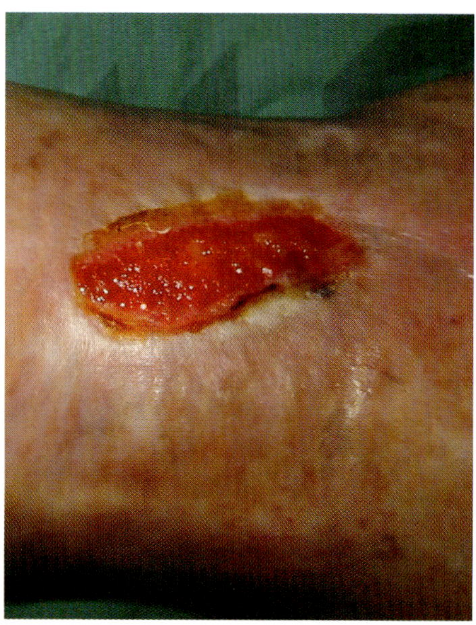

Fig. 10.2. A red, clean ulcer

cellulitis (or erysipelas) requires administration of systemic antibiotics [27].

Note that where diabetic ulcers are concerned, one should distinguish between non-limb-threatening infections and infections which are limb threatening. In non-limb-threatening infections the erythema surrounding the ulcer is less than 2 cm in diameter and there are no signs of systemic toxicity or significant ischemia. Limb-threatening infections are characterized by a more extensive involvement of surrounding tissues, accompanied by systemic toxicity or significant ischemia [10, 28]. They require hospitalization and the administration of intravenous antibiotics, based on bacteriologic data.

The physician should be alert to changes in the appearance of the ulcer which may indicate initial processes of infection: thicker (purulent or seropurulent) secretions, an offensive odor characteristic of anaerobic bacteria, or the smell of *Pseudomonas* strains.

10.3.2 Clean Ulcers

A 'clean' ulcer is red, and is covered by healthy granulation tissue (Fig. 10.2). This is the so-called 'ideal' ulcer a physician would like to achieve, with the best chances for complete healing.

Systemic antibiotics, or topical antimicrobial preparations (whether antibiotics or antiseptics), are not to be used for clean ulcers. Other available advanced dressings and other topical agents are detailed in Chap. 20.

10.3.3 The Broad Spectrum Between Clean Ulcers and Infected Ulcers

There is a spectrum of presentations that extends from the 'classical' clean ulcers to heavily infected ulcers [7, 29]. Somewhere between those two extremes there is a group of ulcers characterized mainly by impaired healing. Some refer to such ulcers as 'locally infected ulcers', while others use the term 'critical colonization'.

The representative ulcer of this group is one that has been in an active healing process and suddenly ceases to progress. Other conditions where one should consider the presence of 'local infection' were detailed by Cutting & Harding in 1994 [29]: deep brown-red granulation tissue that gradually becomes friable and tends to bleed easily [10]; wound breakdown; abnormal smell; localized pain that does not correspond to the clinical entity. Venous ulcers, for example, tend to be painless. Severe pain is expected in ischemia, vasculitis, or certain infections. In our view, most of these ulcers fall into the group of non-healing 'unclean' ulcers, described below.

10.3.4 Non-Healing 'Unclean' Ulcers

The third group comprises cutaneous ulcers that are not clean, yet do not meet the practical definition of infected ulcers, as explained above. Although such an 'unclean' ulcer does not show evidence of 'active' infection (such as cellulitis in the surrounding tissue), it may be secreting a little seropurulent fluid or have yellowish/gray slough on its surface (Fig. 10.3).

Note that we refer here to ulcers that are not in the process of active and progressive healing.

It is reasonable to assume that these findings represent a mild degree of bacterial infection that interferes with the processes of wound healing, even though there are no clear signs of clinical infection. (Some suggest that this condition is similar, in certain respects, to that of a debilitated elderly patient in whom pneumonia may manifest without fever.)

These 'unclean' ulcers, when not in the process of healing, pose several questions regarding the preferred mode of therapy, as described below.

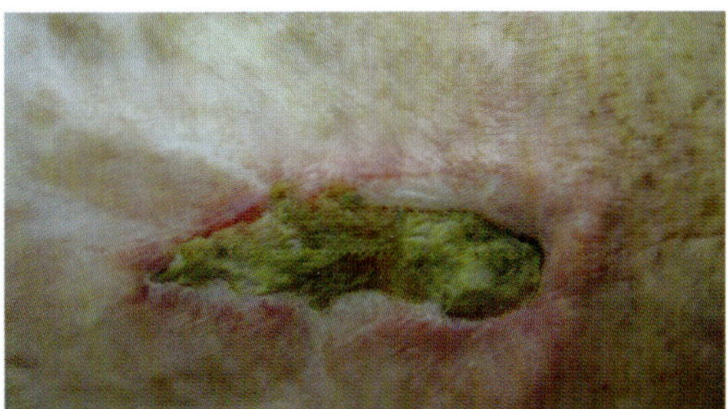

Fig. 10.3. An 'unclean ulcer' with slough on the surface. The mild redness of the surrounding skin does not represent cellulitis, but only reactive erythema

10.4 Systemic Antibiotics for Cutaneous Ulcers

10.4.1 General

Administration of systemic antibiotics for cutaneous ulcers is indicated for 'infected ulcers', namely, in cases of overt infection in the surrounding tissues such as cellulitis or erysipelas, or the presence of purulent secretions on an ulcer bed.

In addition, one should consider administration of systemic antibiotics in the following cases:

- Ulcers contaminated with *Streptococcus pyogenes* (group A) strains (even without overt signs of infection) due to the risk of local invasiveness or the risk of development of acute glomerulonephritis [7, 24]
- Skin grafts transplanted onto cutaneous ulcers which may become infected by *Staphylococcus aureus* or *Pseudomonas* strains, with subsequent significant damage to the grafts. In these cases, some recommend a more liberal administration of systemic antibiotics [24].

Apart from the above conditions, administration of systemic antibiotics for cutaneous ulcers is not currently accepted [10, 22, 30, 31].

Some physicians highly recommend that administration of antibiotics for infected wounds and cutaneous ulcers should be somewhat longer as compared with the usual duration of most antibiotic therapies; they should be given for two weeks or even more, subject to the patient's general condition, type of antibiotic, and clinical course. There are no sufficient data supporting this approach in the literature, and this suggestion is based on clinical experience only.

Antibiotics are not to be given for clean, red ulcers. Similarly, antibiotics should not be applied to ulcers in an already active healing stage, even if their surface is not optimal. The question of whether systemic antibiotics may enhance repair of stagnant, non-healing 'unclean ulcers' has been examined in several clinical studies, as detailed below.

10.4.2 Clinical Studies

Currently, the data are very sparse on the issue of antibiotic treatment in the healing of chronic cutaneous ulcers. There have been few studies documenting the effect of systemic antibiotics on leg ulcers which are not infected. Note that in most of the studies presented below there is no accurate description of the treated ulcers; when an ulcer is defined as 'not infected', it is not clear whether it was covered by slough, by secretions, or presented as a clean, red ulcer.

Alinovi et al. [32] studied two groups of patients with chronic venous ulcers without clinical signs of infection: 24 patients were treated with standard topical treatment and 23 with standard topical treatment plus a 10-day course of systemic antibiotics, based on bacteriologic culture and sensitivity tests. No statistical difference in the rate of healing was found between the two groups.

Huovinen et al. [33] treated 31 patients suffering from 'uncomplicated' venous ulcers, defined as ulcers without cellulitis or osteomyelitis. The patients were treated with either ciprofloxacin (750 mg twice daily), trimethoprim (160 mg twice daily), or placebo (twice daily), for 12 weeks. Complete healing was achieved in 42% of patients treated with ciprofloxacin (five of 12), in 33% of those treated with trimethoprim (three of nine), and in 30% in the placebo group (three of ten). The differences between the groups were not statistically significant at 16 weeks, neither regarding complete healing nor regarding reduction in ulcer size.

Chantelau et al. [34] conducted a double-blind, placebo-controlled study involving 44 diabetic patients with neuropathic forefoot ulcers. In addition to standard topical therapy, they received 500 mg amoxicillin plus 125 mg clavulanic acid, three times a day, and this was compared with placebo. The antibiotic was given for 6–20 days but was discontinued when it proved unsuitable according to bacteriologic specimens. This study demonstrated no beneficial effect of systemic antibiotics as compared with placebo.

Note that the authors stated that all the ulcers, except one, were infected. However, they did not define the diagnostic criteria for 'infection'. It may be assumed, however, that these ulcers were not accompanied by active cellulitis, since in such cases it would not have been possible to administer placebo treatment to these patients.

On the other hand, Valtonen et al. [35] reported that oral ciprofloxacin, given over a three month period, was clinically advantageous in patients with chronic leg ulcers of mixed etiologies and infected by *Pseudomonas aeruginosa* or other aerobic gram-negative rods. Improved healing was demonstrated in 18 patients treated with oral ciprofloxacin combined with standard therapy, compared with eight patients in the control group, treated only with standard therapy.

Levamisole, an antihelmintic drug, is thought to have a certain antibacterial effect, as well as an immunostimulatory influence. In a double-blind, placebo-controlled study evaluating its effect on leg ulcers it was found to have a better cure rate compared with placebo [36].

To the best of our knowledge, no other research studies have been conducted to evaluate the effect of systemic antibiotics on cutaneous ulcers.

10.4.3 Arguments Against the Use of Systemic Antibiotics for Non-Healing 'Unclean' Cutaneous Ulcers

There are certain arguments against systemic antibiotics in non-healing 'unclean' ulcers:

- The above-mentioned studies: Results of the studies presented above do not support the use of systemic antibiotics.

- Wound sterility as an unnecessary goal: An ulcer does not have to be sterile in order to heal. Attempting to achieve wound sterility may be considered an unnecessary goal. Acute wounds, heavily colonized with microorganisms, tend to heal if an optimal environment is provided [37, 38]. Chronic cutaneous ulcers treated by occlusive hydrocolloid dressings [39, 40] have been shown to improve, even though the presence of bacteria on the ulcer bed was confirmed by swab cultures. In our experience, similar findings are usually observed in cases of ulcers treated by cultured keratinocyte grafting or by composite grafts.
- Selection of resistant strains: The main argument against the use of antibiotics for cutaneous ulcers is the subsequent selection of resistant strains. The sharp increase in the prevalence of resistant bacteria, widely documented in the medical literature [41–46], has become one of the major threats in modern medicine. Currently, methicillin-resistant *Staphylococcus aureus* or resistant strains of *Pseudomonas* are being identified in cutaneous ulcers at an ever-increasing rate [47].

10.4.4 Arguments Supporting the Use of Systemic Antibiotics for Non-Healing 'Unclean' Cutaneous Ulcers

There is some evidence supporting the use of antibiotics for 'unclean' cutaneous ulcers. Contamination or colonization of ulcers has been shown to delay healing [9, 10]. Research studies document a correlation between the number of bacteria, impaired healing, and clinical signs of infection [13, 48]. Reducing the number of bacteria in cutaneous ulcers has been shown to

have a favorable influence on ulcer healing [49]. Recently, there has been increasing evidence to indicate that impaired healing in chronic ulcers may be attributed to the presence of gram-positive anaerobic cocci, even in cases without clinical evidence of infection [18, 50].

In addition, a comment regarding the clinical studies examining this issue should be noted: In all the research studies described above, the main goal of the investigators was to achieve complete cure. In our opinion, the purpose of antibiotic treatment is not to obtain complete cure (although it would be desirable); but to enable the ulcer to become a 'red-clean' ulcer. Then cure can be be achieved using advanced modalities such as keratinocyte grafts, composite grafts, or topical application of growth factors.

All the research studies mentioned above were conducted in the 1980s. At that time, more advanced treatments to enhance the process of wound healing were not available.

In view of the above, most of the research studies evaluating the efficacy of certain systemic antibiotics have become somewhat outdated, even if they were randomized, double-blind, and controlled. The result that should be measured in studies nowadays is the efficiency in cleaning the ulcer and its preparation for a definite treatment, and not the achievement of a total cure.

Nevertheless, there is no substantial evidence at present to support the administration of systemic antibiotics for cutaneous ulcers, unless clinical signs of infection are present. (Apart from the two cases pointed out at section 10.4.1.)

10.5 Topical Preparations for Infected Cutaneous Ulcers and 'Unclean' Ulcers

Antibiotic and antiseptic topical preparations can appear in many forms: ointments, creams, solutions, etc., the choice of which depends on the clinical appearance of the ulcer. In the case of profuse secretion, frequent wet dressings of antibiotic or antiseptic solutions are preferred to dry out the wound. When there is no excessive discharge, one may use topical medication in the form of a cream. A dry wound, covered by a black eschar, may be treated by ointments. This issue is discussed in detail in Chap. 20.

> Obviously, there is no reason to use antibiotic and antiseptic preparations on clean ulcers. If used at all, their use should be limited to:
> - 'Unclean' ulcers
> - 'Adjuvant' topical therapy for infected ulcers, in addition to systemic antibiotics

Similar to the use of systemic antibiotics for cutaneous ulcers, the use of topical preparations is also a controversial issue. We discuss below the implications of using antibiotic topical preparations and antiseptic topical preparations on cutaneous ulcers.

10.5.1 Topical Antibiotics

Arguments for and against the use of topical antibiotic preparations on cutaneous ulcers do not differ, in essence, from those mentioned above regarding systemic antibiotics. The main consideration here is also the selection of resistant strains [51, 52]. In fact, this is the main reason many physicians consider the use of topical antibiotics to be bad practice. However, certain aspects unique to the use of topical antibiotics should be noted.

■ **Reaching the Target Organ.** The main advantage of using topical antibiotic preparations as opposed to the administration of systemic antibiotics stems from the fact that the actual site of application is the target organ itself. Therefore, high concentrations of the drug can be applied while avoiding systemic adverse effects [21].

■ **Paucity of Clinical Studies.** In contrast to the issue of systemic antibiotics and cutaneous

ulcers, or antiseptic preparations and cutaneous ulcers, there are very few data available concerning the value of topical antibiotics. The current view is that there is no substantial evidence to support the use of topical antibiotics for the treatment of cutaneous ulcers [30], and some physicians strongly advise against their use on cutaneous ulcers [53]. However, since clinical studies examining this issue are scarce [30], one cannot establish a therapeutic policy based on available data.

Topical antibiotic preparations may decrease the bulk of contaminating bacteria and clean the ulcer, thus preparing it for advanced treatment modalities. Therefore, topical antibiotics should not be used on cutaneous ulcers with the purpose of achieving complete cure, but should be considered a preparatory stage for more advanced therapies.

■ **Role of Topical Antibiotics in Minor Skin Trauma.** Double-blind controlled studies have demonstrated that topical antibiotics may reduce the incidence of staphylococcal and streptococcal infection of minor skin trauma [54, 55]. In many cases, the direct trigger for ulceration in venous insufficiency or in peripheral arterial disease is, in fact, some kind of external physical injury. The use of topical antibiotic preparations may be considered, therefore, in the immediate period after wounding (within the range of a few days) to prevent secondary infection and the development of a chronic ulcer. Note that the short-term use of topical antibiotics in the community has not been linked to bacterial resistance to the same extent to which its long-term use in hospitals has [56].

10.5.2 Topical Antiseptics

The main argument against the use of antiseptics for cutaneous ulcers is their potential toxicity to the host's tissues. While the toxicity of antibiotics tends to be selective – directed mainly against bacteria by virtue of a specific mechanism of action – the toxicity of antiseptics is non-selective and directed against any living tissue. In other words, the damage is not only to the pathogenic microorganisms but also to the host's cells [20]. Tissues surrounding the wound bed are damaged, with a subsequent delay in the wound-healing process.

Alexander Fleming stated in 1919 that "the antimicrobial action of antiseptics should be weighed against their potential toxic effects on tissues" [57]. This approach is still valid today. An old saying among surgeons suggests that solutions that cannot be tolerated in the eye should not be used in the abdominal cavity or on a surgical wound. The same approach may be applied to cutaneous ulcers.

The potential damage that antiseptics can cause has been demonstrated in the past on animal models [58]. In the past two decades this has been repeatedly confirmed and subjected to quantification and more accurate assessment, using keratinocyte and fibroblast cultures [59–62].

Antiseptics such as chlorhexidine or povidone iodine have been found to be cytotoxic to human keratinocytes after 15 min exposure, while antibiotics such as fusidic acid, imipeneme, vancomycin, amikacin, and piperacillin were not found to be toxic to human keratinocytes following an exposure of 48 h [60].

Several other research studies have produced similar findings demonstrating the toxicity of antiseptics as compared with the relatively mild effects of antibiotics [63–65].

In spite of the above, one should keep in mind that most, if not all studies indicating toxicity of various antiseptics have been based on *in vitro* models or laboratory animal models of acute wounds. The implication of these data with respect to the use of topical antiseptics on chronic cutaneous ulcers may require further research.

10.5.3 Allergic Reactions to Topical Antibiotics and Antiseptics

Topical antibiotics or antiseptics may cause contact dermatitis when used on leg ulcers [66–68]. Consequently, ulcers affected by contact dermatitis may deteriorate, with a further delay in wound repair. These reactions are more frequent following the application of antibiotics [66–72], but reactions to antiseptics such as povidone iodine [73–76], chlorhexidine [77], or silver sulfadiazine [78, 79] may occur as well. In some cases, the sensitivity is due not to the active ingredient but to the vehicle or preservatives incorporated in the preparation.

Nevertheless, in most cases, contact sensitivity does not create a severe clinical condition, provided that an appropriate diagnosis was made. Local itching and mild redness around the ulcer are reliable indicators of a sensitivity reaction which should alert the physician to the diagnosis and call for discontinuation of the offending agent. Usually, such a condition tends to improve significantly following the application of alternative topical therapy, together with the use of a mild steroid preparation.

10.5.4 When to Consider the Use of Antiseptics or Topical Antibiotic Preparations

Antiseptics may be applied topically to an unclean' or infected ulcer in order to clean the ulcer and prepare it for more advanced treatment modalities. However, when antiseptics are used, a certain delay in the wound healing process can be expected.

There is a fine line between killing bacteria and causing host-tissue toxicity, which should be taken into consideration whenever antiseptics are used. In 1984, Van Den Hoogenband published an article supporting this approach [80]. He demonstrated improved healing in ulcers treated by silver sulfadiazine cream prior to skin grafting, compared with ulcers treated by skin grafting alone.

Topical antibiotics, even though some physicians strongly advise against their use in cutaneous ulcers [53], may be of value in cases where other therapeutic modalities have failed to clean a sloughy/exudative/unclean ulcer. Sometimes, a course of topical antibiotics for a few days may clean an ulcer, thereby enabling the use of an advanced therapeutic modality such as composite grafting, or a topical preparation containing growth factors.

10.6 Guidelines for the Use of Topical Antibiotics and Antiseptic Preparations in the Management of Cutaneous Ulcers

As stated above, the use of topical antibiotics or antiseptics in the treatment of cutaneous ulcers is still controversial. Further research studies should be carried out to evaluate their efficiency. However, if one decides to use these preparations (e.g., for an unresponsive ulcer), the following guidelines are recommended.

10.6.1 Avoid Toxic Antiseptics

It would be better not to use antiseptics that are documented as being relatively toxic, such as chlorhexidine [60, 81] and hexachlorophene [82, 83]. Acetic acid has also been found to be toxic to fibroblasts, even in quite low concentrations [59]. Milder antiseptics that may be used, such as iodine or chlorine compounds, are detailed in Chap. 11.

Hydrogen peroxide has been reported as being toxic in a few *in vitro* studies [59, 84]. Nevertheless, some suggest considering its use [85]. A reasonable recommendation would be to consider short-term treatment with hydrogen peroxide when dealing with recalcitrant cutaneous ulcers, when other modes of treatment have failed to clean them adequately.

Note: The degree of damage an antiseptic preparation does to host tissue depends on the compound being used, its concentration, and the presence of other ingredients in the preparation. For example, surfactants, which may have detrimental effects on human tissues [86], are sometimes combined with certain other antiseptic agents such as povidone-iodine. Alcoholic solutions may have a detrimental effect as well.

10.6.2 Base Selection of Antibiotics on Clinical Grounds

If you decide to use topical antibiotics, base the choice of drug on:
- Color and type of secretions
- The ulcer's etiology (for example, anaerobes may be present in diabetic ulcers)
- Bacteriologic cultures and the antibiotic-susceptibility pattern (antibiogram)

Characteristics of secretions with identification of the causative bacteria are detailed in Chap. 7. A discussion on the various ways to obtain culture specimens can be found in Addendum A to this chapter.

In addition, a bacterial swab may provide some useful data regarding the bacterial antibiotic-susceptibility pattern. Note that certain antibacterial agents may be more effective against specific strains of bacteria, e.g., silver sulfadiazine against *Pseudomonas* strains, although a selection of resistant strains has been documented [87, 88].

10.6.3 Consider Carefully the Type of Antibiotic Preparation

When using topical antibiotics, it is better to use – as a first-line choice – an antibiotic preparation that is not likely to be needed later on systemically, for example, in case of cellulitis. Using certain antibiotics topically may result in bacterial resistance to the drugs. Chloramphenicol, for example, is used less frequently nowadays as a systemic drug; hence, its topical use does not have implications regarding its systemic administration. In the case of staphylococcal infection, topical mupirocin would be a reasonable choice, since systemic administration of this drug is not possible.

10.6.4 Take a Careful History Regarding Allergic Reactions

Ascertain that the patient has not previously developed an allergic reaction to the preparation intended for use.

10.6.5 Avoid Spreading Infection

When dressings are changed, take particular care not to spread infection to the surrounding environment (as discussed in detail in the Appendix to this book). With respect to virulence and the resistance of microorganisms found in medical centers, as well as the risk of cross-infection, it is advisable to avoid the use of topical antibiotics in an inpatient setting.

10.6.6 Cleanse and Debride the Ulcer

Before considering the use of topical antibiotic or antiseptic, remember that frequent cleansing of the ulcer or wound with saline or Ringer's lactate solution is a very effective method of removing bacteria. In addition, necrotic tissue on an ulcer is a fertile culture medium for bacteria, so debridement is an essential initial step in its management.

10.6.7 Final Comment

In view of all the possible shortcomings of antiseptic and antibacterial preparations, they should not be prescribed indiscriminately. They should be used judiciously and intelligently and in the appropriate situations, as outlined above.

10.7 Addendum A: Collection and Identification of Pathogenic Bacteria

Identification of bacteria present within a cutaneous ulcer may provide valuable information and serve as a guide to the most appropriate therapeutic approach. In addition, it is possible to obtain information on the antibiotic-susceptibility pattern (antibiogram) of the offending microorganism.

The quality of the specimen is the most important factor determining the accuracy of identification. Contamination by normal flora should be avoided. Similarly, specimens that have been exposed to air are no longer reliable for the identification of anaerobic bacteria.

Culture specimens from a cutaneous ulcer may be collected by the following methods:

10.7.1 Swabbing

Using a swab is the most common way to collect bacteriologic specimens. Taking samples at the deepest point of the ulcer margin, close to healthy skin, is recommended [24]. The specimen should not be obtained from an ulcer covered with residues of antibacterial or antiseptic preparation. Ideally, swabbing should be done after the ulcer has been cleansed gently with saline or Ringer's lactate solution.

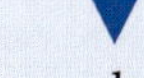

Some do not recommend the use of swabs from ulcers, raising the following arguments:

- Results obtained by swabs reflect, in fact, indiscriminate colonization of bacteria on the surface, rendering the isolation and accurate identification of the actual pathogenic bacteria impossible [25, 89, 90].
- Swabs do not enable appropriate transport of anaerobes for two reasons: (a) Air is trapped in the interstices of the cotton wall [25]; (b) The transport gel medium of a swab is not a suitable breeding ground for their survival.

However, studies on the microbiologic identification of infected diabetic ulcers [91–93] have revealed a relatively high correlation between swabs and deep-tissue biopsy. Examining microflora of limb-threatening diabetic foot infections, Pellizzer et al. [94] demonstrated similar results, but suggested that deep-tissue biopsy may be more sensitive than swabbing for the monitoring of infected foot ulcers that are still active after two weeks of appropriate treatment.

Stephens et al. [18] examined chronic venous ulcers without clinical evidence of infection. The findings of superficial swabs were shown to reflect those obtained by deep-tissue biopsy with respect to the presence of aerobic bacteria. However, they also demonstrated that swabs do not provide reliable data as to the presence of anaerobic cocci in deep tissue.

10.7.2 Deep-Tissue Biopsy

In a full-thickness biopsy, microflora from deep tissue can be obtained. In addition, strict anaerobic isolation techniques can be employed, making accurate identification of anaerobes possible.

Deep tissue biopsy is done after initial debridement has been performed and superficial debris has been cleansed [7].

Note that the use of deep biopsy harbors a relative risk of causing the infection to penetrate deeper. This should be taken into account, especially when dealing with ulcers adjacent to bony tissue.

10.7.3 Needle Aspiration

If there is a sufficient amount of material such as pus or seropurulent fluid, it can be drawn from the depth of the ulcer with a sterile needle and syringe [24, 25]. On the other hand, puncture of tissue with a needle may not be desirable (unless a collection of fluids has been found) since it may cause the infection to penetrate deeper. The information provided regarding the value of needle aspiration in cutaneous ulcers tends to be contradictory [95–97].

10.7.4 Curettage

With curettage, a piece of tissue is removed by a sterile blade, preferably from the deep area after the ulcer has been debrided. Specimens that have been obtained by curettage from the base

of infected diabetic ulcers tend to correlate better with the results obtained by deep-tissue biopsy, compared with findings based on swabs or needle aspiration [97].

10.7.5 Conclusion

The method of choice for obtaining culture specimens still has to be determined. For all practical purposes, however, the most suitable method should be determined according to certain parameters such as the etiology of the ulcer, its depth, extent of the infection, and the suspected microorganism present.

For the time being, a reasonable approach is based on the depth of the ulcer. When one is dealing with a superficial ulcer, a swab can be expected to reflect the content of microflora. If the ulcer presents a minimal degree of infection, it would be unjustified to use invasive procedures such as a deep biopsy, especially in cases in which the ulcer is adjacent to a bone. In contrast, a deep biopsy is required in deeply infected ulcers. Culturing of bone specimens, when needed, can be obtained by percutaneous biopsy or by surgical excision.

When relying on swabs, it must be kept in mind that insufficient information is provided regarding anaerobic bacteria [18].

Note that semi-quantitative or quantitative culture techniques may be used. This enables the physician to: (a) evaluate the extent of actual bacterial burden, based on the traditional definition of infection, i.e., more than 10^5 bacteria per gram of tissue [4, 13, 98]; (b) identify the offending microorganism, assuming that the bacterium present in high concentration is, in fact, the main pathogen.

Using one of the above-mentioned techniques may also provide some useful information regarding the bacterial antibiotic-susceptibility pattern. It is advisable to repeat the procedure every few days, ensuring that bacteria are not developing a resistance to the antibiotic given.

In any case, the method of sampling should be discussed and agreed upon with the local microbiologic laboratory. Similarly, it is highly important that the interpretation of the microbiologic results take place only in conjunction with the clinical findings.

10.8 Addendum B: Biofilms

Recent evidence indicates that bacteria may be present in chronic wounds not only in a free-floating form, but also in the form of biofilms [7, 99]. Biofilms are accumulations of microorganisms (one or more species) within an extracellular polysaccharide matrix.

Topical and systemic antibiotics cannot easily penetrate the biofilms. Moreover, the biofilm environment provides bacteria with optimal conditions for gene transfer with subsequent increased resistance and virulence. The presence of biofilms may partly explain the chronicity of certain infections [100, 101].

It may be assumed that future research will provide a better understanding of the nature of biofilms and may assist in the treatment of chronic ulcers. It may involve the determination of appropriate and accurate regimens for the administration of systemic antibiotics, together with the development of ways to improve the penetration and/or the efficacy of topical antibiotics.

References

1. Dagher FJ, Alongi SV, Smith A: Bacterial studies of leg ulcers. Angiology 1978; 29:641–653
2. Friedman SA, Gladstone JL: The bacterial flora of peripheral vascular ulcers. Arch Dermatol 1969; 100:29–32
3. Eriksson G, Eklund AE, Kallings LO: The clinical significance of bacterial growth in venous leg ulcers. Scand J Infect Dis 1984; 16:175–180
4. Robson MC: Wound infection. A failure of wound healing caused by an imbalance of bacteria. Surg Clin North Am 1997; 77:637–650
5. Robson MC, Stenberg BD, Heggers JP: Wound healing alterations caused by infection. Clin Plast Surg 1990; 17:485–492
6. Reed BR, Clark RA: Cutaneous tissue repair: Practical implications of current knowledge. 2. J Am Acad Dermatol 1985; 13:919–941
7. Kirsner RS, Martin LK, Drosou A: Wound microbiology and the use of antibacterial agents. In: Rovee D, Maibach HI (eds) The Epidermis in Wound Healing, 1st edn. Boca Raton: CRC Press. 2004; pp 153-182
8. Madsen SM, Westh H, Danielsen L, et al: Bacterial colonization and healing of venous leg ulcers. APMIS 1996; 104:895–899
9. Halbert AR, Stacey MC, Rohr JB, et al: The effect of bacterial colonization on venous leg ulcer healing. Australas J Dermatol 1992; 33:75–80
10. Browne A, Dow G, Sibbald RG: Infected wounds; definitions and controversies. In: Falanga V (ed) Cutaneous Wound Healing, 1st edn. London: Martin Dunitz. 2001; pp 203–219
11. Osterholm MT, Hedberg CW, Moore KA: Epidemiologic principles. In: Mandell GL, Bennett JE, Dolin R (eds) Mandell, Douglas, and Bennett's Principles and Practice of Infectious Diseases. 5th edn. Philadelphia: Churchill Livingstone. 2000; pp 156–167
12. Murray PR, Rosenthal KS, Koyabayashi GS, Pfaller MA: Mechanisms of bacterial pathogenesis. In: Medical Microbiology, 3rd edn. St. Louis: Mosby. 1998; pp 152–159
13. Robson MC, Heggers JP: Bacterial quantification of open wounds. Mil Med 1969; 134:19–24
14. Harkess N: Bacteriology. In: McCulloch JM, Kloth LC, Feedar JA (eds) Wound Healing: Alternatives in Management, 2nd edn. Philadelphia: F.A. Davis Company. 1995; pp 60–86
15. Irvin TT: Collagen metabolism in infected colonic anastomoses. Surg Gynecol Obstet 1976;143:220–224
16. Baroni A, Gorga F, Baldi A, et al: Histopathological features and modulation of type IV collagen expression induced by Pseudomonas aeruginosa lipopolysaccharide (LPS) and porins on mouse skin. Histol Histopathol 2001; 16:685–692
17. Nagano T, Hao JL, Nakamura M, et al: Stimulatory effect of pseudomonal elastase on collagen gedradation by cultured keratocytes. Invest Ophthalmol Vis Sci 2001; 42:1247–1253
18. Stephens P, Wall IB, Wilson MJ, et al: Anaerobic cocci populating the deep tissues of chronic wounds impair cellular wound healing responses *in vitro*. Br J Dermatol 2003; 148:456–466
19. Chambers HF: Antimicrobial agents: General considerations. In: Hardman JG, Limbird LE, Gilman AG (eds) Goodman & Gilman's. The Pharmacological Basis of Therapeutics, 10th edn. New York: McGraw-Hill. 2001; pp 1143–1170
20. Brooks GF, Butel JS, Morse SA: Antimicrobial chemotherapy. In: Jawetz, Melnick & Adelberg's Medical Microbiology. 21st edn. Stamford, Conn.: Appleton & Lange. 2001; pp 144–175
21. Tunkel AR: Topical antibacterials. In: Mandell GL, Bennett JE, Dolin R (eds) Mandell, Douglas, and Bennett's Principles and Practice of Infectious Diseases, 5th edn. Philadelphia: Churchill Livingstone. 2000; pp 428–435
22. Cavanagh PR, Buse JB, Frykberg RG, et al: Consensus development conference on diabetic foot wound care. Diabetes Care 1999; 22:1354–1360
23. Parish LC, Witkowski JA: The infected decubitus ulcer. Int J Dermatol 1989; 28:643–647

24. Niedner R, Schopf E: Wound infections and antibacterial therapy. In: Westerhof W (ed) Leg Ulcers: Diagnosis and Treatment. Amsterdam: Elsevier. 1993; pp 293–303

25. Lipsky BA, Berendt AR: Principles and practice of antibiotic therapy of diabetic foot infections. Diabet Met Res Rev 2000; 16 [Suppl 1]: S42–S46

26. Robson MC: Wound Infection: a failure of wound healing caused by an imbalance of bacteria. Surg Clin North Am 1997; 77: 637–650

27. Tsao H, Swartz MN, Weinberg AN, Johnson RA: Soft tissue infections; erysipelas, cellulitis and gangrenous cellulitis. In: Freedberg IM, Eisen AZ, Wolff K, Austen KF, Goldsmith LA, Katz SI and Fitzpatrick TB (eds) Fitzpatrick's Dermatology in General Medicine, 5th edn. New York: McGraw-Hill. 1999; pp 2213– 2231

28. Swartz MN: Cellulitis and subcutaneous tissue infections. Mandell GL, Bennett JE, Dolin R (eds) Mandell, Douglas, and Bennett's Principles and Practice of Infectious Diseases, 5th edn. Philadelphia: Churchill Livingstone. 2000; pp 1037–1057

29. Cutting KF, Harding KG: Criteria to identify wound infection. J Wound Care 1994; 3: 198–201

30. O'Meara SM, Cullum NA, Majid M, et al: Systematic review of antimicrobial agents used for chronic wounds. Br J Surg 2001; 88: 4–21

31. Filius G, Gyssens IC: Impact of increasing antimicrobial resistance on wound management. Am J Clin Dermatol 2002; 3: 1–7

32. Alinovi A, Bassissi P, Pini M: Systemic administration of antibiotics in the management of venous ulcers. A randomized clinical trial. J Am Acad Dermatol 1986; 15: 186–191

33. Huovinen S, Kotilainen P, Jarvinen H, et al: Comparison of ciprofloxacin or trimethoprim therapy for venous leg ulcers: results of a pilot study. J Am Acad Dermatol 1994; 31: 279–281

34. Chantelau E, Tanudjaja T, Altenhofer F, et al: Antibiotic treatment for uncomplicated neuropathic forefoot ulcers in diabetes: a controlled trial. Diabet Med 1996; 13: 156–159

35. Valtonen V, Karppinen L, Kariniemi AL: A comparative study of ciprofloxacin and conventional therapy in the treatment of patients with chronic lower leg ulcers infected with Pseudomonas aeruginosa or other gram-negative rods. Scand J Infect Dis 1989; 60 [Suppl]: 79–83

36. Morias J, Peremans W, Campaert H, et al: Levamisole tratment in ulcus cruris. A double-blind placebo-controlled study. Arzneimittelforschung 1979; 29: 1050– 1052

37. Hutchinson JJ, McGuckin M: Occlusive dressings: a microbiologic and clinical review. Am J Infect Control 1990; 18: 257–268

38. Thomson PD, Smith DJ Jr: What is infection? Am J Surg 1994; 167 [Suppl]: 7S–11S

39. Friedman SJ, Su WP: Management of leg ulcers with hydrocolloid occlusive dressing. Arch Dermatol 1984; 120: 1329–1336

40. Gilchrist B, Reed C: The bacteriology of chronic venous ulcers treated with occlusive hydrocolloid dressing. Br J Dermatol 1989; 121: 337–344

41. Opal SM, Mayer KH, Medeiros AA: Mechanisms of bacterial antibiotic resistance. In: Mandell GL, Bennett JE, Dolin R (eds) Mandell, Douglas, and Bennett's Principles and Practice of Infectious Diseases. 5th edn. Philadelphia: Churchill Livingstone. 2000; pp 236–253

42. Wenzel RP, Edmond MB: Managing antibiotic resistance. N Engl J Med 2000; 343: 1961–1963

43. Gold HS, Meollering RC Jr: Antimicrobial-drug resistance. N Engl J Med 1996; 335: 1445–1453

44. Hart CA: Antibiotic resistance: an increasing problem? Br Med J 1998; 316: 1255–1256

45. Colsky AS, Kirsner RS, Kerdel FA: Analysis of antibiotic susceptibilities of skin wound flora in hospitalized dermatology patients. The crisis of antibiotic resistance has come to the surface. Arch Dermatol 1998; 134: 1006–1009

46. Gould IM: A review of the role of the antibiotic policies in the control of antibiotic resistance. J Antimicrob Chemother 1999; 43: 459–465

47. Roghmann MC, Siddiqui A, Plaisance K, et al: MRSA colonization and the risk of MRSA bacteremia in hospitalized patients with chronic ulcers. J Hosp Inf 2001; 47: 98–103

48. Skog E, Arnesjo B, Troeng T, et al: A randomized trial comparing cadexomer iodine and standard treatment in the out-patient management of chronic venous ulcers. Br J Dermatol 1983; 109: 77–83

49. Lookingbill DP, Miller SH, Knowles RC: Bacteriology of chronic leg ulcers. Arch Dermatol 1978; 114: 1765–1768

50. Wall IB, Davies CE, Hill KE, et al: Potential role of anaerobic cocci in impaired human wound healing. Wound Repair Regen 2002; 10: 346–353

51. Wyatt TD, Ferguson WP, Wilson TS, et al: Gentamycin resistant Staphylococcus aureus associated with the use of topical gentamicin. J Antimicrob Chemother 1977; 3: 213–217

52. Rahman M, Noble WC, Cookson B: Mupirocin-resistant Staphylococcus aureus (letter). Lancet 1987; 2: 387

53. Eriksson G: Local treatment of venous leg ulcers. Acta Chir Scand 1988; 544 [Suppl]: 47–52

54. Leyden JJ, Kligman AM: Rationale for topical antibiotics. Cutis 1978; 22: 515–520, 522–528

55. Leyden JJ, Sulzberger MB: Topical antibiotics and minor skin trauma. Am Fam Phys 1981; 23: 121–125

56. Langford JH, Benrimoj SI: Clinical rationale for topical antimicrobial preparations. J Antimicrob Chemother 1996; 37: 399–402

57. Fleming A: The action of chemical and physiological antiseptics in a septic wound. Br J Surg 1919; 7: 99–129

58. Brennan SS, Leaper DJ: The effect of antiseptics on the healing wound: a study using the rabbit ear chamber. Br J Surg 1985; 72: 780–782

59. Lineaweaver W, McMorris S, Soucy D, et al: Cellular and bacterial toxicities of topical antimicrobials. Plst Reconst Surg 1985; 75:394–396

60. Damour O, Hua SZ, Lasne F, et al: Cytotoxicity evaluation of antiseptics and antibiotics on cultured human fibroblasts and keratinocytes. Burns 1992; 18:479–485

61. Smoot EC 3rd, Kucan JO, Roth A, et al: In vitro toxicity testing for antibacterials against human keratinocytes. Plast Reconst Surg 1991; 87:917–924

62. Cooper ML, Laxer JA, Hansbrough JF: The cytotoxic effects of commonly used topical antimicrobial agents on human fibroblasts and keratinocytes. J Trauma 1991; 31:775–784

63. Leyden JJ, Bartelt NM: Comparison of topical antibiotic ointments, a wound protectant, and antiseptics for the treatment of human blister wounds contaminated with Staphylococcus aureus. J Fam Pract 1987; 24:601–604

64. Tatnall FM, Leigh IM, Gibson JR: Comparative study of antiseptic toxicity on basal keratinocytes, transformed human keratinocytes and fibroblasts. Skin Pharmacol 1990; 3:157–163

65. Boyce ST, Warden GD, Holder IA: Noncytotoxic combinations of topical antomocrobial agents for use with cultured skin substitutes. Antimic Agents Chemother 1995; 39:1324–1328

66. Rietchel RL, Fowler JF: The role of age, sex and color of skin in contact dermatitis. In: Rietchel RL, Fowler JF (eds) Fisher's Contact Dermatitis, 4th edn. Baltimore: Williams & Wilkins. 1995; pp 41–65

67. Dooms-Goossens A, Degreef H, Parijs M, et al: A retrospective study of patch test results from 163 patients with stasis dermatitis or leg ulcers. Dermatologica 1979; 159:93–100

68. Wilson CL, Cameron J, Powell SM, et al: High incidence of contact dermatitis in leg-ulcer patients – implications for management. Clin Exp Dermatol 1991; 16:250–253

69. Fraki JE, Peltonen L, Hopsu-Havu VK: Allergy to various components of topical preparations in stasis dermatitis and leg ulcer. Contact Dermatitis 1979; 5:97–100

70. Zaki I, Shall L, Dalziel KL: Bacitracin: a significant sensitizer in leg ulcer patients? Contact Dermatitis 1994; 31:92–94

71. Lindemayr H, Drobil M: Eczema of the lower leg and contact allergy. Hautarzt 1985; 36:227–231

72. Reichert-Penetrat S, Barbaud A, Weber M, et al: Leg ulcers. Allergologic studies of 359 cases. Ann Dermatol Venereol 1999; 126:131–135

73. Nishioka K, Seguchi T, Yasuno H, et al: The results of ingredient patch testing in contact dermatitis elicited by povidone-iodine preparations. Contact Dermatitis 2000; 42:90–94

74. Erdmann S, Hertl M, Merk HF: Allergic contact dermatitis from povidone-iodine. Contact Dermatitis 1999; 40:331–332

75. Niedner R: Cytotoxicity and sensitization of povidone-iodine and other frequently used unti-infective agents. Dermatology 1997; 195:89–92

76. Waran KD, Munsick RA: Anaphylaxis from povidone-iodine. Lancet 1995; 345:1506

77. Reynolds NJ, Harman RR: Allergic contact dermatitis from chlorhexidine diacetate in a skin swab. Contact Dermatitis 1990; 22:103–104

78. Degreef H, Dooms-Goossens A: Patch testing with silver sulfadiazine cream. Contact Dermatitis 1985; 12:33–37

79. McKenna SR, Latenser BA, Jones LM, et al: Serious silver sulphadiazine and mafenide acetate dermatitis. Burns 1995; 21:310–312

80. Van Den Hoogenband HM: Treatment of leg ulcers with split- thickness skin grafts. Dermatol Surg Oncol 1984; 10:605–608

81. Gasset AR, Ishii Y: Cytotoxicity of chlorhexidine. Can J Ophthalmol 1975; 10:98–100

82. Faddis D, Daniel D, Boyer J: Tissue toxicity of antiseptic solutions. A study of rabbit articular and periarticular tissues. J Trauma 1977; 17:895–897

83. Kimbrough RD: Review of the toxicity of hexachlorophene. Arch Environ Health 1971; 23:119–122

84. Disinfectants and preservatives. In: Kathleen Parfitt (ed) Martindale – The Complete Drug Reference. 32nd edn. London: Pharmaceutical Press. 1999; pp 1116–1117

85. Drosou A, Falabella A, Kirsner RS: Antiseptics on wounds: An area of controversy. Wounds 2003; 15:149–166

86. Eaglstein WH, Falanga V: Chronic wounds. Surg Clin North Am 1997; 77:689–700

87. Monafo WW, Freedman B: Topical therapy for burns. Surg Clin North Am 1987; 67:133–145

88. Pirnay JP, De Vos D, Cochez C, et al: Molecular epidemiology of Pseudomonas aeruginosa colonization in a burn unit: persistence of a multidrug-resistant clone and a silver sulfadiazine-resistant clone. J Clin Microbiol 2003; 41:1192–1202

89. Wilson MJ, Weightman AJ, Wade WG: Applications of molecular ecology in the characterization of uncultured microorganisms associated with human disease. Rev Med Microbiol 1997; 8:91–101

90. Caputo GM, Cavanagh PR, Ulbrecht JS, et al: Assessment and management of foot disease in patients with diabetes. N Engl J Med 1994; 331:854–860

91. Slater R, Ramot Y, Rapoport M: Diabetic foot ulcers: principles of assessment and treatment. Isr Med Assoc J 2001; 3:59–62

92. Slater R, Lazarovitch Z, Boldur I, et al: Culturing the infected diabetic foot ulcer: swabs versus tissue specimens. In: Israel Diabetes Annual: Proceedings of the 18th meeting of the Israel Diabetes Association. Tel Aviv, Israel, 2001

93. Basak S, Dutta SK, Gupta S, et al: Bacteriology of wound infection: evaluation by surface swab and quantitative full thickness wound biopsy culture. J Indian Med Assoc 1992; 90:33–34

94. Pellizzer G, Strazzabosco M, Presi S, et al: Deep tissue biopsy vs. superficial swab culture monitoring in the microbiological assessment of limb-threatening diabetic foot infection. Diabet Med 2001; 18:822–827

95. Wheat LJ, Allen SD, Henry M, et al: Diabetic foot infections: Bacteriologic analysis. Arch Intern Med 1986; 146:1935–1940
96. Lee PC, Turnidge J, McDonald PJ: Fine-needle aspiration biopsy in diagnosis of soft tissue infections. J Clin Microbiol 1985; 22:80–83
97. Sapico FL, Witte JL, Canawati HN, et al: The infected foot of the diabetic patient: quantitative microbiology and analysis of clinical features. Rev Infect Dis 1984; 6:S171–S176
98. Buchanan K, Heimbach DM, Minshew BH, et al: Comparison of quantitive and semiquantitative culture techniques for burn biopsy. J Clin Microbiol 1986; 23:258–261
99. Bello YM, Falabella AF, DeCaralho H, et al: Infection and wound healing. Wounds 2001; 13:127–131
100. Davis SC, Mertz PM, Eaglstein WH: The wound environment: implications from research studies for healing and infection. In: Krasner D, Rodeheaver G, Sibbald G (eds) Chronic Wound Care, 1st edn. Wayne, PA: HMP Communications. 2001; pp 253–263
101. Potera C: Forging a link between biofilms and disease. Science 1999; 283:1837–1839

Topical Antibacterial Agents **11**

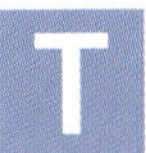

> he germ is nothing; the terrain is everything.
>
> (Attributed to Louis Pasteur on his deathbed, 1895)
>
> 

Contents

11.1 Overview

This chapter reviews topical antibacterial preparations used for cutaneous ulcers. The preparations discussed below are antiseptics. As stated in the previous chapter, these compounds exhibit non-selective toxicity, directed against any living tissue. The damage is not only to the pathogenic microorganisms but also, to a variable extent, to the host's cells. The degree of toxicity of these compounds is determined by the nature and concentration of their active ingredients, or by the presence or absence of additional substances such as surfactants or alcohol. Of the substances discussed, the only one that cannot be considered a pure antiseptic agent is silver sulfadiazine, since it contains an antibiotic component – sulfadiazine.

This chapter discusses the information and hypotheses relating to antiseptics and their mode of action, indication for use, and clinical guidelines. Substances having a high degree of toxicity and not recommended for use on cutaneous ulcers, such as chlorhexidine [1, 2], hexachlorophene [3, 4], or surfactants [5], will not be discussed. Other substances (e.g., hydrogen peroxide) will be mentioned, although their use on cutaneous ulcers is controversial.

11.2 Oxidizing Agents

11.2.1 Hydrogen Peroxide

The active oxidant form, which has a detrimental effect on living tissues, is not hydrogen peroxide itself but rather the free hydroxyl radicals formed by its decomposition [6]. Hydrogen peroxide, in concentrations of 3–6%, is effective against bacteria. At higher concentrations it kills other organisms, including spores. However, it should not be used on tissues at those concentrations, since it may cause irritating burns to skin and mucous membranes [7].

In fibroblast culture studies, 3% hydrogen peroxide solution was more toxic to fibroblasts than to bacteria [8]. It inhibited keratinocyte migration and proliferation when used in low concentrations [9].

A few studies have suggested that hydrogen peroxide has a beneficial effect on wound healing. Tur et al. [10] showed that topical use of hydrogen peroxide on ischemic ulcers of guinea pigs might enhance blood recruitment to the ulcer site and adjacent skin, as well as to distant sites. Nevertheless, in view of the toxicity involved, in most cases the use of hydrogen peroxide on cutaneous ulcers should be avoided. Its use may be considered in difficult-to-heal ulcers that other modes of treatment have failed to clean adequately.

Recently, a topical preparation (Crystacide®) was developed in which 1% hydrogen peroxide is integrated in a network of lipid crystals combined with two monoglycerides – monoleurine and monomyristine. This product has been shown to have some antibacterial activity [11]. This form of oxidative agent may reduce the toxicity against host tissue while maintaining its antibacterial effect. More studies are required to evaluate whether this type of preparation may have beneficial effects on cutaneous ulcers.

11.2.2 Potassium Permanganate

Potassium permanganate is available as purple crystals, soluble in water. The preparation is used for soaking the treated area, or a cloth soaked in potassium permanganate may be applied repeatedly to the wound. The solution should be diluted to a concentration of 0.01% (1 in 10,000 solution) so as to achieve a light pink color [12].

Higher concentrations of potassium permanganate are not recommended and may damage the ulcer tissue. Very high concentrations of potassium permanganate may be caustic. An excessively high concentration can be detected, since it stains the nails. Reports of fatalities following ingestion of potassium permanganate attest to its toxicity [13, 14].

11.3 Iodines

Iodine in its various chemical forms has been used for two centuries in the management of wounds. Iodine can penetrate cell walls of microorganisms and is active against bacteria, viruses, and fungi. Its effect is attributed to the disruption of proteins and nucleic acids [15].

11.3.1 Povidone-Iodine

Povidone-iodine is a complex of iodine with povidone and is the most widely used form of iodine as an antiseptic. This complex provides a reservoir of iodine, with a gradual release of iodine to the target tissue. For management of wounds or chronic skin ulcers, povidone-iodine is available as a solution or as an ointment, in concentrations of 4–10% [16].

The principles of management of cutaneous ulcers (as described in Chap. 20) also apply to povidone-iodine. In solution form, it should be used for secreting wounds, while the ointment is intended for dry wounds, or for chronic ulcers covered by dry crust. The effectiveness of povidone-iodine wanes after a few hours, so the dressing needs to be replaced twice daily [17].

At lower concentrations, povidone-iodine is also available as a surgical scrub or skin cleanser, with 0.75% iodine incorporated in a detergent base [18].

Several studies have demonstrated the potential toxicity of povidone-iodine to human keratinocytes and fibroblasts [8, 19, 20]. One-percent povidone-iodine was found to be toxic to human fibroblasts when added to in vitro cultures. However, in a concentration of 1:1000, bactericidal activity was still demonstrated, with no evidence of human-fibroblast toxicity [8].

Contact sensitivity may occur following the use of povidone-iodine [21–23], although it is less frequent compared with neomycin, a commonly used topical antibiotic [24]. Acute generalized urticaria-angioedema has been reported following the topical use of povidone-iodine [25], and anaphylaxis has occurred following vaginal application [26]. In any patient, inflammatory changes of the skin around the ulcer, accompanied by itching, necessitate immediate discontinuation of the treatment.

Numerous clinical trials have been performed on the effectiveness of povidone-iodine on cutaneous ulcers, yielding conflicting results, several of which are discussed below.

Pierard-Franchimont et al [27] compared the effect of povidone-iodine solution with hydrocolloid with that of hydrocolloid alone, as well as with elastic stockings. There was no statistically significant difference in wound healing between the two groups after eight weeks of treatment.

A unique study was published in 2002 by Fumal et al. [28], involving 51 patients who each had at least two chronic leg ulcers of similar nature. The wound beds were described as dull and dark red with dispersed yellowish foci. In 17 of the patients, one of the two ulcers was treated with hydrocolloid dressings and saline rinsing three times a week, while the second ulcer was treated similarly with povidone-iodine solution applied underneath the hydrocolloid dressing. They measured the surface areas of the ulcers after three and six weeks of treatment. The use of povidone-iodine significantly improved the rate of healing and lowered the time required to achieve complete healing of the ulcers.

The effect of povidone-iodine dressings was compared with that of hydrocolloid dressings. No statistically significant difference in healing was found between the two groups after 56 days of treatment [29].

11.3.2 Other Iodine Compounds

Other formulations of iodine have been studied, such as iodoform, a slow-release iodine preparation [16], and cadexomer-iodine gel, which contains microspheres that are intended to absorb bacteria and exudate, while slowly releasing iodine into the wound. This issue is detailed in Chap. 8.

■ **Toxicity of Iodine Compounds.** As stated in the previous chapter, there is not always a clear concordance between *in vitro* results and the actual clinical outcome when antiseptic substances are applied to human chronic ulcers.

This is especially applicable to advanced forms of iodine compounds such as cadexomer-iodine®. Recent evidence suggests that low-concentration slow-release formulations of iodine do not present a significant risk of toxicity. Avoiding their use based on the results of *in vitro* studies of the past, therefore, is evidently not justified [30, 31].

11.4 Chlorines

Hypochlorites are common chlorine-releasing compounds, widely used in the management of cutaneous ulcers. They have a wide spectrum of antimicrobial activity against bacteria, fungi, and viruses.

It is not clear how chlorine compounds exert their antimicrobial activity. Possible mechanisms involve the denaturation of proteins, the inactivation of nucleic acids, and the inactivation of certain key enzymatic reactions within the cell [15, 32].

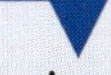

Chlorine compounds commonly used are:
- Eusol
- Dakin's solution
- Milton's solution

Eusol (Edinburgh University Solution of Lime) consists of a chlorinated lime and boric-acid solution containing 0.25% chlorine [33]. Sodium hypochlorite solutions such as Dakin's solution or Milton's solution, diluted up to 0.5% of available chlorine [34], are used on cutaneous ulcers.

All chlorine compounds were toxic to human tissue when tested on keratinocyte or fibroblast cultures [19, 20]. When applied to open wounds that were healing by secondary intention, Eusol was shown to prolong the acute inflammatory response [35]. Brennen et al. [36] demonstrated the pronounced detrimental effect of Eusol on granulation tissue in animal models following its application to healing tissue. In light of the above, chlorine compounds should be used on cutaneous ulcers for limited periods of time only, the purpose being to cleanse the ulcer bed.

11.5 Silver

11.5.1 General Comments

Silver and silver compounds, known for their antibacterial effect, have been used in medicine since the nineteenth century [37, 38]. Silver nitrate and later silver sulfadiazine have been used in recent decades as the treatments of choice for burns.

The bacteriostatic properties of silver ions were evaluated in vitro by Deltch et al. [39] using a woven nylon cloth coated with metallic silver. The antibacterial effects were shown to be proportional to the concentration of silver ions around the organisms tested. In vivo tests [40–42] have demonstrated the antibacterial effect of silver in a variety of organisms, including *Staphylococcus aureus*, *Esherichia coli*, *Pseudomonas aeruginosa*, and *Proteus mirabilis*. The bacteriocidal action of silver is proportional to the amount of silver and its rate of release [38]. Silver denatures nucleic acids, thereby inhibiting bacterial replication [43, 44].

Compared to the situation with antibiotic substances, bacteria show a relatively low tendency to develop resistance to silver or silver compounds [45, 46]. Furthermore, silver is effective against *Candida* species [38, 47] by interfering with the normal synthesis of the yeast cell wall. Wright et al. reported the effectiveness of topical silver against fungal infections in burns [48].

There is also evidence that silver ions can damage host tissue by interfering with fibroblast proliferation, thus possibly impairing wound-healing processes [49–51]. Data on the possible toxicity of silver sulfadiazine are discussed below.

Currently, silver compounds may be used in the treatment of cutaneous ulcers in the form of silver sulfadiazine. Novel modes of dressings incorporating silver have been introduced, such as Actisorb (discussed in Chap. 8).

11.5.2 Silver Sulfadiazine

Silver sulfadiazine (SSD) is prepared as a water-soluble cream in a concentration of 1%. It is composed of silver nitrate and sodium sulfadiazine, both having antibacterial qualities [52].

SSD is commonly used in the management of burns and cutaneous ulcers. It seems to be effective against a wide range of pathogenic bacteria, including *Staphylococcus aureus*, *Esherichia coli*, *Proteus*, *Enterococci* and, to some extent, *Pseudomonas* strains [52–54]. However, the presence of *Pseudomonas* strains resistant to silver sulfadiazine has been documented [54]. SSD has some effect against methicillin-resistant *Staphylococcus aureus* [55, 56]. As is the case with other silver compounds, SSD also shows a certain degree of activity against some yeast and fungi [52, 53].

■ **Contraindications.** In cases of documented sensitivity to sulfa compounds or G6PD deficiency, SSD is contraindicated. In addition, since sulfonamides are known to be possible inducers of kernicterus, silver sulfadiazine is contraindicated in pregnancy or during the first 2 months of life.

■ **Adverse Effects.** When SSD is used for cutaneous ulcers, the most common side effect is allergic contact dermatitis, manifested by redness and itching [57, 58]. In most cases, the sensitivity is to the vehicle component and not to the active ingredient. Usually, these reactions are well tolerated and can be easily managed by avoiding topical application or by using steroid topical preparations, if needed. Other adverse effects of SSD have been reported following its use for widespread burns, including transient leukopenia [59, 60] and methemoglobinemia [61].

■ **Silver Sulfadiazine and Cutaneous Ulcers.** SSD is applied twice a day to cutaneous ulcers, and care must be taken to remove all traces of the substance from the ulcer bed when changing the dressing. Following the topical use of SSD a proteinaceous gel forms over the wound surface area, which must be distinguished from a purulent discharge.

■ **Silver Toxicity.** Not surprisingly, as with other antiseptic compounds, the antimicrobial activity of silver is associated with some degree of toxicity to host tissues. *In vitro* studies of keratinocyte cultures have demonstrated significant toxicity against human keratinocytes [20, 51]. *In vivo* studies on the effect of SSD on epithelialization have shown contradictory results. In most studies, in fact, SSD has not been found to delay epithelialization [62–64]. A significant delay in wound contraction following the use of SSD has been documented [64, 65].

■ **Clinical Studies.** Several clinical studies on cutaneous ulcers comparing the effect of SSD with that of saline cleansing plus non-adherent dressing showed no statistically significant differences in wound healing [66]. However, other studies did show a beneficial effect of SSD.

Bishop et al. [67] conducted a prospective, randomized study on the healing of venous ulcers, comparing the effect of SSD with that of tripeptide-copper complex or placebo. SSD was found to be significantly more effective than the other two preparations in reducing the ulcer area.

Van den Hoogenenband documented better healing results of chronic leg ulcers treated by split-thickness skin grafting when silver sulfadiazine had been applied over a period of five days before the grafting procedure [68].

The unique study quoted above in reference to povidone-iodine [28] also included an arm involving the use of SSD: In 17 of the patients who had two chronic leg ulcers of similar nature, one of the two ulcers was treated with hydrocolloid dressings and saline rinse, while the other ulcer was treated similarly, but with the addition of SSD applied underneath the hydrocolloid dressing. They measured the surface areas of the ulcers after three and six weeks of treatment. Those ulcers treated with SSD showed a modest improvement over those treated with hydrocolloid alone.

■ **Final Comment.** The information presented above should be considered when SSD is applied; it should be used for only a limited period of time. Most of the antibacterial substances in this chapter should be used for limited periods of time, basically with the aim of cleansing the wound and protecting against infection. Once the ulcer is clean, more definitive treatment should be used.

Examples of dressings containing silver:
- Acticoat with Silcryst® nanocrystals – Smith & Nephew
- Actisorb plus® – Johnson & Johnson (a charcoal dressing)
- Actisorb silver 220® – Johnson & Johnson (a charcoal dressing)
- Aquacel AG® – Convatec
- Contreet foam® – Coloplast
- Contreet hydrocolloid® – Coloplast

11.6 Other Antiseptics

11.6.1 Antiseptic Dyes

Antiseptic dyes have been used for many years to disinfect wounds and chronic skin ulcers [69]. Substances such as **gentian violet** (crystal violet) or **brilliant green** are known to have antibacterial properties against gram-positive and gram-negative bacteria. Gentian violet was reported to be effective in the eradication of methicillin-resistant *Staphylococcus aureus* strains from pressure ulcers [70]. Brilliant green was also shown to be especially effective against dermatophytes and yeasts [69].

However, both substances have been found to be potent inhibitors of wound healing. Neidner at al. [71] found that both dyes reduced granulation tissue formation to 5% of the normal amount. There are also reports of significant tissue damage caused by gentian violet, and of its inhibitory effect on wound healing [72–74]. In addition, necrotic skin reactions have been documented following the use of gentian violet [75], and there have been reports of a possible carcinogenic effect of antiseptic dyes [75, 76]. Therefore, these dyes are contraindicated in the treatment of cutaneous ulcers.

Among other antiseptic dyes are eosin, a fluorescent dye, used in a concentration of 0.5%, which has an antibacterial effect and does not interfere with wound healing [69]. Fuchsin is a mixture of rosaniline and pararosaniline. It has an antimycotic effect [69] and is used only in the form of 'solutio castellani cum colore'.

There are no evidence-based clinical data regarding the use of eosin or fuchsin on cutaneous ulcers.

11.6.2 Burow's Solution

Burow's solution, named after Karl August von Burow (1809–1874), has been used since the nineteenth century [77]. At present, it is employed mainly as a local otological preparation for the treatment of discharging ear. In its diluted form, it may be applied to the skin as a wet dressing to oozing areas, including secreting cutaneous ulcers [78, 79]. It is composed of aluminum acetate, prepared from aluminum sulfate and acetic acid, and purified water. It contains about 0.65% aluminum salts [78]. The solution must be freshly prepared and used within a few days.

The solution is said to have an antiseptic effect, which may be attributed to its acidity. Being hygroscopic, it can absorb secretions. This quality further supports its use on secreting cutaneous ulcers.

In vitro studies have demonstrated that Burow's solution may have a certain inhibitory effect on bacteria such as *Pseudomonas aeruginosa*, *Staphylococcus aureus*, and *Proteus mirabilis* [80], as well as on species of fungi and yeasts [81].

In a double-blind, randomized study comparing the effect of Burow's solution with that of gentamicin sulfate in the treatment of otorrhea, no significant difference was observed between the preparations. In contrast to gentamicin, however, development of resistant organisms was not found following treatment with Burow's solution [82]. At present, there are no adequate data regarding the efficacy of Burow's solution on cutaneous ulcers.

11.7 Conclusion

Under certain circumstances, one may consider using the substances discussed in this chapter to cleanse cutaneous ulcers. Be aware, however, of possible damage to the wound tissues, or possible impairment of wound healing that may follow the use of these substances.

There may be a price to pay in order to control infection and achieve a cleaner ulcer. Therefore, this treatment is meant to be used for only short periods of time, and once the ulcer is clean, other forms of treatment should be employed.

References

1. Damour O, Hua SZ, Lasne F, et al: Cytotoxicity evaluation of antiseptics and antibiotics on cultured human fibroblasts and keratinocytes. Burns 1992; 18: 479–485
2. Gasset AR, Ishii Y: Cytotoxicity of chlorhexidine. Can J Ophthalmol 1975; 10: 98–100
3. Faddis D, Daniel D, Boyer J: Tissue toxicity of antiseptic solutions. A study of rabbit articular and periarticular tissues. J Trauma 1977; 17: 895–897
4. Kimbrough RD: Review of the toxicity of hexachlorophene. Arch Environ Health 1971; 23: 119–122
5. Eaglstein WH, Falanga V: Chronic wounds. Surg Clin North Am 1997; 77: 689–700
6. Murray PR, Rosenthal KS, Kobayashi GS, et al: Sterilization, disinfection, and antisepsis. In: Murray PR, Rosenthal KS, Kobayashi GS, Pfaller MA (eds) Medical Microbiology, 3rd edn. St. Louis: Mosby. 1988; pp 74–78
7. Disinfectants and preservatives. In: Kathleen Parfitt (ed) Martindale – The Complete Drug Reference, 32nd edn. London: Pharmaceutical Press. 1999; pp 1116–1117
8. Lineaweaver W, McMorris S, Soucy D, et al: Cellular and bacterial Toxicities of topical antimicrobials. Plast Reconstr Surg 1985; 75: 394–396
9. O'Toole EA, Goel M, Woodley DT: Hydrogen peroxide inhibits human keratinocyte migration. Dermatol Surg 1996; 22: 525–529
10. Tur E, Bolton L, Constantine BE: Topical hydrogen peroxide treatment of ischemic ulcers in the guinea pig: blood recruitment in multiple skin sites. J Am Acad Dermatol 1995; 33: 217–221
11. Christensen OB, Anehus S: Hydrogen peroxide cream: an alternative to topical antibiotics in the treatment of impetigo contagiosa. Acta Derm Venereol (Stockh) 1994; 74: 460–462
12. Disinfectants and preservatives. In: Kathleen Parfitt (ed) Martindale – The Complete Drug Reference, 32nd edn. London: Pharmaceutical Press. 1999; pg 1123
13. Southwood T, Lamb CM, Freeman J: Ingestion of potassium permanganate crystals by a three-year-old boy. Med J Aust 1987; 146: 639–640
14. Middleton SJ, Jacyna M, McClaren D, et al: Haemorrhagic pancreatitis – a cause of death in severe po-

tassium permanganate poisoning. Postgrad Med J 1990; 66:657–658

15. Rutala WA: Antisepsis, disinfection, and sterilization in hospitals and related institutions. In: Murray PR, Baron EJ, Pfaller MA, Tenover FC, Yolken RH (eds) Manual of Clinic Microbiology, 6th edn. Washington: ASM Press. 1995; pp 227–245

16. Disinfectants and preservatives. In: Kathleen Parfitt (ed): Martindale – The Complete Drug Reference, 32nd edn. London: Pharmaceutical Press. 1999; pp 1123–1124

17. Georgiade NG, Harris WA: Open and closed treatment of burns with povidone iodine. Plast Reconstr Surg 1973; 52:640–644

18. Burks RI: Povidone-iodine solution in wound treatment. Phys Ther 1998; 78:212–218

19. Smoot EC 3rd, Kucan JO, Roth A, et al: In vitro toxicity testing for antibacterials against human keratinocytes. Plast Reconstr Surg 1991; 87:917–924

20. Cooper ML, Laxer JA, Hansbrough JF: The cytotoxic effects of commonly used topical antimicrobial agents on human fibroblasts and keratinocytes. J Trauma 1991; 31:775–784

21. Kozuka T: Patch testing to exclude allergic contact dermatitis caused by povidone-iodine. Dermatology 2002; 204:96–98

22. Nishioka K, Seguchi T, Yasuno H, et al: The results of ingredient patch testing in contact dermatitis elicited by povidone-iodine preparations. Contact Dermatitis 2000; 42:90–94

23. Erdmann S, Hertl M, Merk HF: Allergic contact dermatitis from povidone-iodine. Contact Dermatitis 1999; 40:331–332

24. Niedner R: Cytotoxicity and sensitization of povidone-iodine and other frequently used unti-infective agents. Dermatology 1997; 195:89–92

25. Lopez Saez MP, de Barrio M, Zubeldia JM, et al: Acute lgE-mediated generalized urticaria-angioedema after application of povidone-iodine. Allergol Immunopathol (Madr) 1998; 26 23–26

26. Waran KD, Munsick RA: Anaphylaxis from povidone-iodine. Lancet 1995; 345:1506

27. Pierard-Franchimont C, Paquet P, Arrese JE, et al: Healing rate and bacterial necrotizing vasculitis in venous leg ulcers. Dermatology 1997; 194:383–387

28. Fumal I, Braham C, Paquet P, et al: The beneficial toxicity paradox of antimicrobials in leg ulcer healing impaired by a polymicrobial flora: a proof of concept study. Dermatology 2002; 204:70–74

29. O'Meara SM, Cullum NA, Majid M, Sheldon TA: Systemic review of antimicrobial agents used for chronic wounds. Br J Surg 2001; 88:4–21

30. Donohue K, Rausch H, Falanga V: Wound bed preparation. In: Rovee DT, Maibach HI (eds) The Epidermis in Wound Healing. Boca Raton, CRC Press. 2004; pp 255-264.

31. Kirsner RS, Martin LK, Drosou A: Wound microbiology and the use of antibacterial agents. In: Rovee DT, Maibach HI (eds) The Epidermis in Wound Healing. Boca Raton: CRC Press. 2004; pp 155-182.

32. Dychdala GR: Chlorine and chlorine compounds. In: Block SS (ed) Disinfection, Sterilization and Preservation. 4th edn. Philadelphia: Lea & Febiger. 1991; pp 131–151

33. Leaper DJ: Eusol: Still awaiting proper clinical trials. Br Med J 1992; 304:930–931

34. Mertz PM, Alvarez OM, Smerbeck RV, et al: A new in vivo model for the evaluation of topical antiseptics on superficial wounds. Arch Dermatol 1984; 120:58–62

35. Brennan SS, Foster ME, Leaper DJ: Antiseptic toxicity in wound healing by secondary intention. J Hosp Infect 1986; 8:263–267

36. Brennan SS, Leaper DJ: The effect of antiseptics on the healing wound: a study using the rabbit ear chamber. Br J Surg 1985; 72:780–782

37. Spadaro JA, Chase SE, Webster DA: Bacterial inhibition by electrical activation of percutaneous silver implants. J Biomed Mater Res 1986; 20:565–577

38. Lansdown AB: Silver I. Its antibacterial properties and mechanism of action. J Wound Care 2002; 11:125–130

39. Deitch EA, Marino AA, Gillespie TE, et al: Silver-nylon: a new antimicrobial agent. Antimicrob Agents Chemother 1983; 23:356–359

40. Colmano G, Edwards SS, Barranco SD: Activation of antibacterial silver coatings on surgical implants by direct current: preliminary studies in rabbits. Am J Vet Res 1980; 41:964–966

41. Tsai WC, Chu CC, Chiu SS, et al: In vitro quantitative study of newly made antibacterial braided nylon sutures. Surg Gynecol Obstet 1987; 165:207–211

42. Chu CC, Tsai WC, Yao JY, et al: Newly made antibacterial braided nylon sutures. I. In vitro qualitative and in vivo preliminary biocompatibility study. J Biomed Mater Res 1987; 21:1281–1300

43. Wysor MS, Zollinhofer RE: On the mode of action of silver sulphadiazine. Pathol Microbiol 1972; 38:296–308

44. Modak SM, Fox CL Jr: Binding of silver sulfadiazine to the cellular components of Pseudomonas aeruginosa. Biochem Pharmacol 1973; 22:2391–2404

45. Lowbury EJ, Babb JR, Bridges K, et al: Topical chemoprophylaxis with silver sulphadiazine and silver nitrate chlorhexidine creams: emergence of sulphonamide-resistant. Gram-negative bacilli. Br Med J 1976; 1:493–496

46. Fuller FW, Parrish M, Nance FC: A review of the dosimetry of 1% silver sulphadiazine cream in burn wound treatment. J Burn Care Rehabil 1994; 15:213–223

47. Wlodkowski TJ, Rosenkranz HS: Antifungal activity of silver sulphadiazine. Lancet 1973; 2:739–740

48. Wright JB, Lam K, Hansen D, et al: Efficacy of topical silver against fungal burn wound pathogens. Am J Infect Control 1999; 27:344–350

49. Hidalgo E, Dominguez C: Study of cytotoxicity mechanisms of silver nitrate in human dermal fibroplasts. Toxicol Lett 1998; 98:169–179

50. Hidalgo E, Bartolome R, Barroso C, et al: Silver nitrate: antimicrobial activity related to cytotoxicity in cultured human fibroblasts. Skin Pharmacol Appl Skin Physiol 1998; 11:140–151

51. McCauley RL, Li YY, Poole B, et al: Differential inhibition of human basal keratinocyte growth to silver sulfadiazine and mafenide acetate. J Surg Res 1992; 52:276–285

52. Antibacterials. In: Kathleen Parfitt (ed) Martindale – The Complete Drug Reference. 32nd edn. London: Pharmaceutical Press. 1999; pp 247, 248

53. Monafo WW, Freedman B: Topical therapy for burns. Surg Clin North Am 1987; 67:133–145

54. Pirnay JP, De Vos D, Cochez C, et al: Molecular epidemiology of Pseudomonas aeruginosa colonization in a burn unit: persistence of a multidrug-resistant clone and a silver sulfadiazine-resistant clone. J Clin Microbiol 2003; 41:1192–1202

55. Yoshida T, Ohura T, Sugihara T, et al: Clinical efficacy of silver sulfadiazine (AgSD: Geben cream) for ulcerative skin lesions infected with MRSA. Jpn J Antibiot 1997; 50:39–44

56. Marone P, Monzillo V, Perversi L, et al: Comparative in vitro activity of silver sulfadiazine, alone and in combination with cerium nitrate, against staphylococci and gram-negative bacteria. J Chemother 1998; 10:17–21

57. Degreef H, Dooms-Goossens A: Patch testing with silver sulfadiazine cream. Contact dermatitis 1985; 12:33–37

58. McKenna SR, Latenser BA, Jones LM, et al: Serious silver sulphadiazine and mafenide acetate dermatitis. Burns 1995; 21:310–312

59. Fuller FW, Engler PE: Leukopenia in non-septic burn patients receiving topical 1% silver sulfadiazine cream therapy: a survey. J Burn Care Rehabil 1988; 9:606–609

60. Thomson PD, Moore NP, Rice TL, et al: Leukopenia in acute thermal injury: evidence against topical silver sulfadiazine as the causative agent. J Burn Care Rehabil 1989; 10:418–420

61. Chou TD, Gibran NS, Urdahl K, et al: Methemoglobinemia secondary to topical silver nitrate therapy – a case report. Burns 1999; 25:549–552

62. Geronemus RG, Mertz PM, Eaglstein WH: Wound healing. The effects of topical antimicrobial agents. Arch Dermatol 1979; 115:1311–1314

63. Glesinger R, Cohen AD, Bogdanov-Berezovsky A, et al: A randomized controlled trial of silver sulfadiazine, biafine, and saline-soaked gauze in the treatment of superficial partial-thickness burn wounds in pigs. Acad Emerg Med 2004; 11:339–342

64. Watcher MA, Wheeland RG: The role of topical agents in the healing of full thickness wounds. J Dermatol Surg Oncol 1989; 15:1188–1195

65. Phillips TJ, Dover JS: Leg ulcers. J Am Acad Dermatol 1991; 25:965–987

66. Blair SD, Backhouse CM, Wright DDI, et al: Do dressings influence the healing of chronic venous ulcers? Phlebology 1988; 3:129–134

67. Bishop JB, Phillips LG, Mustoe TA, et al: A prospective randomized evaluator-blinded trial of two potential wound healing agents for the treatment of venous stasis ulcers. J Vasc Surg 1992; 16:251–257

68. Van Den Hoogenband HM: Treatment of leg ulcers with split- thickness skin grafts. J Dermatol Surg Oncol 1984; 10:605–608

69. Niedner R, Schopf E: Wound infections and antibacterial therapy. In: Westerhof W (ed) Leg Ulcers: Diagnosis and Treatment. Amsterdam: Elsevier. 1993; pp 293– 303

70. Saji M, Taguchi S, Uchiyama K, et al: Efficacy of gentian violet in the eradication of methicillin-resistant Staphylococcus aureus from skin lesions. J Hosp Infect 1995; 31:225–228

71. Niedner R, Schopf E: Inhibition of wound healing by antiseptics. Br J Dermatol 1986; 115 [Suppl]:41–44

72. Mobacken H: Gentian violet and wound repair. J Am Acad Dermatol 1986; 15:1303

73. Bjornberg A, Mobacken H: Necrotic skin reactions caused by 1% gentian violet and brilliant green. Acta Derm Vevereol 1972; 52:55–60

74. Mobacken H, Zederfeldt B: Influence of a cationic triphenylmethane dye on granulation tissue growth in vivo. An experimental study in rats. Acta Derm Venereol 1973; 53:167–172

75. Balabanova M, Popova L, Tchipeva R: Dyes in dermatology. Clin Dermatol 2003; 21:2–6

76. Disinfectants and preservatives. In: Kathleen Parfitt (ed) Martindale – The Complete Drug Reference, 32nd edn. London: Pharmaceutical Press. 1999; pp 1111–1112

77. Goldwyn RM: Carl August Burow. Plast Reconstr Surg 1984; 73:687–690

78. Wilkinson JD: Formulary of topical applications. In: Champion RH, Burton JL, Ebling FJC (eds) Rook/Wilkinson/Ebling Textbook of Dermatology. 5th edn. Oxford: Blackwell Scientific Publications. 1992; pp 3122

79. Supplementary drugs and other substances. In: Kathleen Parfitt (ed) Martindale – The Complete Drug Reference, 32nd edn. London: Pharmaceutical Press. 1999; pp 1547

80. Thorp MA, Kruger J, Oliver S, et al: The antibacterial activity of acetic acid and Burow's solution as topical otologic preparations. J Laryngol Otol 1998; 112:925– 928

81. Stern JC, Shah MK, Lucente FE: In vitro effectiveness of 13 agents in otomycosis and review of the literature. Laryngoscope 1988; 98:1173–1177

82. Clayton MI, Osborne JE, Rutherford D, et al: A double-blind, randomized, prospective trial of a topical antiseptic versus a topical antibiotic in the treatment of otorrhoea. Clin Otolaryngol 1990; 15:7–10

Skin Grafting

12

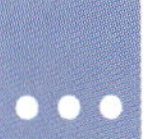

> skin for skin and all that a man has he will give for his life.
>
> *(Job II: 4)*

Contents

12.1 Introduction

Attempts to develop skin substitutes that may function as normal, healthy integument have been made for many years in the treatment of burns, surgical wounds, cutaneous ulcers, and other skin defects. The accepted term for skin substitutes originally derived from living tissues is 'biological dressings'. This term is used regardless of whether the substitutes contain living cells or not.

The classic, simple technique of applying biologic dressings is to use autologous split-thickness or full-thickness skin grafts, surgically excised from the patient's own healthy skin. Skin grafting is known to have been used some 3000 years ago in India [1–3] and there are isolated reports of its use during the nineteenth century [1–3]. The first documentation of skin grafting in humans in the 'early modern' medical literature is attributed to Reverdin in 1869 [4]. The procedure of grafting became commonly accepted, especially for burns, following the invention of the dermatome by Padgett and Hood, reported in 1939 [5].

Grafting autologous skin is still a commonly accepted method of covering a cutaneous surface denuded by a variety of causes, such as cutaneous ulcers [6–14].

Possible forms of skin grafting are as follows:

- Autograft (or 'autologous graft'): a graft originating from one part of the body and transplanted onto another area (from patient's own healthy skin)
- Isograft (or 'isogeneic graft'): Isografting usually relates to laboratory animals belonging to the same species and sharing an identical genetic makeup. In human beings, an isograft is any sort of graft transferred from one genetically identical twin to the other.
- Allograft (or 'allogeneic graft'; previously termed 'homograft'): a graft from one person to another, who do not have identical genetic characteristics; in general, it is transferred from one individual to another of the same species
- Xenograft (syn. 'heterograft'): a graft taken from an individual of one species and transplanted onto an individual of another species. (The term *zoograft* has a similar meaning and refers to a graft from an animal to a human.)

It follows that the most common type of skin grafts today are autografts. These will be dealt with in this chapter. The use of allografting is becoming more and more common, both in the form of allogeneic keratinocyte grafting and as composite grafting. That topic will be covered in Chap. 13. There is also use of xenografts, i.e., skin grafts from an animal – commonly a pig – which may have some use as a temporary biologic dressing, to be applied to extensively denuded areas, such as in large burn wounds.

12.2 Split-Thickness Skin Graft and Full-Thickness Skin Graft

The graft may be in the form of a split-thickness skin graft or a full-thickness skin graft. A split-thickness skin graft contains epidermis and a certain amount of dermis, while a full-thickness skin graft contains epidermis and the whole dermis (Figs. 12.1, 12.2)

A full-thickness skin graft offers better protection from trauma. It does not contract as much as a split-thickness skin graft and generally looks more natural after healing; thus, it is often used for aesthetic reasons. However, a full-thickness graft requires a well-vascularized recipient bed. Because of this limitation, it is not commonly used in cutaneous ulcers. On the other hand, a split-thickness skin graft results in a better 'take', even when applied to tis-

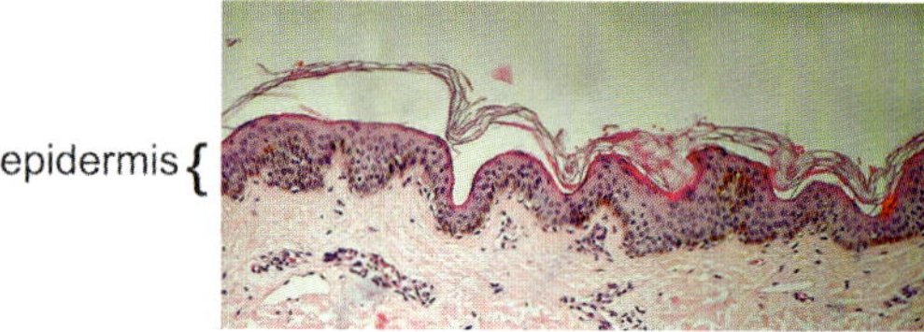

Fig. 12.2. Histological representation of a split-thickness skin graft

sue in which vascularization is not optimal and relatively reduced (Fig. 12.3). This feature makes it more appropriate for use in the management of cutaneous ulcers.

The thicker the graft, the smaller the extent of contraction of the grafted wound. Similarly, wounds covered with thin split-thickness skin grafts contract less than open wounds [15].

12.3 Preparing a Cutaneous Ulcer for Grafting

Grafting should be done only onto a viable wound surface. Prior to the application of the skin graft, the ulcer bed should be debrided to remove any necrotic tissue. Vital granulating tissue should be exposed, thereby enabling cells

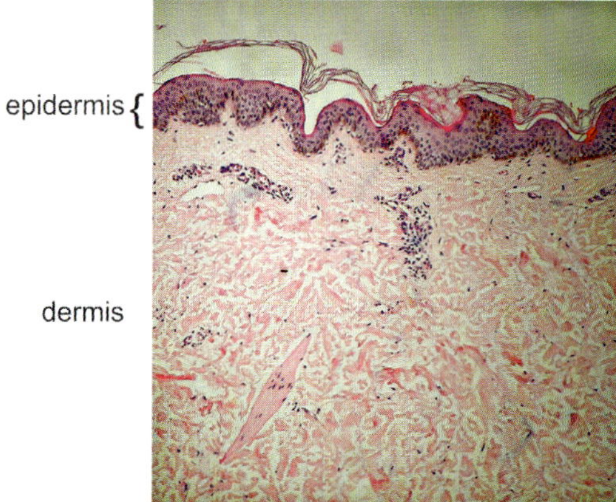

Fig. 12.1. Histological representation of a full-thickness skin graft

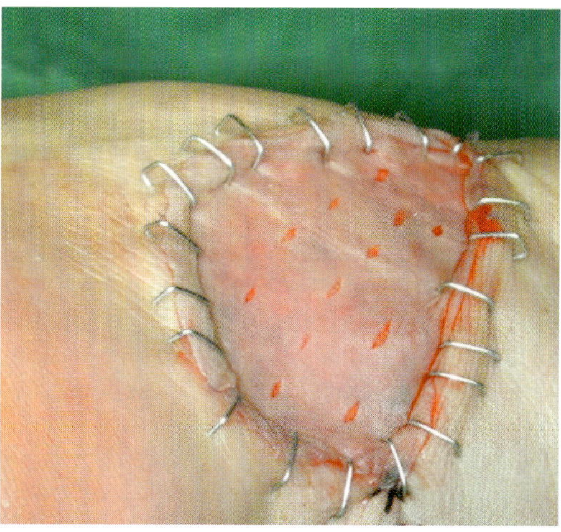

Fig. 12.3. A split-thickness graft is placed on a cutaneous ulcer. Longitudinal incisions in the graft were made in order to facilitate drainage of secretions and prevent their accumulation under the graft, which would prevent its 'taking'

in the graft to attach to the ulcer's surface and its blood supply. Note that the presence of more than 10^5 bacteria per gram of tissue should be regarded as infection (see Chap. 10).

12.4 Forms of Autologous Grafting

A simple autograft, applied as a layer, whether done with a dermatome, a scalpel, or a special grafting knife, may provide appropriate biological coverage. However, it must be remembered that the harvesting of an autograft results in a wound in the healthy donor skin, analogous to a second-degree burn. The donor wound, apart from being painful, may require a considerable amount of effort and time to heal. Therefore, several techniques have been developed to reduce the required surface area of the donor skin.

Techniques in use for applying autologous grafts are:

- Taking one sheet of grafted skin to cover all the denuded area: A split-thickness graft is harvested with a dermatome; a full-thickness graft is usually obtained using a small scalpel.
- Small pieces: One way of decreasing the required area of donor skin is to apply smaller pieces of donor skin, instead of one large sheet that covers the entire area of the ulcer. These grafts are placed onto the ulcer bed at regular intervals, to allow drainage of secretions.
- Pinch grafting was documented as early as 1869 by Reverdin [4, 16]. The skin is anesthetized, a small portion is lifted up on the point of a needle, and the top is cut off with a scalpel. Pinch grafts should be of full thickness, 3–5 mm in diameter. The grafts are evenly placed on the ulcer bed, with free spaces of 5 to 10 mm between each of the grafts. Pinch grafting has been documented several times in the past 20 years

as a possible treatment method for chronic skin ulcers [17–23].

- Punch grafts, obtained by using a punch biopsy instrument, represent another modification of full-thickness autografting. This procedure enables a smaller area of donor skin to be used, assuming that epithelialization will take place and advance peripherally from each punch. The punch method is still used [24]. The punch grafts, which may be 3–5 mm in diameter, are placed onto the ulcer's surface at regular intervals.
- Mesh grafting (Fig. 12.4): A mechanical device is used to cut multiple slits in the graft, thereby allowing it to be stretched, so that it can expand and cover a larger surface area. This procedure is commonly used for burns, where large areas of donor grafts may be needed, but not for cutaneous ulcers.

Ahnlide and Bjellerup [17] used pinch grafting for 145 therapy-resistant leg ulcers. Three months following the procedure, the average healing rate was 36%. Poskitt et al. [23] presented a randomized trial comparing autologous pinch grafting (25 patients) with porcine der-

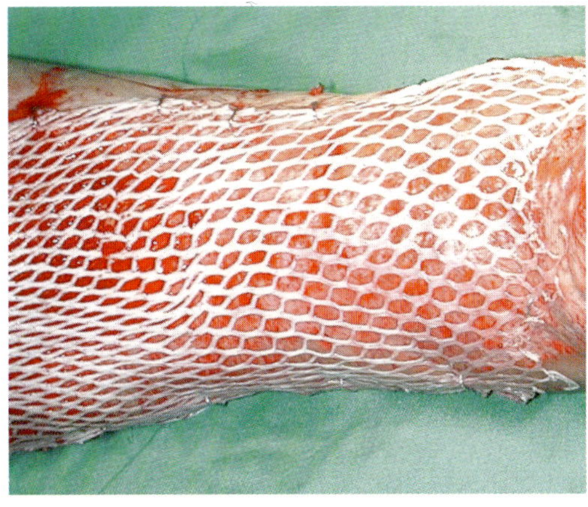

Fig. 12.4. Mesh grafting

mis dressings (28 patients). Sixty-four percent (64%) of ulcers treated by autologous pinch grafting were healed at six weeks and 74% by 12 weeks, compared with ulcers treated by porcine dermis, where healing rates were 29% and 46%, respectively, after 6 and 12 weeks.

While pinch grafting and punch grafting are usually intended for relatively small ulcers, some suggest that mesh grafting may be used for larger ulcers. Kirsner et al. [9] documented 29 patients with 36 leg ulcers of various etiology, treated by meshed split-thickness skin grafts. The grafts were harvested with a Padget dermatome and expanded through meshing to one and a half times their original size. The initial 'take' of the grafts was recorded as 'excellent'. At a mean follow-up of 11 months (three months to three years) 52% of ulcers were healed.

The information above covers simple autografts. More advanced forms such as cultured keratinocyte grafting and tissue engineering are discussed in Chap. 13.

12.5 Conclusion

In a comprehensive Cochrane review, Jones and Nelson [6] suggest that further research is needed to compare the beneficial effects of 'simple' skin grafting with those of other modes of treatment intended for venous leg ulcers. This conclusion may actually be implemented for other types of cutaneous ulcers as well.

The 'take' of the graft and the final result depend on the ulcer's condition in terms of vascularization, absence of infection, and appropriate preparation of the ulcer bed, as well as on the patient's general condition.

In our experience, a skin graft may provide suitable coverage for a cutaneous ulcer, resulting in healing. However, in some cases, the graft does not 'take' well for the same reasons that resulted in the ulceration in the first place (e.g., poor vascularization) and the ulcer does not heal. Moreover, even in cases where closure of a cutaneous ulcer is achieved by skin grafting, the final clinical result is not satisfactory – in most cases because there is no adequate proliferation of granulation tissue (Fig. 12.5). The original ulcer site usually remains as a depression

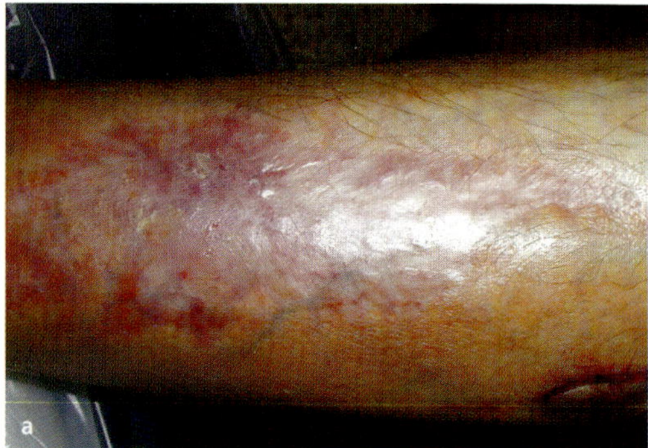
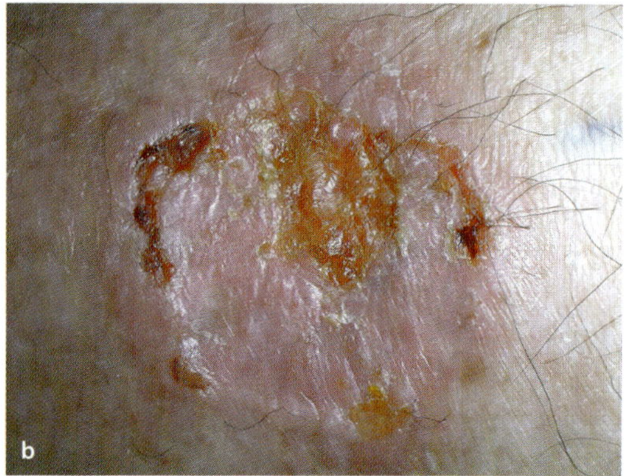

Fig. 12.5. Cutaneous ulcers following grafting and partial (**b**) and complete (**a**) healing. Note that the area is slightly depressed due to decreased production of granulation tissue during active stages of healing

in the skin, with inadequate subcutaneous tissue covered by a thin, very vulnerable cutaneous layer. Hence, autologous skin grafting of cutaneous ulcers is commonly followed by re-ulceration.

In view of the above, advanced modalities such as keratinocyte grafting, composite grafts, or preparations containing growth factors, which may stimulate proliferation of granulation tissue, may be used (see Chaps. 13, 14, and 15). The use of advanced modalities (e.g., growth factors) may indeed result in complete healing of a treated ulcer, even without skin grafting. However, in many cases this stimulus will not suffice for healing and closure – especially with relatively large chronic ulcers. It may well be that the solution to the problem of certain ulcers will lie in a combination of such advanced modalities together with skin grafting.

References

1. Ratner D: Skin grafting. From here to there. Dermatol Clin 1998; 16:75–90
2. Hauben DJ, Baruchin A, Mahler D: On the history of the free skin graft. Ann Plast Surg 1982; 9:242–245
3. Kelton PL: Skin grafts and skin substitutes. Selected Readings in Plastic Surgery 1982; 9:1–23
4. Reverdin JL: Greffe epidermique, experience faite dans le service de monsieur le docteur Guyon, a l'Hopital Necker. Bull Imp Soc Chir Paris 1869; 10: 511–515
5. Padgett EC: Skin grafting in severe burns. Am J Surg 1939; 43:626
6. Jones JE, Nelson EA: Skin Grafting for venous leg ulcers (Cochrane Review). The Cochrane Library, issue 4. 2000; Oxford: Update Software
7. Fisher JC: Skin grafting. In: Georgiade GS, Riefkohl R, Levin LS (eds): Plastic, Maxillofacial and Reconstructive Surgery. 3rd edn. Baltimore: Williams & Wilkins. 1996; pp 13–18
8. Kirsner RS, Eaglstein WH, Kerdel FA: Split-thickness skin grafting for lower extremity ulcerations. Dermatol Surg 1997; 23:85–91
9. Kirsner RS, Mata SM, Falanga V, et al: Split-thickness skin grafting of leg ulcers. Dermatol Surg 1995; 21: 701–703
10. Berretty PJ, Neumann HA, Janssen de Limpens AM, et al: Treatment of ulcers on legs from venous hypertension by split-thickness skin grafts. J Dermatol Surg Oncol 1979; 5:966–970
11. Michaelides P, Camisa C: The treatment of ulcers on legs with split- thickness skin grafts : report of a simple technique. J Dermatol Surg Oncol 1979; 5: 961–965
12. Van den Hoogenband HM: Treatment of leg ulcers with split-thickness skin grafts. J Dermatol Surg Oncol 1984; 10:605–608
13. Harrison PV: Split-skin grafting of varicose leg ulcers: a survey and the importance of assessment of risk factors in predicting outcome from the procedure. Clin Exp Dermatol 1988; 13:4–6
14. Ruffieux P, Hommel L, Saurat JH: Long-term assessment of chronic leg ulcer treatment by autologous skin grafts. Dermatology 1997; 195:77–80
15. Rudolph R: The effect of skin graft preparation on wound contraction. Surg Gynecol Obstet 1976; 142: 49–56
16. Reverdin JL: Sur la greffe epidermique. Arch Gen Med Paris 1872; 19:276–303
17. Ahnlide I, Bjellerup M: Efficacy of pinch grafting in leg ulcers of different aetiologies. Acta Derm Venereol 1997; 77:144–145
18. Steele K: Pinch grafting for chronic venous leg ulcers in general practice. J R Coll Gen Pract 1985; 35: 574–575
19. Christiansen J, Ek L, Tegner E: Pinch grafting of leg ulcers. A retrospective study of 412 treated ulcers in 146 patients. Acta Derm Venereol (Stockh) 1997; 77: 471–473
20. Millard LG, Roberts MM, Gatecliffe M: Chronic leg ulcers treated by the pinch graft method. Br J Dermatol 1977; 97:289–295
21. Oien RF, Hansen BU, Hakansson A: Pinch grafting of leg ulcers in primary care. Acta Derm Venereol (Stockh) 1998; 78:438–439
22. Ceilley RI, Rinek MA, Zuehlke RL: Pinch grafting for chronic ulcers on lower extremities. J Dermatol Surg Oncol 1977; 3:303–309
23. Poskitt KR, James AH, Lloyd-Davies ER, et al: Pinch skin grafting or porcine dermis in venous ulcers: a randomised clinical trial. Br Med J 1987; 294: 674–676
24. Mol MA, Nanninga PB, Van Eendenburg JP, et al: Grafting of venous leg ulcers. An intraindividual comparison between cultured skin equivalents and full thickness skin punch grafts. J Am Acad Dermatol 1991; 24:77–82

Skin Substitutes and Tissue-Engineered Skin Equivalents

13

Contents

13.1 Overview

The accepted term for skin substitutes that are originally derived from living tissues, whether they contain living cells when applied to the wound surface or not, is 'biological dressings'. In view of the limitations of skin grafting, as discussed in the previous chapter, a variety of substitutes have been developed. We distinguish herein between 'non-living' substitutes, which do not contain living cells, and those containing living cells, termed 'living' skin substitutes.

The products described below may be considered 'tissue-engineered' skin, according to the accepted definition, namely, skin products composed mainly of cells, skin products composed of extracellular matrix materials, or a combination of both [1, 2]. We shall focus our discussion mainly on skin products intended to be used for skin ulcers.

13.2 'Non-Living' Skin Substitutes

13.2.1 General Functions

Under the heading 'non-living skin substitutes' we include biological dressings originally derived from living tissues, but which, when applied to denuded cutaneous areas, do not contain living cells (see Table 13.1). A variety of non-living skin substitutes have been used in the treatment of burns and surgical wounds. Non-living skin substitutes function as highly effective biological dressings. They fulfill the main purposes of an optimal dressing, i.e., provision of a moist environment, prevention of water loss (indeed, dermal skin substitutes were primarily developed for the treatment of burns), and protection against external infections or trauma. Their use is usually accompanied by significant pain reduction.

Moreover, several research studies suggest that a layer of acellular dermis may serve as a template for the regeneration of a viable dermis [3–5]. Several types, described below, have been discussed in the literature. They have been proposed for use mainly in surgical wounds or burns and their efficacy in cutaneous ulcers has yet to be validated. Some are in current clinical use and some are still under research.

13.2.2 Allogeneic Cadaver Skin

Allogeneic cadaver skin may be used as a biological dressing. Devitalization of the allograft obviates its antigenic effect. The graft can be preserved by various techniques, such as cryopreservation with glycerol [6] or by freeze-drying [7]. Another possibility is to produce an

Table 13.1. Non-living skin substitutes

Non-living skin substitutes	Commercial products	Comments
Products processed from fresh cadaver skin	AlloDerm®	Cadaver skin and xenografts are not widely used by commercial companies, but rather by laboratories and skin banks in medical centers
Naturally occurring collagen matrix (processed xenografts)	CollatamFascie® E-Z-derm® Integra® Oasis® SkinTemp®	These products may be regarded as modifications of xenografts (manufactured from bovine or porcine tissue)
Synthetic collagen dressings	Biobrane® Fibracol Plus® Promogran®	Promogran also contains oxidized regenerated cellulose to neutralize the matrix metalloproteinases in the ulcer bed

acellular dermal matrix by the removal of the epidermis and the cells in the dermis [3]. Chakarbarty et al. [8] used ethylene oxide sterilization followed by immersion of the skin in 1 mol/l sodium chloride for eight h to achieve acellularization. The current clinical use of cryopreserved or acellular allografts is mainly in the management of burn wounds [9–12].

There are few reports on the use of allogeneic cadaver skin substitutes as an option for the treatment of chronic cutaneous ulcers. In 1999, Snyder et al. [13] documented treatment with cadaveric allografts in 27 patients with 34 leg ulcers of various etiologies. In 65% of patients the ulcers healed by secondary intention, and the average healing time was 113.9 days.

13.2.3 Xenografts

The most common source of xenografts (syn.: heterografts or zoografts) is porcine skin, since it is similar to human skin. Sterility is achieved by irradiation [14]; thus, the graft is actually non-living. The use of xenografts is well documented for burns, surgical wounds, and cutaneous ulcers [15–22]. The products defined as naturally occurring collagen matrix, described below, are actually processed xenografts.

13.2.4 Naturally Occurring Collagen Matrix and Collagen-Containing Dressings

Collagen has unique biologic and physical properties that, with appropriate processing and manufacturing, make it an ideal dressing product. Collagen is found in abundance in supporting tissues such as skin, fascia, tendons, and bones. Its structure is organized and aligned, and it forms strong fibers [23].

Certain scientific observations lend further support to the medical use of collagen in the management of wounds and wound healing:
- A collagen matrix may serve as a skeleton or scaffolding on which the new tissue gradually forms [24, 25].
- It has been suggested that attachment of fibroblasts to the implanted collagen enhances new collagen synthesis in the healing wound [26].
- A collagen matrix can efficiently provide the basic requirements of a dressing. Being tough in texture, it protects the ulcer and its surroundings from mechanical trauma. Its

permeability may vary depending on its method of manufacture, but in most cases it can provide a moist environment, which is desirable for the healing process.

The following discussion distinguishes between two forms of collagen dressings. The first relates to the use of collagen in its native form, i.e., as a naturally occurring collagen matrix, while the second relates to synthetic dressings that contain collagen.

13.2.4.1 Naturally Occurring Collagen Matrix

The use of natural collagen matrix represents a relatively advanced modification of the biological dressing. In practice, the products described below are sheets of xenografts (porcine or bovine) that have been processed to make them suitable for use on denuded skin areas.

There are several advantages to such products:

- The collagen is in its natural form, which preserves the normal structure and alignment of the fibers (as opposed to dressings containing collagen, which have undergone more complex processing). The manufacturers claim that the former product acts as a more natural scaffolding, which 'takes' better to the wound surface.
- Some of these products may contain growth factors that signal host cells within the wound bed to attach and proliferate on the collagen template [27].

In this group of biological dressings, more advanced modifications have been developed using non-living skin substitutes, whose structure is that of a cross-linked matrix of collagen. A graft composed of bovine collagen matrix with chondroitin-6 sulfate covered by a silicone layer (Integra®), has been shown to have a beneficial effect on burn wounds at an initial stage; a meshed autograft is applied a few weeks later [9, 25]. Another product, composed of lyophilized type-1 bovine collagen (SkinTemp®), has been used for surgical wound healing by secondary intention [28]. Bovine collagen products are thought to form a network-like architectural structure, which enhances organization of fibroblasts and newly forming collagen bundles. Degradation products of bovine collagen are considered to act as chemotactic factors, which further enhance wound repair processes [29, 30]. Another product (CollatamFascie®) is a type-1 collagen derived from bovine Achilles tendons, which has been shown to enhance healing in acute wounds and chronic cutaneous ulcers [14].

An acellular collagen matrix derived from porcine small intestine (Oasis®) has been introduced as a substitute skin covering [31, 32]. The intestine is processed to remove the serosal, smooth-muscle, and mucosal layers while retaining the submucosa. The final product is an acellular, collagenous sheet. Brown-Etris et al. [33] reported on 15 patients with leg ulcers treated with acellular matrix derived from porcine small intestinal submucosa. Wound closure was reported in seven patients within 4–10 weeks.

E-Z-derm® is another biosynthetic acellular dressing made of xenogeneic collagen matrix. It is made of porcine collagen that has been chemically cross-linked with an aldehyde. This process is claimed to impart durability to the product, enabling its storage at room temperature.

13.2.4.2 Collagen-Containing Dressings

In dressings containing collagen, the collagen has undergone more complex processing (as compared with naturally occurring collagen), so that in essence the product is synthetic. In spite of the theoretical advantages of using collagen as a dressing, results of initial experiments using collagen dressings were disappointing [34–36].

Other early developments of dressing materials containing collagen peptides were laminates such as Biobrane®. This consisted of a laminate of silicone rubber with nylon, linked with porcine collagen peptides [37]. Biobrane® was found to be an effective dressing material that provided adequate covering for surgical or burn wounds [38–40].

Another collagen-containing dressing, Fibracol®, was relatively effective in the treatment of diabetic foot ulcers when compared with regular gauze moistened with normal saline [41], and in the treatment of pressure ulcers, compared with calcium-sodium alginate dressings [42].

Recently, a new collagen-containing dressing was introduced (Promogran®). In addition to bovine collagen (55%), with its above-mentioned advantages, Promogran® also contains oxidized regenerated cellulose (45%). The latter is said to bind (and thereby neutralize) matrix metalloproteinases in the ulcer bed, thus obviating their proteolytic effects on the growth factors and matrix proteins (Fig. 13.1). Ghatnekar et al. [43] found that Promogran®, combined with good wound care, was more cost-effective than good wound care alone in the treatment of diabetic foot ulcers. Veves et al. [44] conducted a randomized, controlled trial comparing Pro-

mogran® and standard treatment with a moistened gauze in the management of diabetic foot ulcers. The results, after 12 weeks of treatment, were not statistically significant. However, among 95 patients with ulcers of less than six months' duration, 43 (45%) of those treated with Promogran® underwent healing, compared with 29 (33%) of those treated by moistened gauze. The beneficial effect of Promogran on venous leg ulcers has also been demonstrated by Vin et al. [45].

13.2.5 Conclusion

At present, non-living skin substitutes are considered to function as efficient biological dressings for cutaneous ulcers. However, the overall impression is that they do not actively stimulate or enhance wound healing, as do living substitutes.

Whether non-living skin replacements contribute further to wound healing, as compared with synthetic dressings, is questionable. Some investigators suggest, as mentioned above, that the acellular dermis may serve as a template for dermal regeneration. Some of these non-living substitutes are said to contain cytokines [27], which may render them more effective than synthetic dressings. Nevertheless, controlled research studies must be undertaken on the various types of non-living skin substitutes before this assumption can be confirmed. By the same token, further studies are needed in order to obtain a more accurate evaluation of the efficacy of newer combinations of collagen-containing dressings.

13.3 'Living' Skin Substitutes

13.3.1 General

Recently, more sophisticated techniques have been developed in an attempt to create skin equivalents and to re-establish the appropriate physiological microenvironment needed for optimal wound repair. In the following discussion, distinctions should be made between sub-

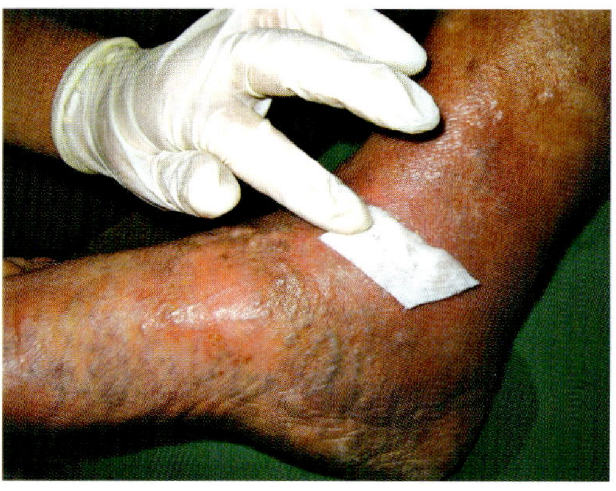

Fig. 13.1. Application of a collagen-containing dressing (Promogran) to a cutaneous ulcer

types of living equivalents, i.e., those containing epidermal components, those containing dermal components, and composite grafts containing both dermal and epidermal components.

13.3.2 Epidermal: Keratinocyte Grafts

The use of viable epidermal cells is thought to contribute to the wound repair process by actively stimulating the ulcer to heal. In 1975, Rheinwald and Green [46] described a method for culturing keratinocytes from single-cell suspensions of human epidermal cells. Their breakthrough opened new vistas in the field of

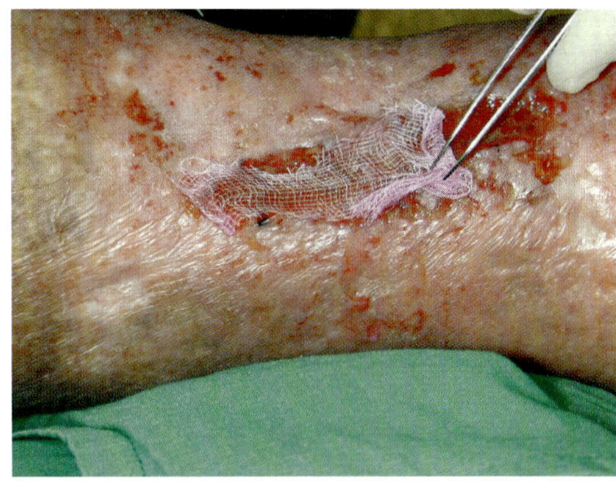

Fig. 13.4. Placing the graft on the ulcer

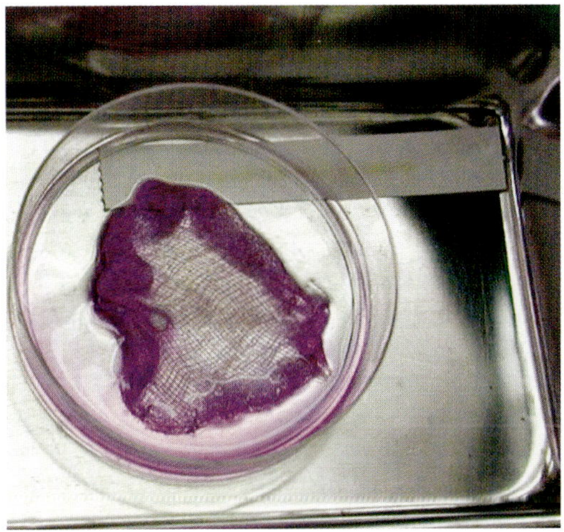

Fig. 13.2. Graft pad containing cultured keratinocytes in a Petri dish

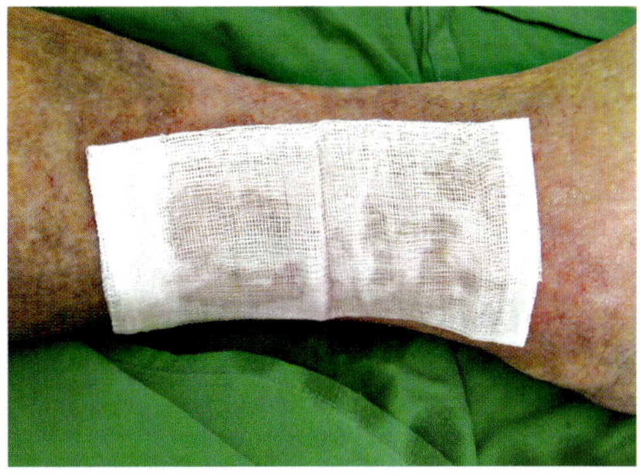

Fig. 13.5. Placing a gauze pad, moistened with saline, on the graft pad

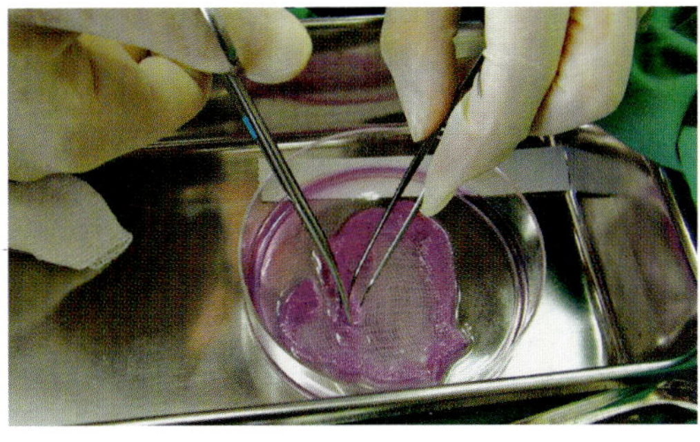

Fig. 13.3. Trimming a graft pad of cultured keratinocytes to the appropriate size preparatory to the grafting

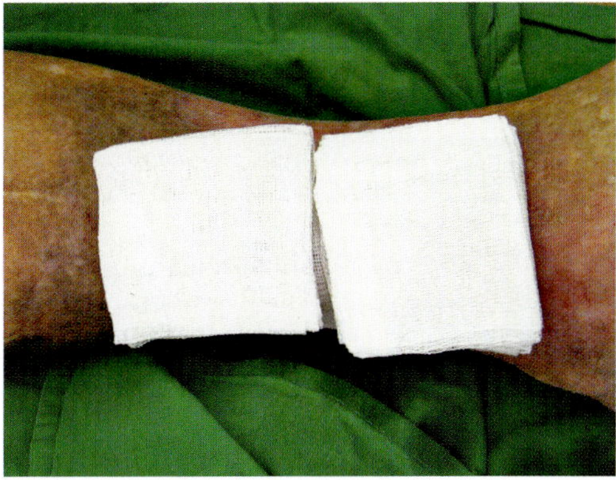

Fig. 13.6. Placing additional gauze pads to protect the graft

skin research and led to clinical applications involving cultured keratinocyte grafting (Fig. 13.2–13.6). At present, it is possible to produce multi-layered stratified skin equivalents that very closely resemble natural skin.

Initially, keratinocyte grafts were autologous grafts derived from the patient's skin on burn wounds [47–54]. They were later introduced in the management of cutaneous leg ulcers [55, 56]. At a still later stage, the method was modified by using allogeneic cultured keratinocyte grafts, derived from the foreskins of newborns [57–62]. The first group of leg ulcer patients treated by allogeneic grafts was described by Leigh et al. [58] in 1987, comprising 51 patients with 70 ulcers of various etiologies. The mean duration of the ulcers prior to the grafting procedure was 16 years. Beneficial effects were manifested either by the appearance of islands of epithelium on the ulcer bed (in 29% of the ulcers) or by enhanced migration of epithelium from the periphery of the ulcer (seen in 44% of the ulcers).

Since then, other studies have shown that topically applied allogeneic keratinocyte grafts accelerate the healing of chronic cutaneous ulcers, with similar findings: significant reduction in the ulcer area within three weeks following grafting, and complete healing of 65–83% of treated ulcers within a few weeks. In most of the ulcers, even those that did not undergo complete healing, granulation tissue formed (with a subsequent decrease in ulcer depth), with enhanced epithelialization and reduction in the ulcer surface area [59–62].

The main advantage of allogeneic keratinocyte grafts compared with autologous keratinocyte grafts lies in the fact that newborn keratinocytes are thought to be more effective in promoting healing. This effect is attributed mainly to the increased secretion of growth factors by younger keratinocytes compared with adult cells (see below) [58, 59, 62–65]. Having said this, it is our experience that even autologous keratinocyte grafts will, in many cases, promote wound healing, as shown by the proliferation of granulation tissue in the ulcer bed and advancing epithelialization.

While neonatal keratinocytes can be prepared from newborn foreskins, refrigerated and used immediately for grafting when needed, the preparation of an autologous keratinocyte graft is a more complex procedure that requires either a biopsy specimen from the patient's skin or a sample of his/her hair follicles, obtained by hair plucking [66, 67]. It takes a period of 2–3 weeks before there is sufficient epithelium to cover the ulcer surface area. This process is carried out either in specialized medical centers or by commercial companies that prepare the autologous grafts for grafting from samples of the patient's skin or hair follicles (see Table 13.2).

■ **Mechanism of Healing.** In view of the fact that patients with cutaneous ulcers report significant pain relief within a few hours of keratinocyte grafting, it seems that the graft functions as a semi-occlusive dressing that prevents dehydration and reduces pain. However, an allogeneic graft does not serve as a permanent

Table 13.2. Living skin substitutes

Living skin substitutes	Commercial product	Comments
Keratinocyte grafts	BioSeed®	Autologous-obtained from skin biopsy
	Epibase®	Autologous-obtained from skin biopsy
	Epicel®	Autologous-obtained from skin biopsy
	Epidex®	Autologous-obtained by plucking hair
Dermal grafting	Dermagraft®	
	Transcyte®	
Composite grafting	Apligraf®	
	OrCel®	

alternative cover over the ulcer, since it remains on the ulcer bed for only a short period. After a few hours, rejection of the graft occurs. The graft is then replaced by autologous cells, as demonstrated by DNA fingerprinting and the disappearance of Y chromosomes in sex-matched grafts [51].

Accumulating evidence suggests that the main factor in wound healing using allogeneic keratinocyte grafts lies in the presence of soluble growth factors produced by transplanted newborn keratinocytes [58, 59, 62–65]. The effect of growth factors is manifested clinically by the formation of healthy granulation tissue on the ulcer bed and the gradual epithelialization of its surface.

■ **Beneficial Effect.** Ideally, in order to assess the efficacy of keratinocyte grafting, one would require patients with symmetrically located (i.e., one on each leg) cutaneous ulcers; one ulcer would be grafted while the other would be treated by placebo in a controlled, double-blind procedure.

In most of the reported studies, this procedure has not been compared with an alternative therapeutic modality. Moreover, some of the studies contain methodological errors. Jones and Nelson [65] have indicated that, not infrequently, research studies have failed to present baseline data such as a history of previous ulceration, which may affect the prognosis. However, the overall impression in the medical literature nowadays is that allogeneic keratinocyte grafting, containing an epithelial component of living keratinocytes does, in fact, enhance wound healing in chronic cutaneous ulcers.

Recently, Bolivar-Flores and Kuri-Harcuch [68] documented complete healing in 10 patients with recalcitrant leg ulcers of various etiologies, using frozen allogeneic keratinocyte grafting.

Three research studies have also compared cultured keratinocyte allografts to control dressings [69–71]. Teepe et al. [69] compared the beneficial effect of cryopreserved allogeneic keratinocyte grafting vs. hydrocolloid dressings in 43 patients with 47 cutaneous ulcers. They demonstrated enhanced healing rates and increased reduction of ulcer size in the grafted group. However, there was no difference between the two groups in the number of healed ulcers at six weeks.

Lindgren et al. [70] did not demonstrate superiority of cryopreserved allogeneic keratinocyte grafting in 15 patients with chronic venous leg ulcers compared with 12 patients in a control group. The authors suggested that this observation (contradicting their previous experiments using fresh keratinocytes) might be attributed to the effect of cryopreservation.

Jones and Nelson [65] summarized the data of the relevant trials in a Cochrane review, and found no demonstrable benefit of allogeneic keratinocyte grafting over control dressings.

In our clinical experience, keratinocyte grafting does provide some degree of improvement in most cases, even in ulcers that do not heal completely. Improvement is manifested by granulation tissue formation, epithelialization advancing from the ulcer margin, and a significant reduction in the ulcer surface area.

In relatively small ulcers of up to 2–3 cm in diameter, the use of allogeneic cultured keratinocytes can provide the 'push' needed to promote complete healing and closure of the lesion. On the other hand, in larger ulcers it is unreasonable, in most cases, to expect complete healing following allogeneic keratinocyte grafting. In this particular situation, one may consider using repeated combinations of allogeneic keratinocyte grafts with autologous grafts taken from the patient himself. Alternatively, one could consider using other advanced modalities, discussed elsewhere in this book (see Chap. 20).

We have found that allogeneic keratinocyte grafting is preferable to surgical autologous split- or full-thickness skin grafts, since the former induces granulation tissue formation, which fills the wound cavity and reduces its depth.

Nowadays, cultured keratinocyte grafting is commercially available and is performed in many medical centers (mainly burn centers). These products are also produced and marketed by commercial companies (See Table 13.2).

13.3.3 Dermal Grafting

Viable dermal substitutes may be considered a step beyond non-viable forms. However, to the best of our knowledge, there are no documented studies comparing the effectiveness of the viable dermal substitute with non-viable dermis.

Dermagraft® is a viable dermal substitute which consists of a bioabsorbable mesh, upon which cryopreserved fibroblasts derived from neonatal foreskins are cultured. The cultured fibroblasts are screened for the presence of infectious organisms.

The neonatal fibroblasts proliferate within the polymer mesh, and secrete dermal matrix proteins (collagens, tenascin, vitronectin) and growth factors [72, 73]. Once the graft has been placed on the wound, it may provide an extracellular matrix and growth factors, synthesized by the transplanted fibroblasts. The mesh consists of biodegradable material which dissolves gradually within 3–4 weeks. As previously mentioned, following dermal grafting (provided the ulcer is ready), keratinocyte grafts can be placed on the fibroblast-containing dermal bed.

Each unit of Dermagraft® is supplied frozen. It is packaged in a clear bag, within a saline-based cryoprotectant, containing 10% dimethylsulfoxide and bovine serum. A Dermagraft piece, measuring 5×7.5 cm, is intended for single-use application.

Studies on diabetic foot ulcers treated with this dermal graft have shown improved healing compared with controls [9, 74–77]. Recently, Marston et al. [78] conducted a randomized, controlled, single-blind, multi-centered study, enrolling 314 patients suffering from chronic diabetic foot ulcers. The efficacy of Dermagraft® (130 patients) was compared with that of a moist saline gauze covering (115 patients). Both groups received standard care such as pressure-reducing footwear. Following 12 weeks of treatment, complete wound closure was achieved in 30% of patients treated with Dermagraft®, compared with 18.3% of patients in the control group.

Another unique randomized, controlled, single-blind, clinical trial was introduced in 1996 by Gentzkow et al. [74]. The rate of complete healing of diabetic foot ulcers was higher in patients treated with Dermagraft® than in patients in the control group. The article also evaluated the desirable frequency of Dermagraft® application, suggesting that a weekly application is better than less frequent applications.

Transcyte® is a product made of neonatal fibroblasts. The cells are cultured on nylon mesh for 4–6 weeks. The product eventually consists of dense cellular tissue (with human matrix proteins) and contains high levels of growth factors. Transcyte® is supplied in a cassette containing two transparent units, each measuring 13×19 cm. The product is intended for burn wounds. To date, the use of Transcyte® on chronic cutaneous ulcers has not been reported.

13.3.4 Composite Grafts

Composite grafts represent a combination of dermal substitute and epidermal grafts. Research has shown that epidermal grafts are more beneficial when applied to a dermal bed. We distinguish here between composite grafts containing devitalized dermis and those with viable dermis in which fibroblasts are embedded.

■ **Composite Grafts Combining Epidermal Cells with Devitalized Dermis.** As described above, a dermal matrix (even acellular dermis) may function as a template for cutaneous regeneration [3, 4]. The addition of allogeneic or autologous cultured keratinocytes may further contribute to healing. Some suggest that the dermal component protects the basal layer of the epidermis and affects the biological processes of epithelial proliferation, differentiation, migration, and wound healing.

In practice, following the absorption and 'take' of acellular dermal grafts such as those mentioned earlier in this chapter (Integra®, SkinTemp®, CollatamFascie®), cultured keratinocytes may be seeded onto these dermal grafts, approximately two weeks after the dermal graft has been applied. However, the beneficial effect of devitalized dermis with epidermal cells is not well documented. More advanced methods, combining dermal components with living fibroblasts, together with cultured keratinocytes, tend to yield better results (see below).

■ **Cutaneous Ulcers Treated by Composite Grafts with Viable Dermis.** The incorporation of viable fibroblasts improves the epidermal response of the grafted skin [78–83]. Most studies described below, using composite grafts, involved improvised products. Some of the composite grafts used were ephemeral and did not manage to penetrate the current pharmaceutical market, while others became the prototype for the composite grafts currently being marketed.

While the general impression of the products discussed in this section is positive, there are insufficient data to assess their efficacy. There are more controlled studies and data related to those in current use (i.e., Apligraf®), described in Chap. 14.

Following are studies on cutaneous ulcers implementing the use of composite grafts that are not commercially available:

- Mol et al. [84] compared the efficacy of punch grafts with that of composite grafts (allogeneic fibroblasts covered by autologous cultured keratinocytes), with both types being applied to the ulcer site in the same patient. The median healing time of ulcers covered by composite grafts was 18 days whereas that of ulcers treated by punch grafts was 15 days.
- Bovine collagen matrix used by Burke et al. [25], as described above, was modified by the incorporation of fibroblasts into the collagen-glycosaminoglycan substrate and by replacing the silastic layer with human keratinocytes. Clinical efficacy was documented in burns [85] and chronic cutaneous ulcers [86].
- Harvima et al. [87] conducted an open study comparing the effect of

cultured allogeneic keratinocytes with that of fibroblast-gelatin sponge placed on the ulcer bed once weekly. This study involved 22 diabetic patients with chronic ulcers and 16 patients with leg or ankle ulcers of different etiologies. From the diabetic group, four randomly selected patients (five ulcers) received combined treatment. The patients were first treated by fibroblast-gelatin sponge, up to the point where the ulcer area was reduced by 50%. These ulcers were then treated with keratinocyte cultures. In general, the treatment was effective. All but one diabetic ulcer healed. Nevertheless, the investigators did not find a significant difference between the cultured keratinocyte treatment alone and the combined treatment.

13.4 Summary

There is a wide range of skin substitutes that can be used in the treatment of chronic cutaneous ulcers. From the current information available, it is difficult to evaluate precisely the efficacy of each of the methods reviewed in this chapter. Some studies lack basic data about the patients, such as the presence of ulceration in the past, or information regarding the clinical appearance of the ulcer. Other studies involved an insufficient number of patients to draw significant conclusions, while others were not controlled.

Nevertheless, the general impression that arises from these studies is that in the treatment of cutaneous ulcers, skin substitutes containing living cells are likely to be superior to skin substitutes that do not contain living cells. This being the case, advanced treatment modalities such as keratinocyte cultures or composite grafts could present a reasonable treatment option when dealing with clean ulcers with relatively healthy granulation tissue.

References

1. Bello YM, Falabella AF, Eaglstein WH: Tissue-Engineered Skin. Current status in wound healing. Am J Clin Dermatol 2001; 2:305–313

2. Eaglstein WH, Falanga V: Tissue engineering for skin: an update. J Am Acad Dermatol 1998; 39: 1007–1010

3. Wainwright DJ: Use of an acellular allograft dermal matrix (AlloDerm) in the management of full thickness burns. Potential as a template for the reconstruction of viable dermis. Burns 1995; 21:243–248

4. Livesey SA, Herndon DN, Hollyoak MA, et al: Transplanted acellular allograft dermal matrix. Transplantation 1995; 60:1–9

5. Gustafson CJ, Kratz G: Cultured autologous keratinocytes on a cell-free dermis in the treatment of full-thickness wounds. Burns 1999; 25:331–335

6. Hussmann J, Russell RC, Kucan JO, et al: Use of glycerolized human allografts as temporary and permanent cover in adults and children. Burns 1994; 20 [Suppl 1]:S61–S66

7. Abbott WM, Hembree JS: Absence of antigenicity in freeze-dried skin allografts. Cryobiology 1970; 6: 416–418

8. Chakrabarty KH, Dawson RA, Harris P, et al: Development of autologous human dermal-epidermal composites based on sterilized human allodermis for clinical use. Br J Dermatol 1999; 141:811–823

9. Phillips TJ: New skin for old: Developments in biological skin substitutes. Arch Dermatol 1998; 134: 344–349

10. Herndon DN: Perspectives in the use of allograft. J Burn Care Rehabil 1997; 18:S6

11. Greenleaf G, Hansbrough JF: Current trends in the use of allograft skin for patients with burns and reflections on the future of skin banking in the United States. J Burn Care Rehabil 1994; 15:428–431

12. Balasubramani M, Kumar TR, Babu M: Skin substitutes: a review. Burns 2001; 27:534–544

13. Snyder RJ, Simonson DA: Cadaveric allograft as adjunct therapy for nonhealing ulcers. J Foot Ankle Surg 1999; 38:93–101

14. Ruszczak Z, Schwartz RA: Modern aspects of wound healing: an update. Dermatol Surg 2000; 26:219–229

15. Davis DA, Arpey CJ: Porcine heterografts in dermatologic surgery and reconstruction. Dermatol Surg 2000; 26:76–80

16. Bromberg BE, Song IC: Homograts and heterografts as skin substitutes. Am J Surg 1966; 112:28–33

17. Culliton P, Kwasnik RE, Novicki D, et al: The efficacy of porcine skin grafts for treating non-healing cutaneous ulcers. Part I: clinical studies. J Am Podiatry Assoc 1978; 68:1–10

18. Elliott RA Jr, Hoehn JG: Use of commercial porcine skin for wound dressings. Plast Reconstr Surg 1973; 52:401–405

19. Ersek RA, Lorio J: The most indolent ulcers of the skin treated with porcine xenografts and silver ions. Surg Gynecol Obstet 1984; 158:431–436

20. Kaplan EG, Kaplan GS, Kaplan DM, et al: Superficial ulcer treatment utilizing hyperbaric oxygen and porcine skin grafts. J Foot Surg 1978; 17:144–149

21. Kudo K, Yokota M, Fujioka Y: Immediate reconstruction using a scalp-forehead flap for the entire upper lip defect with the application of lyophilized porcine skin to surgical wounds. A case report of a malignant melanoma in the upper lip and oral mucosa. J Maxillofac Surg 1983; 11:275–278

22. Poskitt KR, James AH, Lloyd-Davies ER, et al: Pinch skin grafting or porcine dermis in venous ulcers: a randomised clinical trial. Br Med J 1987; 294:674–676

23. Piez KA: Structure and assembly of the native collagen fibril. Connect Tissue Res 1982; 10:25–36

24. Dedhar S, Ruoslahti E, Pierschbacher MD: A cell surface receptor complex for collagen type I recognizes the Arg-Gly-Asp sequence. J Cell Biol 1987; 104: 585–593

25. Burke JF, Yannas IV, Quinby WC Jr, et al: Successful use of a physiologically acceptable artificial skin in the treatment of extensive burn injury. Ann Surg 1981; 194:413–428

26. Postlethwaite AE, Seyer JM, Kang AH: Chemotactic attraction of human fibroblasts to type I, II, and III collagens and collagen-derived peptides. Proc Natl Acad Sci USA 1978; 75: 871–875

27. Voytik-Harbin SL, Brightman AO, Kraine MR, et al: Identification of extractable growth factors from small intestinal submucosa. J Cell Biochem 1997; 67: 478–491

28. Kolenik SA 3rd, McGovern TW, Leffell DJ: Use of a lyophilized bovine collagen matrix in postoperative wound healing. Dermatol Surg 1999; 25:303–307

29. Motta G, Ratto GB, De Barbieri A, et al: Can heterologous collagen enhance the granulation tissue growth? An experimental study. Ital J Surg Sci 1983; 13:101–108

30. Leipziger LS, Glushko V, DiBernardo B, et al: Dermal wound repair: role of collagen matrix implants and synthetic polymer dressings. J Am Acad Dermatol 1985; 12:409–419

31. Hodde JP, Badylak SF, Brightman AO, et al: Glycosaminoglycan content of small intestinal submucosa: A bioscaffold for tissue replacement. Tissue Engineering 1996; 2:209–217

32. McPherson TB, Badylak SF: Characterization of Fibronectin derived from porcine small intestinal submucosa. Tissue Engineering 1998; 4:75–83

33. Brown-Etris M, Punchello M, Shields D: Final report on a pilot study to evaluate porcine small intestinal submucosa as a covering for partial thickness wounds. WOCN 32nd Annual Conference. June 2000; Toronto

34. Mian E, Martini P, Beconcini D, et al: Healing of open skin surfaces with collagen foils. Int J Tissue React 1992; 14 [Suppl]:27–34

35. Lorenzetti OJ, Fortenberry B, Busby E, et al: Influence of microcrystalline collagen on wound healing. I. Wound closure of normal excised and burn excised wounds of rats, rabbits and pigs. Proc Soc Exp Biol Med 1972; 140:896–900

36. Chvapil M: Considerations on manufacturing principles of a synthetic burn dressing: a review. J Biomed Mater Res 1982; 16: 245–263

37. Phillips TJ, Dover JS: Leg Ulcers. J Am Acad Dermatol 1991; 25: 965–987

38. Zapata- Sirvent R, Hansbrough JF, Carroll W, et al: Comparison of Biobrane and Scarlet red dressings for treatment of donor site wounds. Arch Surg 1985; 120: 743–745

39. McHugh TP, Robson MC, Heggers JP, et al: Therapeutic efficacy of Biobrane in partial- and full-thickness thermal injury. Surgery 1986; 100: 661–664

40. Zachary L, Heggers JP, Robson MC, et al: The use of topical antimicrobials combined with Biobrane in burn wound infections. J Trauma 1982; 22: 833–836

41. Donaghue VM, Chrzan JS, Rosenblum BI, et al: Evaluation of a collagen-alginate wound dressing in the management of diabetic foot ulcers. Adv Wound Care 1998; 11: 114–119

42. Alvarez O, Fahey C, Papantonio C, et al: Experience with a collagen-alginate wound dressing in the management of chronic venous ulcers. Symposium on Advanced Wound Care and Medical research forum on Wound Repair. 1999

43. Ghatnekar O, Willis M, Persson U: Cost-effectiveness of treating deep diabetic foot ulcers with Promogran in four European countries. J Wound Care 2002; 11: 70–74

44. Veves A, Sheehan P, Pham HT: A randomized, controlled trial of Promogran (a collagen/oxidized regenerated cellulose dressing) vs standard treatment in the management of diabetic foot ulcers. Arch Surg 2002; 137: 822–827

45. Vin F, Teot L, Meaume S: The healing properties of Promogran in venous leg ulcers. J Wound Care 2002; 11: 335–341

46. Rheinwald JG, Green H: Serial cultivation of strains of human epidermal keratinocytes: The formation of keratinizing colonies from single cells. Cell 1975; 6: 331–343

47. O'Connor NE, Mulliken JB, Banks-Schlegel S, et al: Grafting of burns with cultured epithelium prepared from autologous epidermal cells. Lancet 1981; 1: 75–78

48. Gallico GG 3rd, O'Connor NE, Compton CC, et al: Permanent coverage of large burn wounds with autologous cultured human epithelium. N Engl J Med 1984; 311: 448–451

49. Teepe RG, Ponec M, Kreis RW, et al: Improved grafting method for the treatment of burns with autologous cultured human epithelium (letter). Lancet 1986; 1: 385

50. Teepe RG, Ponec JA, Kempenaar B: Clinical, histological and ultrastructural aspects of cultured epithelium. In: Proceedings of the International Symposium on the clinical Use of Cultured Epithelium in Surgery and Dermatology. Leiden, March, 1987

51. De Luca M, Albanese E, Bondanza S, et al: Multicentre experience in the treatment of burns with autologous and allogenic cultured epithelium, fresh or preserved in a frozen state. Burns 1989; 15: 303–309

52. Eldad A, Burt A, Clarke JA, et al: Cultured epithelium as a skin substitute. Burns Incl Therm Inj 1987; 13: 173–180

53. Bettex-Galland M, Slongo T, Hunziker T, et al: Use of cultured keratinocytes in the treatment of severe burns. Z Kinderchir 1988; 43: 224–228

54. Gao ZR, Hao ZQ, Nie LJ, et al: Coverage of full skin thickness burns with allograft inoculated with autogenous epithelial cells. Burns Inc Therm Inj 1986; 12: 220–224

55. Hefton JM, Caldwell D, Biozes DG, et al: Grafting of skin ulcers with cultured autologous epidermal cells. J Am Acad Dermatol 1986; 14: 399–405

56. Leigh IM, Purkis PE: Culture grafted leg ulcers. Clin Exp Dermatol 1986; 11: 650–652

57. Teepe RG, Keobrugge EJ, Ponec M, et al: Fresh versus cryopreserved cultured allografts for the treatment of chronic skin ulcers. Br J Dermatol 1990; 122: 81–89

58. Leigh IM, Purkis PE, Navsaria HA, et al: Treatment of chronic venous ulcers with sheets of cultured allogeneic keratinocytes. Br J Dermatol 1987; 117: 591–597

59. Phillips TJ, Gilchrest BA: Cultured allogeneic keratinocyte grafts in the management of wound healing: prognostic factors. J Dermatol Surg Oncol 1989; 15: 1169–1176

60. Beele H, Naeyaert JM, Goeteyn M, et al: Repeated cultured epidermal allografts in the treatment of chronic leg ulcers of various origins. Dermatologica 1991; 183: 31–35

61. Marcusson JA, Lindgren C, Berghard A: Allogeneic cultured keratinocytes in the treatment of leg ulcers. Acta Derm Venereol (Stockh) 1992; 72: 61–64

62. De Luca M, Albanese E, Cancedda R, et al: Treatment of leg ulcers with cryopreserved allogeneic cultured epithelium. A multicenter study. Arch Dermatol 1992; 128: 633– 638

63. Stanulis- Praeger BM, Gilchrest BA: Growth factor responsiveness declines during adulthood for human skin-derived cells. Mech Ageing Dev 1986; 35: 185–198

64. Sauder DN, Stanulis-Praeger BM, Gilchrest BA: Autocrine growth stimulation of human keratinocytes by epidermal cell-derived thymocyte activating factor: Implications for skin aging. Arch Dermatol Res 1988; 280: 71–76

65. Jones JE, Nelson EA: Skin grafting for venous leg ulcers (Cochrane Review). In: The Cochrane Library, Issue 4, 2000. Oxford: Update Software

66. Limat A, Mauri D, Hunziker T: Successful treatment of chronic leg ulcers with epidermal equivalents generated from cultured autologous outer root sheath cells. J Invest Dermatol 1996; 107: 128–135

67. Limat A, French LE, Blal L, et al: Organotypic cultures of autologous hair follicle keratinocytes for the treatment of recurrent leg ulcers. J Am Acad Dermatol 2003; 48: 207–214

68. Bolivar-Flores YJ, Kuri-Harcuch W: Frozen allogeneic human epidermal cultured sheets for the cure of complicated leg ulcers. Dermatol Surg 1999; 25: 610–617

69. Teepe RG, Roseeuw DI, Hermans J, et al: Randomized trial comparing cryopreserved cultured epidermal allografts with hydrocolloid dressings in healing chronic venous ulcers. J Am Acad Dermatol 1993; 29:982–988

70. Lindgren C, Marcusson JA, Toftgard R: Treatment of venous leg ulcers with cryopreserved cultured allogeneic keratinocytes: a prospective open controlled study. Br J Dermatol 1998; 139:271–275

71. Duhra P, Blight A, Mountford E, et al: A randomized controlled trial of cultured keratinocyte allografts for chronic venous ulcers. J Dermatol Treat 1992; 3: 189–191

72. Jones I, Currie L, Martin R: A guide to biological skin substitutes. Br J Plast Surg 2002; 55: 185–193

73. Hansbrough JF, Morgan J, Greenleaf G, et al: Development of a temporary living skin replacement composed of human neonatal fibroblasts cultured in Biobrane, a synthetic dressing material. Surgery 1994; 115: 633–644

74. Gentzkow G, Iwasaki SD, Hershon KS, et al: Use of Dermagraft: a cultured human dermis to treat diabetic foot ulcers. Diabetes care 1996; 19:350–354

75. Pollak RA, Edington H, Jensen JL, et al: A human dermal replacement for the treatment of diabetic foot ulcers. Wounds 1997; 9:175–183

76. Hanft JR, Surprenant MS: Healing of chronic foot ulcers in diabetic patients treated with a human fibroblast-derived dermis. J Foot Ankle Surg 2002; 41: 291–299

77. Hansbrough J: Status of cultured skin replacement. Wounds 1995; 7:130–136

78. Marston WA, Hanft J, Norwood P, et al: The efficacy and safety of Dermagraft in improving the healing of chronic diabetic foot ulcers. Diabetes Care 2003; 26: 1701–1705

79. Bell E, Ehrlich HP, Sher S, et al: Development and use of a living skin equivalent. Plast Reconstr Surg 1981; 67:386–392

80. MacKenzie IC, Fusenig NE: Regeneration of organized epithelial structure. J Invest Dermatol 1983; 81: 189S–194S

81. Cuono CB, Langdon R, Birchall N, et al: Composite autologous-allogeneic skin replacement: Development and clinical application. Plast Reconstr Surg 1987; 80:626–637

82. Bell E, Ehrlich HP, Buttle DJ, et al: Living tissue formed in vitro and accepted as skin-equivalent tissue of full thickness. Science 1981; 211:1052–1054

83. Krejci NC, Cuono CB, Langdon RC, et al: In vitro reconstitution of skin: Fibroblasts facilitate keratinocyte growth and differentiation on acellular reticular dermis. J Invest Dermatol 1991; 97:843–848

84. Mol MA, Nanninga PB, van Eendenburg JP, et al: Grafting of venous leg ulcers. An intraindividual comparison between cultured skin equivalents and full-thickness skin punch grafts. J Am Acad Dermatol 1991; 24:77–82

85. Hansbrough JF, Dore C, Hansbrough WB: Clinical trials of a living dermal tissue replacement placed beneath meshed, split thickness skin grafts on excised burn wounds. J Burn Care Rehabil 1992; 13: 519–529

86. Boyce ST, Glatter R, Kitzmiller WJ: Case studies: Treatment of chronic wounds with cultured skin substitutes: a pilot study. Ostomy Wound Manage 1995; 41:26–28, 30, 32

87. Harvima IT, Virnes S, Kauppinen L, et al: Cultured allogeneic skin cells are effective in the treatment of chronic diabetic leg and foot ulcers. Acta Derm Venereol (Stockh) 1999; 79:217–220

Human Skin Equivalents: When and How to Use

14

Contents

14.1 General Structure and Mechanism of Action

The term 'human skin equivalents' (HSE) refers to living composite grafts composed of a dermal component containing human living fibroblasts and an epidermal component containing living keratinocytes. HSE is also referred to as 'graftskin', 'bio-engineered tissue', 'bilayered cellular matrix' or 'bilayered skin substitute'.

The manufacturing of HSE is based on an original idea mooted by Bell [1] in 1981. Two available commercial HSE products are FDA approved: Apligraf® and OrCel®. Apligraf® is the product with which the most experience has been gathered in the treatment of cutaneous ulcers. Therefore, most of the following discussion is based on research studies investigating Apligraf®. Further types of commercial composite grafts are expected to be available in forthcoming years. As described in Chap. 13, some studies have been carried out with HSE products not in commercial use and intended for research purposes only.

HSE products manufactured *in vitro* from neonatal foreskins represent a modification of allogeneic grafting. They have an internal dermal layer containing living human fibroblasts and an external epidermal layer containing living keratinocytes. Histologically, the currently available HSE products do not contain Langerhans' cells, macrophages, melanocytes, lymphocytes, blood vessels, or hair follicles [2, 3].

Having the above-mentioned qualities, an HSE product functions as an effective biological dressing, providing an optimal environment for wound repair. Its dermal layer may serve as a structural template for dermal generation. Fibroblasts incorporated in the dermal layer, as well as the epidermal cells, induce secretion of growth factors, by which HSE are considered to exert their healing effect [4–7]. In fact, positive immunostaining has been shown within the dermal component of Apligraf® for platelet-derived growth factor (PDGF), transforming growth factor-beta (TGF-β), and basic fibroblast growth-factor (FGF-2) [4]. OrCel®, according to the manufacturer, contains several growth factors including fibroblast growth factor (FGF), granulocyte-macrophage colony stimulating factor (GM-CSF), and keratinocyte growth factor (KGF). It has been suggested that the new allogeneic cells incorporated in HSE may initiate a cascade of growth factors produced within the treated ulcer [5, 8].

Apligraf® has also been shown to produce certain antibacterial peptides, such as human β-defensin 2, a substance active against gram-negative bacteria, yeasts, and fungi [4]. In any case, the allogeneic cells do not survive on the transplanted ulcer bed, although their rejection may be delayed in conditions of abnormal immune status [9].

14.2 Product Description

14.2.1 Apligraf®

The supporting internal dermal layer of Apligraf® consists of living human fibroblasts embedded in a bovine type-1 collagen. The external epidermal layer contains living keratinocytes. The behavior of Apligraf® is similar to that of human skin, and its epidermal layer is able to produce differentiated stratum corneum. *In vitro*, it demonstrates self-healing capacities following injury.

Each unit of Apligraf® is kept in a sealed polyethylene bag in a plastic dish, over a layer of an agar-like material. The product should be kept in the sealed bag until used, within a temperature range of 20°–31°C, in order to ensure its viability. Each sheet is manufactured as a circular disc measuring 7.5 cm in diameter and is 0.75 mm thick.

According to the manufacturer's information, the agar-based Apligraf® medium contains agarose, L-glutamine, hydrocortisone, bovine serum albumin, bovine insulin, human transferrin, triiodothyronine, ethanolamine, O-phosphoryletanolamine, adenine, selenious acid, DMEM powder, HAM's F-12 powder, sodium bicarbonate, calcium chloride, and water for injection. All components of the product undergo thorough screening for various potential infectious agents, including viruses (HIV and hepatitis A, B, and C), bacteria (such as syphilis), and fungi [3]. The cells are also screened for identification of chromosomal abnormalities and biochemical defects. The product is packed so that its dermal, glossy layer is placed face down on the agar substrate, while its epidermal (dull) layer faces up.

14.2.2 OrCel®

The product OrCel® is made of two separate compartments of a porous, type-I bovine collagen sponge. It contains cultured allogeneic keratinocytes and fibroblasts, both originating from human neonatal foreskin [10]. It measures approximately 6×6 cm (36 cm²).

The donor's cells are screened for viruses (HTLV I and II, Hepatitis B, HIV I and II, EBV and HHV-6), bacteria, fungi, yeast, mycoplasma, and tumorigenicity. The final product should fulfill the required criteria as to morphology, cell density, cell viability, sterility, and physical container integrity.

14.3 Indications

HSE products induce repair in ulcers that have been considered recalcitrant to conventional therapy.

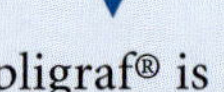

Apligraf® is FDA approved for the conditions listed below, i.e., for venous ulcers and diabetic ulcers:

- Venous ulcers that fulfill the following criteria:
  - Of partial or full thickness
  - Non-infected
  - Not showing significant improvement following one month of conventional therapy
- Diabetic ulcers that fulfill the following criteria:
  - Of full thickness
  - Non-infected
  - With neuropathic etiology
  - Not showing significant improvement following three weeks of conventional therapy
  - Not extending into tendons, muscles or bones
  - Located on the plantar, medial, or lateral aspects of the foot (excluding the heel)

However, Apligraf® has also been reported as beneficial for other types of cutaneous ulcers, such as those caused by polyarteritis nodosa, those due to sarcoidosis, and epidermolysis bullosa lesions [11–13]. Apligraf® has also been used for excised burn wounds [14].

> Currently, OrCel® is FDA approved for:
> - Split-thickness donor sites of burn patients
> - Surgical wounds and donor sites associated with mitten-hand deformities secondary to recessive dystrophic epidermolysis bullosa

Note that OrCel® has recently been reported to be beneficial in the treatment of diabetic neuropathic foot ulcers [15] (see Table 14.1).

14.4 Instructions for Use

The main principles described below are based on our experience with Apligraf®. However, similar techniques should be implemented when dealing with other HSE products. The instructions also apply, at least in their main principles, to dermal grafting products (such as Dermagraft®). There are unique guidelines for the grafting of each product, and manufacturers' instructions should be followed precisely and thoroughly.

14.4.1 Preparing the Ulcer Bed

The product should be applied onto a clean, viable granulation tissue. Debridement is required in order to obtain an optimal substrate for grafting.

> The ulcer bed should be prepared as follows:
> - Prior to debridement, the ulcer should be cleansed thoroughly with a saline solution.
> - Any necrotic tissue present should be removed by scalpel and forceps. Shaving the ulcer's surface until a minor degree of bleeding can be seen is required to create an optimal, vascular substrate for the HSE treatment [8, 16]. The principles that apply here are the same as those for preparing the ulcer bed for the application of preparations containing growth factors [17].
> - Shaving the upper layer of the ulcer bed, superficially and horizontally, may be performed with a scalpel or with a fine curette. A fine curette can be used for the removal of layers near the ulcer's margin – its shape enabling an accurate outlining. Debridement of the ulcer's margin is extremely important, since peripheral epithelialization can be stimulated by this procedure. This issue is detailed in Chap. 9.
> - Bleeding following debridement may be dealt with by applying gentle pressure with a sterile gauze. Following debridement, the ulcer should be cleansed with saline or Ringer's lactate solution.

14.4.2 Steps to Take Prior to Applying the Product to the Ulcer Bed

Check the expiry date of the product to be used. Assure that the product has been kept under appropriate conditions prior to grafting (temperature range according to manufacturer's instructions). Note: Products should be used within a limited period following removal from their packaging (i.e., 15 min for Apligraf®).

14.4.3 Grafting Procedure

Grafting should be done as follows:
- The technique demands attention to absolute sterility. Sterile gloves should be worn. The plastic tray, after its removal from its protective polyethylene cover, should be placed on a sterile surface (Fig. 14.1).
- The HSE sheet should be fenestrated, with its epidermal side facing down, to enable drainage of secretions from the ulcer bed. The HSE should be trimmed to conform to ulcer size.
- Ascertain that the right side of the graft (its dermal layer) is placed in direct contact with the wound bed (Fig. 14.2).
- After the HSE sheet has been placed on the wound bed, it should be straightened and smoothed using a saline-moistened cotton applicator (Fig. 14.3), in order to achieve continuous contact between the HSE layer and the wound bed, without wrinkles or folds. Alternatively, Apligraf® can be meshed, thereby allowing the product to expand and to cover a larger ulcer area.

14.4.4 Dressing the HSE Layer

Once the graft has been correctly applied, it should be covered with a non-adherent primary dressing, followed by a cotton gauze dressing (Fig. 14.4).

The treated area is now bandaged. The use of sutures or staplers to attach the graft sheet to the ulcer bed is not recommended, since these cause unnecessary tissue damage and increase the risk of local infection in the treated area. For the same reasons, it is not recommended to use an occluding substance such as vaseline over the HSE layer.

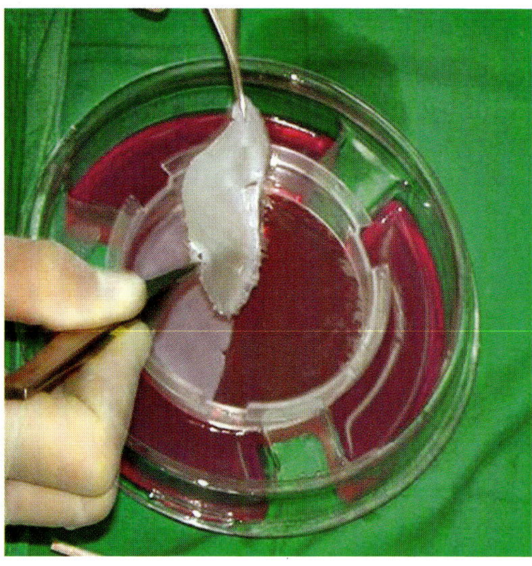

Fig. 14.1. Lifting the HSE sheet prior to its application onto the ulcer

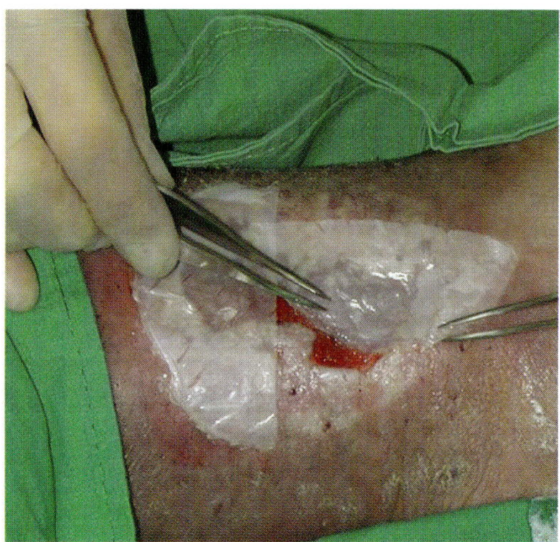

Fig. 14.2. The HSE sheet is placed onto the ulcer bed

14.4.5 Following Grafting

Frequency of dressing replacement will depend on the amount of secretions from the ulcer. If, based on a swab culture, there is evidence of colonization by 'notorious' bacteria (*Pseudomonas aeruginosa*, methicillin-resistant *Staphylococcus aureus*), frequent examination of the treated ul-

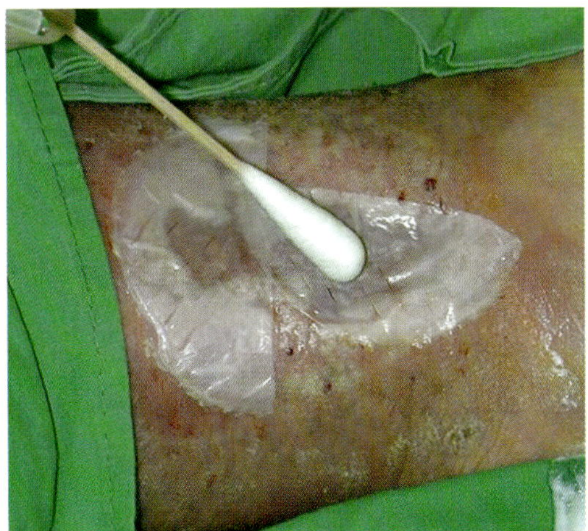

Fig. 14.3. Straightening and smoothing the Apligraf

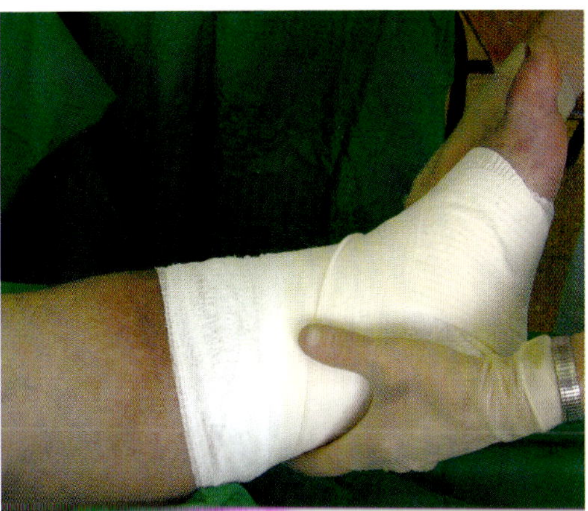

Fig. 14.4. Dressing the treated area

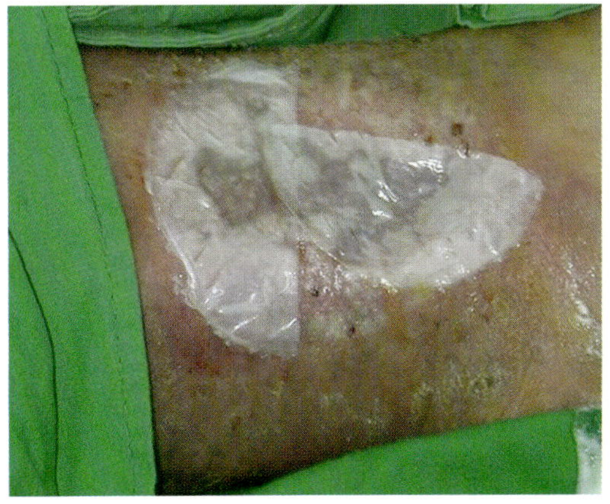

Fig. 14.5. One day after the application of Apligraf®

cer is recommended. Additional applications of HSE may be used according to the progress of healing.

14.5 Contraindications

HSE products are contraindicated under the following conditions:
- For infected wounds/ulcers
- For patients known to be hypersensitive to bovine collagen
- For patients known to be hypersensitive to substances contained in the preserving/shipping medium

OrCel® may contain traces of penicillin, streptomycin, gentamicin, and amphotericin B. It should therefore be avoided in patients with known allergies to these drugs.

In any case, current indications and contraindications of each product should be verified and updated according to manufacturers' guidelines and regulations as determined by medical/legal authorities of each country.

14.6 Efficacy

The efficacy of HSE products which have been applied to chronic cutaneous ulcers, as examined in several clinical trials, is detailed in Table 14.1. Figures 14.5–14.7 illustrate the progress of an ulcer following the application of Apligraf®.

14.7 Concluding Remark

Human skin equivalents represent an advanced mode of therapy that may be used for cutaneous ulcers. Their use is intended for relatively clean ulcers. HSE has been found to be effective in difficult-to-heal ulcers of long duration.

Table 14.1. Efficacy of HSE products applied to chronic ulcers

Study	Year	Design	Participants	Duration	Intervention	Outcome
APLIGRAF®						
Falanga et al. [2]	1998	• randomized • controlled • open-label • multi-centered	• 309 patients suffering from chronic venous ulcers • 293 patients were treated, from which • 275 patients were evaluated	• 8 weeks of treatment • 6 months follow-up, plus • 6 months safety evaluation	• 146 patients: Apligraf® with compression therapy • 129 patients: external dressing containing zinc-oxide paste with compression therapy	• 63% of ulcers treated with Apligraf® healed, vs • 49% in the control group
Falanga et al. [18]	1999	• randomized • controlled • open-label • multi-centered	• 120 patients with difficult-to-heal venous ulcers of long duration (more than 1 year)	• 8 weeks treatment • 6 months follow-up	• 72 patients: Apligraf® with compression therapy • 48 patients: external dressing containing zinc-oxide paste with compression therapy	• 47% of ulcers treated with Apligraf® achieved complete wound closure vs • 19% in the control group
Pham et al. [19]	1999	• randomized • controlled • open-label	• 33 with diabetic foot ulcers	• 12 weeks (treatment with Apligraf® within first four weeks)	• 16 patients: Apligraf® • 17 patients: woven gauze kept moist by saline	• 75% of ulcers treated with Apligraf® achieved complete wound closure (12 patients), vs • 41% in the control group (7 patients) • The median time for ulcer closure was 38.5 days for Apligraf® vs 91 days in the control group
ORCEL®						
Lipkin et al. [15]	2003	• randomized • controlled • open-label • multi-centered	• 40 patients with chronic, neuropathic, diabetic foot ulcers	• 12 weeks	• 20 patients: OrCel® with standard care (moist saline gauze cover) • 20 patients: standard care alone	• 35% of treated ulcers achieved complete healing (7 of 20 wounds), vs • 20% in the control group (4 out of 20 wounds)

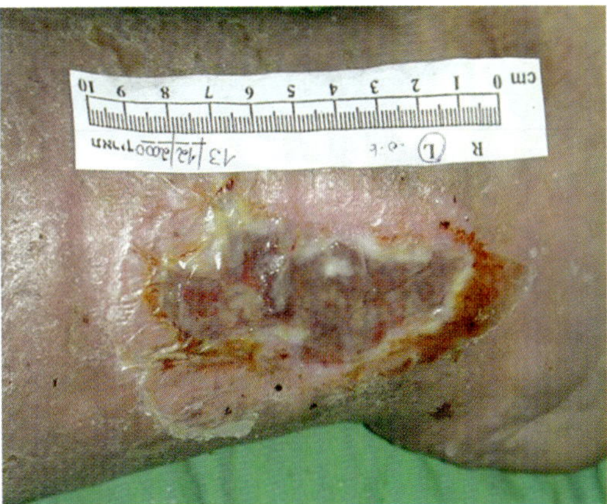

Fig. 14.6. After eight days

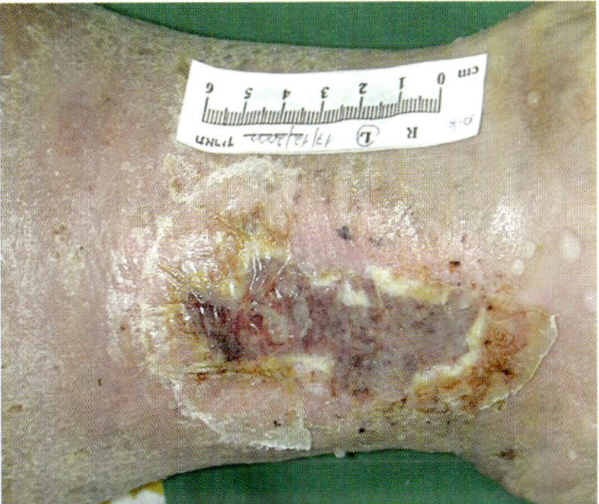

Fig. 14.7. After 12 days

References

1. Bell E, Ehrlich HP, Buttle DJ, et al: Living tissue formed *in vitro* and accepted as skin-equivalent tissue of full thickness. Science 1981; 211:1052–1054
2. Falanga V, Margolis D, Alvarez O, et al: Rapid healing of venous ulcers and lack of clinical rejection with an allogeneic cultured human skin equivalent. Arch Dermatol 1998; 134:293–300
3. Wilkins LM, Watson SR, Prosky SJ, et al: Development of a bilayered living skin construct for clinical applications. Biotechnol Bioeng 1994; 43:747–756
4. Schmid P: Apligraf – phenotypic characteristics and their potential implications for the treatment of diabetic foot ulcers. A satellite symposium at the 36th annual meeting of the European association for the study of diabetes (EASD). Jerusalem, September 2000
5. Phillips TJ, Manzoor J, Rojas A, et al: The longevity of a bilayered skin substitute after application to venous ulcers. Arch Dermatol 2002; 138:1079–1081
6. Navsaria HA, Myers SR, Leigh IM, et al: Culturing skin *in vitro* for wound therapy. Trends Biotechnol 1995; 13:91–100
7. Martin P, Hopkinson-Woolley J, McCluskey J: Growth factors and cutaneous wound repair. Prog Growth Factor Res 1992; 4:25–44
8. Falanga V: How to use Apligraf to treat venous ulcers. Skin & Aging 1999; 7:30–36
9. Fine JD: Skin bioequivalents and their role in the treatment of inherited epidermolysis bullosa. Arch Dermatol 2000; 136:1259–1260
10. Still J, Glat P, Silverstein P, et al: The use of a collagen sponge/living cell composite material to treat donor sites in burn patients. Burns 2003; 29:837–841
11. Pennoyer JW, Susser WS, Chapman MS, et al: Ulcers associated with polyarteritis nodosa treated with bioengineered human skin equivalent (Apligraf). J Am Acad Dermatol 2002; 46:145
12. Streit M, Bohlen LM, Braathen LR: Ulcerative sarcoidosis successfully treated with apligraf. Dermatology 2001; 202:367–370
13. Falabella AF, Valencia IC, Eaglstein WH, et al: Tissue-engineered skin (Apligraf) in the healing of patients with epidermolysis bullosa wounds. Arch Dermatol 2000; 136:1225–1230
14. Waymack P, Duff RG, Sabolinski M: The effect of a tissue engineered bilayered living skin analog, over meshed split-thickness autografts on the healing of excised burn wounds. Burns 2000; 26:609–619
15. Lipkin S, Chaikof E, Isseroff Z, et al: Effectiveness of bilayered cellular matrix in healing of neuropathic diabetic foot ulcers: results of a multicenter pilot trial. Wounds 2003; 15:230–236
16. Brem H, Balledux J, Sukkarieh T, et al: Healing of venous ulcers of long duration with a bilayered living skin substitute: results from a general surgery and dermatology department. Dermatol Surg 2001; 27:915–919
17. Steed DL, Donohoe D, Webster MW, et al: Effect of extensive debridement and treatment on the healing of diabetic foot ulcers. J Am Coll Surg 1996; 183:61–64
18. Falanga V, Sabolinski M: A bilayered living skin construct (Apligraf) accelerates complete closure of hard to heal venous ulcers. Wound Repair Regen 1999; 7:201–207
19. Pham HT, Rosenblum BI, Lyons TE, et al: Evaluation of a human skin equivalent for the treatment of diabetic foot ulcers in a prospective, randomized, clinical trial. Wounds 1999; 11:79–86

Growth Factors

15

Contents

15.1 Overview

The identification of topical growth factors and the development of their use in treating chronic ulcers of the skin represents a major breakthrough of recent years in the field of wound healing. Advanced dressing modalities have been reviewed in previous chapters. However, while various dressing materials are intended to provide an optimal environment for the healing of an ulcer, growth factors can do much more.

Growth factors actually provide a significant stimulus for the healing of cutaneous ulcers: They not only function as an external cover that may provide optimal conditions for repair, but also actually initiate and enhance the wound healing process. The effect of certain therapeutic modalities in wound healing involving living cell grafting, such as cultured keratinocyte grafts or composite grafts, is attributed, in part, to the stimulation of various cells within the treated ulcer to secrete endogenous growth factors, thereby enhancing the healing process [1–5].

15.2 What Are Growth Factors?

Growth factors are a specific subgroup of cytokines, whose main activity is the induction of mitosis. They are secreted by a wide range of cells including macrophages, fibroblasts, endothelial cells, and platelets [6].

Many cytokines have been identified as having a role in wound healing. These include platelet-derived growth factor (PDGF), fibroblast-derived growth factor (FGF), epidermal growth factor (EGF), tumor necrosis factor (TNF), granulocyte-macrophage colony-stimulating factor (GM-CSF), insulin-like growth factor (IGF), transforming growth factors (TGF) α and β, and many others.

Growth factors exert their effect on cells through cell-surface receptors. They may bind to one or several receptors. In the process of wound healing, endogenous growth factors coordinate cellular migration including chemotaxis of inflammatory cells. They have a mitogenic effect on epithelial cells, by inducing their proliferation and differentiation with enhancement of epithelial regeneration. They also exert a mitogenic effect on mesodermal cells, manifested as stimulated angiogenesis and granulation tissue formation. Growth factors also influence and regulate the degradation and formation of collagen [6–15].

Note that the current terminology used for growth factors does not adequately present an accurate description of their biological activity. In most cases, the original naming of each growth factor is associated with the circumstances of its biochemical identification, derived from what has been considered previously as its 'source cell'.

The equivocal terminology associated with growth factors in the scientific literature exists, in fact, to a much wider extent. Thus, apart from being secreted by platelets, platelet-derived growth factor (PDGF) is also secreted by a wide range of cells including macrophages, fibroblasts, and endothelial cells.

Various peptides that activate cellular reactions similar to those of growth factors may be called *interleukins* or *colony-stimulating factors*; yet, by the same token, it would also be scientifically justified to refer to these peptides as growth factors.

15.3 Beneficial Effects of Growth Factors on Acute Wounds and Chronic Cutaneous Ulcers

In animal models, research studies have shown that growth factors may enhance the process of healing in acute wounds [12, 16–21]. Several studies have demonstrated the beneficial effects of growth factors on the healing of acute wounds in human beings, i.e., split-thickness donor sites [22, 23] or punch wounds to normal skin [24].

Preparations containing growth factors are used mainly for chronic cutaneous ulcers. Current evidence indicates that in chronic cutaneous ulcers, for reasons that are not fully understood, the process of wound healing is arrested. Hence, a chronic ulcer remains in an ongoing inflammatory phase, rather than proceeding through the phases of healing, as occurs in a 'healthy' acute wound [25, 26].

Studies of wound fluid in chronic cutaneous ulcers have revealed an increased protease activity with the breakdown of growth factors [27–31]. The reduced activity of growth factors in chronic ulcers may partly explain why these ulcers sometimes fail to heal. The use of preparations containing growth factors in the treatment of chronic cutaneous ulcers may overcome this stagnatory state, thereby stimulating the repair process and facilitating wound healing.

Today, advances in molecular biology have enabled the production of large amounts of growth factors by recombinant DNA technologies. Hence, specific growth factors may be used to enhance wound healing. In this process, there is interaction between various growth factors and the induction of stimulatory or inhibitory effects. Therefore, a specific growth factor may act at several stages in the course of healing of an ulcer or a wound. However, when used individually, certain growth factors have not been found not to promote healing in practice, since they affect only specific sites in the chain of processes. A few cytokines, such as TGF β, GM-CSF, and PDGF have been known to influence several key steps in the wound healing process [6, 7, 12, 13, 32–36]. Currently, only PDGF is commercially available. Hence, PDGF will be discussed in detail below.

15.4 Recombinant Human Platelet-Derived Growth Factor: rhPDGF (Becaplermin)

Initial observations have demonstrated that a platelet-derived growth factor (PDGF), stored in α granules of circulating platelets, is released following injury as part of the process of blood clotting. However, in the human body, PDGF is secreted by a wide range of cells, including macrophages, fibroblasts, and endothelial cells. It regulates numerous aspects of wound healing including chemotaxis of inflammatory cells and mitogenesis in mesodermal and epithelial cells and enhances epithelial regeneration [36–39].

Of the growth factors currently under investigation, PDGF has shown beneficial effects in phase III clinical trials, and it is the only one commercially available (Regranex gel®). The commercial topical preparation is produced using recombinant DNA technology. The gene for the β chain of PDGF is inserted into the yeast *Saccharomyces cerevisiae* – a process that enables production of high amounts of this compound [40]. It is manufactured in tubes of 7.5 g or 15 g as an aqueous-based sodium carboxymethyl cellulose topical gel containing 0.01% recombinant human PDGF.

In clinical use, PDGF has been shown to increase the formation of granulation tissue (manifested by the continuous flattening of relatively deep cutaneous ulcers) and the concurrent coverage of the wound surface by layers of regenerative epithelium. Several research studies [41–46] in which it was compared with a placebo gel have shown it to be of benefit in diabetic foot ulcers. In 1997, it was approved for clinical use in North America and in the European Union for treating diabetic neuropathic ulcers of the lower extremities.

Currently, there are many ongoing studies investigating the effect of PDGF on other types of wounds and chronic ulcers. Promising results of its use in the management of pressure ulcers [47–49] and radiation ulcers [50] have also been reported. Recently, Wieman documented the beneficial effect of PDGF, together with good wound care based on compression therapy, in the treatment of patients with chronic venous leg ulcers [51].

pathic diabetic ulcers that had been present for more than eight weeks. Following 20 weeks of treatment with recombinant human PDGF, 50% of the treated ulcers healed, compared with a 35% healing rate in the control group treated with a placebo preparation. In addition, the time needed to achieve complete wound closure was reduced by 32%.

In another study, Steed et al. [42] also demonstrated the efficacy of rhPDGF. Twenty-nine of 61 patients (48%) with diabetic neuropathic ulcers treated with rhPDGF healed within 20 weeks, compared with a healing rate of 25% (14 of 57 patients) in placebo-treated ulcers.

In 1999, Smiell et al. [44] summarized the combined results of four multicenter, randomized studies that evaluated the efficacy of rhPDGF. A total of 922 patients with diabetic ulcers in the lower legs were treated once a day with a topical preparation containing either 100 µg/g rhPDGF, 30 µg/g rhPDGF, or placebo. Patients were treated until complete healing was achieved, or for a period of 20 weeks. A program of good ulcer care was given to all treatment groups, including initial sharp debridement (and additional debridement if necessary throughout the research project), a non-weight-bearing regimen, systemic antibiotics when needed (for infected wounds), and moist saline dressings. The 100-µg/g rh PDGF preparation was shown to significantly decrease the time to achieve complete healing compared with the placebo gel.

Other research studies indicating the beneficial effect of PDGF on diabetic ulcers have also been published [45, 46]. Note that PDGF has been shown to have a beneficial effect not only on chronic cutaneous ulcers, but also on acute wounds. Cohen and Eaglestein [24] conducted a double-blind controlled study, in which PDGF was applied to punch biopsy wounds on normal skin of healthy volunteers and was found to speed up the healing rate of the treated wounds.

15.5 Research Studies Using Recombinant Human PDGF

Wieman et al. [41] conducted a multicenter, double-blind, placebo-controlled study in 1998 that included 382 patients with chronic neuro-

15.6 PDGF: Indications and Contraindications

PDGF is intended for use only on a clean (or a relatively clean) ulcer. In any case, superficial debridement is needed (see below). For the time being, it has been approved for use only on non-infected diabetic foot ulcers.

Contraindications to the use of PDGF, as presented by the manufacturer are:
— Infected ulcers
— Known hypersensitivity to a component of the preparation (e.g., the parabens)
— Neoplasm in the application site

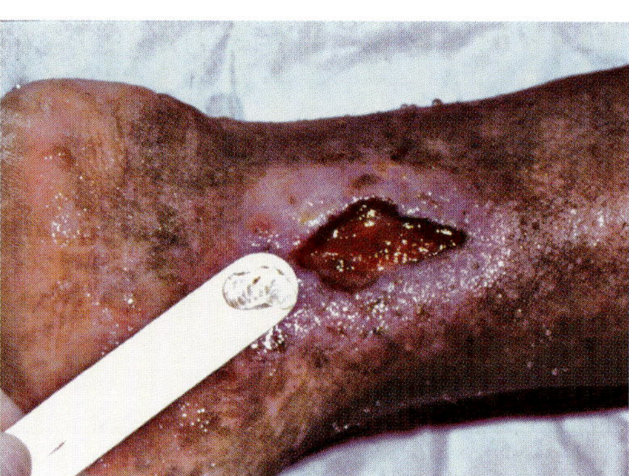

Fig. 15.1. Application of the preparation onto the ulcer's surface with a tongue depressor

15.7 Mode of Using PDGF Gel Preparation

The ulcer should be thoroughly rinsed prior to the application of a PDGF preparation. The superficial outer layer of a cutaneous ulcer should be debrided and removed prior to the application of PDGF gel. Debridement should extend (very superficially) to viable healthy tissue until a minor degree of bleeding (pinpoint bleeding) is achieved, and vital granulating tissue is exposed (see Chap.9, Section 9.4.1.1). This creates a more vascular bed, providing a better substrate for the wound-healing process. In addition, the superficial debridement removes a fibrin superficial layer (which, although almost invisble, may still prevent the preparation from coming into direct contact with the ulcer bed).

In a retrospective study conducted by Steed et al. [52], better healing rates were achieved in centers where ulcers were debrided more frequently. Some suggest that superficial, very delicate debridement may be repeated every 7–10 days; however, extreme care should be taken not to remove the newly forming epithelial layer.

After any minor bleeding has ceased, a very thin layer (approximately 0.2 cm thick) of PDGF gel is applied to the ulcer. The preparation should be spread over the ulcer surface with an application device, such as a tongue depressor, in order to obtain an even and continuous layer (Fig. 15.1). Subsequently, the wound should be covered with gauze.

The amount of preparation required depends on the ulcer's surface area. The manufacturer's directions suggest that each square inch of surface area requires a length of approximately 2/3 - inch of gel preparation, squeezed from a standard tube (7.5 g or 15 g). In metric terms, each square centimeter of the ulcer's surface area requires a length of 0.25 cm of gel preparation from a standard tube. The physician should re-evaluate the required amount of preparation needed, depending on the current surface area, every 1–2 weeks.

The preparation should be changed once daily; provided that the previously applied preparation is rinsed off with normal saline solution each time. Note that PDGF gel should be kept in the refrigerator. Room temperature may damage the preparation. It should not be kept in the freezer.

15.8 Topical Use of Other Growth Factors

Although PDGF is the only growth factor that has been licensed for use, other growth factors have been shown to be effective when used on experimental wounds or cutaneous ulcers. In view of the large extent of this issue, we discuss below only growth factors whose effects have been documented on humans. For example, in randomized, double-blind placebo-controlled research studies, Robson et al. [53] have demonstrated a beneficial effect of recombinant basic fibroblast growth factor (FGF) on patients with stage III/IV pressure sores. FGF has also been shown to accelerate wound healing in burns, split-thickness skin graft donor-site wounds, and chronic cutaneous ulcers [23]. Similarly, topically applied recombinant human keratinocyte growth factor-2 was shown to accelerate the healing of venous ulcers [54].

Other studies have examined the effect of various growth factors including TGF-β, insulin-like growth factors, and interleukin-1-β on acute wounds and chronic cutaneous ulcers [55, 56]. Nevertheless, at present, the two growth factors that have been studied the most intensively (in addition to PDGF) are GM-CSF and EGF.

15.8.1 Granulocyte-Macrophage Colony-Stimulating Factor

In vivo research studies have shown that rhGM-CSF may enhance wound healing by affecting several healing mechanisms, including the induction of myofibroblast differentiation, the mobilization of white blood cells, and the stimulation of proliferation and migration of epithelial cells [32, 57].

■ **Perilesional GM-CSF.** A few case reports have suggested that using perilesional rhGM-CSF on chronic cutaneous ulcers may be effective [58– 60]. More solid evidence may be derived from two randomized, double-blind, placebo-controlled studies. Da Costa et al. [61] documented the effect of rhGM-CSF injected subcutaneously adjacent to the ulcer margin in 25 patients with chronic venous ulcers. In eight of 16 (50%) patients treated with GM-CSF, there was complete healing within eight weeks, compared with a healing rate of 11% (one of nine) in control patients, treated with injections of saline solution.

In another double-blind, placebo-controlled study conducted by Da Costa et al. [62], 60 patients with chronic venous leg ulcers were treated by perilesional injections of rhGM-CSF. Complete healing was achieved within 12–14 weeks in 57% of patients treated with a 200-mg

preparation of GM-CSF and in 61% of patients treated with a 400-mg preparation of GM-CSF, but in only 19% of the placebo group.

■ **Topical GM-CSF.** The most convincing study documenting the beneficial effect of topical GM-CSF has been provided by Jaschke et al. [63], in which 52 venous ulcers were treated with a topical preparation containing 0.5–1.0 g/cm 2–3 times weekly. Ninety percent of the ulcers healed completely, with an average healing time of 19 weeks. Several other studies have also given credence to the hypothesis that topical GM-CSF is of benefit [64–66].

15.8.2 Epidermal Growth Factor

Epidermal growth factor (EGF) is a single polypeptide chain consisting of 53 amino acids originating mainly from macrophages and monocytes. It was the first growth factor isolated from urine, saliva, breast milk, and amniotic fluid; this was followed by its biochemical identification [67–69]. Initial animal studies conducted in the 1980s showed that EGF induces epidermal proliferation and angiogenesis [70, 71].

In 1989, Brown et al. [22] conducted a randomized, double-blind study on 12 patients, each with two skin graft donor sites. In each patient, one donor site was treated with silver-sulfadiazine, while the other was treated with silver-sulfadiazine containing EGF. There was improved healing at the donor sites treated with the silver-sulfadiazine/EGF combination, compared with those treated with silver-sulfadiazine only.

In 1992, Falanga et al. [72] used an aqueous solution of 10 g/ml human recombinant EGF, applied twice daily to venous ulcers. The preparation was applied for up to 10 weeks or until complete healing was achieved. Of the 18 patients treated with the EGF solution, complete healing was achieved in six (35%), while only two of the 17 patients (11%) in the control group were healed completely. The median reduction in ulcer size was 73% in the EGF group, compared with 33% in the control group. Though the above data look promising, there have been no well-documented studies of EGF since 1992.

Other members of the EGF family are ligands of the receptor EGF-R that share similar proliferative activity in the epidermis. These are transforming growth factor α (TGF-α), amphiregulin, and heregulin. Yet, for the time being, EGF is the only member of this group whose effects on wounds and ulcers have been documented.

15.9 Anti-Infective Effects of Growth Factors

In addition to their effect on healing, growth factors may also possess certain features that assist human tissues in coping with infection. Some aspects of this issue are obvious: Through induction of angiogenesis, for example, and improved vascularization of affected tissues, the ability to overcome infection is increased.

There may be other ways in which growth factors enhance the immune function of patients. For example, granulocyte colony-stimulating factor (G-CSF) has been shown to have a beneficial effect on foot infection in diabetic patients, which is attributed to improvement in neutrophil function [73]. De Lalla et al. [74] demonstrated that the administration of G-CSF for three weeks as an adjunctive therapy in limb-threatening diabetic foot infections was associated with better clinical outcomes, i.e., fewer cases of infection leading to the need to amputate the affected limb. The question as to whether growth factors actually secrete any active anti-bacterial substances requires further research.

15.10 Summary and Future Research

Advances in the field of molecular biology have enabled the production of highly purified recombinant human proteins. For the time being, PDGF is the only growth factor commercially available. Its beneficial effects on cutaneous ulcers have been demonstrated in numerous clinical trials. In addition to PDGF, several other growth factors are currently being investigated.

Future research may focus on:
- Combining growth factors with skin grafts, various skin substitutes, and tissue engineering products
- Matching and adapting growth factors to specific types of cutaneous ulcers or wounds, depending on their etiology or clinical appearance
- Identifying and using the anti-infective potential that certain growth factors may possess, thereby extending their use to infected cutaneous ulcers

References

1. Leigh IM, Purkis PE, Navsaria HA, et al: Treatment of chronic venous ulcers with sheets of cultured allogenic keratinocytes. Br J Dermatol 1987; 117:591–597
2. Phillips TJ, Gilchrest BA: Cultured allogenic keratinocyte grafts in the management of wound healing: prognostic factors. J Dermatol Surg Oncol 1989; 15:1169–1176
3. Stanulis-Praeger BM, Gilchrest BA: Growth factor responsiveness declines during adulthood for human skin-derived cells. Mech Ageing Dev 1986; 35:185–198
4. Sauder DN, Stanulis-Praeger BM, Gilchrest BA: Autocrine growth stimulation of human keratinocytes by epidermal cell-derived thymocyte activating factor: Implications for skin ageing. Arch Dermatol Res 1988; 280:71–76
5. Phillips TJ, Manzoor J, Rojas A, et al: The longevity of a bilayered skin substitute after applications to venous ulcers. Arch Dermatol 2002; 138:1079–1081
6. Harding K: Introduction to growth factors. In: Meeting the challenge of managing the diabetic foot: use of growth factor therapy. Proceedings from a symposium preceding the 35th Annual Meeting of the European Association for the Study of Diabetes. Antwerp. 1999; pp 31–40
7. Falanga V, Shen J: Growth factors, signal transduction and cellular responses. In: Falanga V (ed) Cutaneous Wound Healing, 1st edn. London: Martin Dunitz. 2001; pp 81–93
8. Robinson CJ: Growth factors: therapeutic advances in wound healing. Ann Med 1993; 25:535–538
9. Lawrence WT, Diegelmann RF: Growth factors in wound healing. Clin Dermatol 1994; 12:157–169
10. Sporn MB, Roberts AB: A major advance in the use of growth factors to enhance wound healing. J Clin Invest 1993; 92:2565–2566
11. Rohovsky S, D'Amore PA: Growth factors and angiogenesis in wound healing. In: Ziegler TR, Pierce GF,

Herndon DN (eds) Growth Factors and Wound Healing: Basic Science and Potential Clinical Applications. Berlin Heidelberg New York: Springer-Verlag. 1997; pp 8–26

12. Greenhalgh DG: The role of growth factors in wound healing. J Trauma 1996; 41:159–167

13. Jaschke E, Zabernigg A, Gattringer C: Recombinant human granulocyte-macrophage colony-stimulating factor applied locally in low doses enhances healing and prevents recurrence of chronic venous ulcers. Int J Dermatol 1999; 38:380–386

14. Declair V: The importance of growth factors in wound healing. Ostomy Wound Manage 1999; 45: 64–68, 70–72, 74

15. Gibbs S, Silva-Pinto AN, Murli S, et al: Epidermal growth factor and keratinocyte growth factor differentially regulate epidermal migration, growth, and differentiation. Wound Rep Reg 2000; 8:192–203

16. Mustoe TA, Pierce GF, Thomason A, et al: Accelerated healing of incisional wounds in rats induced by transforming growth factor β. Science 1987; 237:1333–1336

17. Leitzel K, Cano C, Marks JG Jr, et al: Growth factors and wound healing in the hamster. J Dermatol Surg Oncol 1985; 11:617–622

18. McGee GS, Davidson JM, Buckley A, et al: Recombinant basic fibroblast growth factor accelerates wound healing. J Surg Res 1988; 45:145–153

19. Hebda PA, Klingbeil CK, Abraham JA, et al: Basic fibroblast growth factor stimulation of epidermal wound healing in pigs. J Invest Dermatol 1990; 95:626–631

20. Wu L, Mustoe TA: Effect of ischemia on growth factor enhancement of incisional wound healing. Surgery 1995; 117:570–576

21. Greenhalgh DG, Sprugel KH, Murray MJ, et al: PDGF and FGF stimulate healing in the genetically diabetic mouse. Am J Pathol 1990; 136:1235–1246

22. Brown GL, Nanney LB, Griffen J, et al: Enhancement of wound healing by topical treatment with epidermal growth factor. N Engl J Med 1989; 321:76–79

23. Fu X, Shen Z, Chen Y, et al: Recombinant bovine basic fibroblast growth factor accelerates wound healing in patients with burns, donor sites and chronic dermal ulcers. Chin Med J (Engl) 2000; 113:367–371

24. Cohen MA, Eaglstein WH: Recombinant human platelet-derived growth factor gel speeds healing of acute full-thickness punch biopsy wounds. J Am Acad Dermatol 2001; 45: 857–862

25. Bello YM, Phillips TJ: Recent advances in wound healing. JAMA 2000; 83: 716–718

26. Konig M, Peschen M, Vanscheidt W: Molecular biology of chronic wounds. In: Hafner J, Ramelet AA, Schmeller W, Brunner UV (eds) Management of Leg Ulcers. Current Problems in Dermatology, vol 27. Basel: Karger. 1999; pp 8–12

27. Castronuovo JJ Jr, Ghobrial I, Giusti AM, et al: Effects of chronic wound fluid on the structure and biological activity of becaplermin (rhPDGF-BB) and becaplermin gel. Am J Surg 1998; 176:61S–67S

28. Pierce GF, Tarpley JE, Tseng J, et al: Detection of platelet-derived growth factor (PDGF)-AA in actively healing human wounds treated with recombinant PDGF-BB and absence of PDGF in chronic nonhealing wounds. J Clin Invest 1995; 96:1336–1350

29. Staiano-Coico L, Higgins PJ, Schwartz SB, et al: Wound fluids: a reflection of the state of healing. Ostomy Wound Manage 2000; 46 [1 A Suppl]:85S–93S

30. Trengove NJ, Stacey MC, MacAuley S, et al: Analysis of the acute and chronic wound environments: the role of proteases and their inhibitors. Wound Rep Reg 1999; 7:442–452

31. Yager DR, Zhang LY, Liang HX, et al: Wound fluids from human pressure ulcers contain elevated matrix metalloproteinase levels and activity compared to surgical wound fluids. J Invest Dermatol 1996; 107: 743–748

32. Kaplan G, Walsh G, Guido LS, et al: Novel responses of human skin to intradermal recombinanat granulocyte/macrophage-colony-stimulating factor: Langerhans cell recruitement, keratinocyte growth, and enhanced wound healing. J Exp Med 1992; 175:1717–1728

33. Kiritsy CP, Lynch AB, Lynch SE: Role of growth factors in cutaneous wound healing: a review. Crit Rev Oral Biol Med 1993; 4:729–760

34. Robson MC, Mustoe TA, Hunt TK: The future of recombinant growth factors in wound healing. Am J Surg 1998; 176(2A Suppl): 80S–82S

35. Limat A, French LE: Therapy with growth factors. In: Hafner J, Ramelet AA, Schmeller W, Brunner UV (eds) Management of Leg Ulcers. Current Problems in Dermatology, vol 27. Basel: Karger. 1999; pp 49–56

36. Wieman TJ: Clinical efficacy of becaplermin (rhPDGF-BB) gel. Am J Surg 1998; 176 [Suppl 2A]:74S–79S

37. Ross R, Raines EW, Bowen-Pope DF: The biology of platelet-derived growth factor. Cell 1986; 46:155–169

38. Lynch SE, Colvin RB, Antoniades HN: Growth factors in wound healing: Single and synergistic effects on partial thickness porcine skin wounds. J Clin Invest 1989; 84:640–646

39. Ross R: Platelet-derived growth factor. Annu Rev Med 1987; 38:71–79

40. Yarborough P, Bennet MS, Cannon B, et al: New Product Bulletin – Regranex® (becaplermin) gel. American Pharmaceutical Association. 1998

41. Wieman TJ, Smiell JM, Su Y: Efficacy and safety of a topical gel formulation of recombinant human platelet-derived growth factor-BB (becaplermin) in patients with chronic neuropathic diabetic ulcers. Diabetes Care 1998; 21:822–827

42. Steed DL: Clinical evaluation of recombinant human platelet-derived growth factor for the treatment of lower extremity diabetic ulcers. Diabetic ulcer study group. J Vasc Surg 1995; 21:71–78

43. D'Hemecourt PA, Smiell JM, Karim MR: Sodium carboxymethylcellulose aqueous-based gel vs. becaplermin gel in patients with nonhealing lower extremity diabetic ulcers. Wounds 1998; 10:69–75

44. Smiell JM, Wieman TJ, Steed DL, et al: Efficacy and safety of becaplermin (recombinant human platelet-derived growth factor-BB) in patients with nonhealing, lower extremity diabetic ulcers: a combined analysis of four randomized studies. Wound Rep Reg 1999; 7:335–346

45. Embil JM, Papp K, Sibbald G, et al: Recombinant human platelet-derived growth factor-BB (becaplermin) for healing chronic lower extremity diabetic ulcers: an open-label clinical evaluation of efficacy. Wound Rep Reg 2000; 8:162–168
46. Mannari RJ, Payne WG, Ochs DE, et al: Successful treatment of recalcitrant diabetic heel ulcers with topical becaplermin (rh PDGF-BB) gel. Wounds 2002; 14:116–121
47. Rees RS, Robson MC, Smiell JM, et al: Becaplermin gel in the treatment of pressure ulcers: a phase II randomized, double-blind, placebo-controlled study. Wound Rep Reg 1999; 7:141–147
48. Kallianinen LK, Hirshberg J, Merchant B, et al: Role of platelet-derived growth factor as an adjunct to surgery in the management of pressure ulcers. Plast Reconstr Surg 2000; 106:1243–1248
49. Robson MC, Phillips LG, Thomason A, et al: Platelet-derived growth factor BB for the treatment of chronic pressure ulcers. Lancet 1992; 339:23–25
50. Wollina U, Liebold K, Konrad H: Treatment of chronic radiation ulcers with recombinant platelet-derived growth factor and a hydrophilic copolymer membrane. J Eur Acad Dermatol Venereol 2001; 15:455–457
51. Wieman TJ: Efficacy and safety of recombinant human platelet-derived growth factor-BB (becaplermin) in patients with chronic venous ulcers: a pilot study. Wounds 2003; 15:257–264
52. Steed DL, Donohoe D, Webster MW, et al: Effect of extensive debridement and treatment on the healing of diabetic foot ulcers. Diabetic ulcer study group. J Am Coll Surg 1996; 183:61–64
53. Robson MC, Phillips LG, Lawrence WT, et al: The safety and effect of topically applied recombinant basic fibroblast growth factor on the healing of chronic pressure sores. Ann Surg 1992; 216:401–408
54. Robson MC, Phillips TJ, Falanga V, et al: Randomized trial of topically applied repifermin (recombinant human keratinocyte growth factor-2) to accelerate wound healing in venous ulcers. Wound Rep Reg 2001; 9:347–352
55. Robson MC, Smith PD: Topical use of growth factors to enhance healing. In: Falanga V (ed) Cutaneous Wound Healing, 1st edn. London: Martin Dunitz. 2001; pp 379–398
56. Nayeri F, Stromberg T, Larsson M, et al: Hepatocyte growth factor may accelarate healing in chronic leg ulcers: a pilot study. J Dermatolog Treat 2002; 13:81–86
57. Groves RW, Schmidt-Lucke JA: Recombinant human GM-CSF in the treatment of poorly healing wounds. Adv Skin Wound Care 2000; 13:107–112
58. Da Costa RM, Aniceto C, Jesus FM, et al: Quick healing of leg ulcers after molgramostim. Lancet 1994; 344:481–482
59. Halabe A, Ingber A, Hodak E, et al: Granulocyte-macrophage colony stimulating factor – a novel therapy in the healing of chronic ulcerative lesions. Med Sci Res 1995; 23:65–66
60. Voskaridou E, Kyrtsonis MC, Loutradi-Anagnostou A: Healing of chronic leg ulcers in the hemoglobinopathies with perilesional injections of granulocyte macrophage colony-stimulating factor. Blood 1999; 93: 3568–3569
61. Da Costa RM, Jesus FM, Aniceto C, et al: Double-blind randomized placebo-controlled trial of the use of granulocyte-macrophage colony- stimulating factor in chronic leg ulcers. Am J Surg 1997; 173: 165–168
62. Da Costa RM, Jesus FM, Aniceto C, et al: Randomized, double-blind, placebo-controlled, dose-ranging study of granulocyte-macrophage colony stimulating factor in patients with chronic venous leg ulcers. Wound Repair Regen 1999; 7:17–25
63. Jaschke E, Zabernigg A, Gattringer C: Low dose recombinant human granulocyte macrophage colony stimulating factor in the local treatment of chronic wounds. Paper presented at: GM-CSF: New Applications for Wound Healing. Sixth European Conference on Advances in Wound Management. Amsterdam: October 2, 1996
64. Raderer M, Kornek G, Hejna M, et al: Topical granulocyte-macrophage colony- stimulating factor in patients with cancer and impaired wound healing [letter]. J Natl Cancer Inst 1997; 89:263
65. Pieters RC, Rojer RA, Saleh AW, et al: Molgramostim to treat SS – sickle cell leg ulcers. Lancet 1995; 345:528
66. Robson MC, Hill DP, Smith PD, et al: Sequential cytokine therapy for pressure ulcers: clinical and mechanistic response. Ann Surg 2000; 231:600–611
67. Starkey RH, Cohen S, Orth DN: Epidermal growth factor: Identification of a new hormone in Human Urine. Science 1975; 189:800–802
68. Tranuzzer RW, Macaulay SP, Mast BA, et al: Epidermal growth factor in wound healing: A model for the molecular pathogenesis of chronic wounds. In: Ziegler TR, Pierce GF, Herndon DN (eds) Growth Factors and Wound Healing: Basic Science and Potential Clinical Applications. Berlin Heidelberg New York: Springer-Verlag. 1997; pp 206–228
69. Carpenter G, Cohen S: Epidermal growth factor. J Biol Chem 1990; 265:7709–7712
70. Laato M, Niinikoski J, Lebel L, et al: Stimulation of wound healing by epidermal growth factor. A dose-dependent effect. Ann Surg 1986; 203:379–381
71. Franklin JD, Lynch JB: Effects of topical applications of epidermal growth factor on wound healing. Experimental study on rabbit ears. Plast Reconstr Surg 1979; 64:766–770
72. Falanga V, Eaglstein WH, Bucalo B, et al: Topical use of human recombinant epidermal growth (h-EGF) in venous ulcers. J Derm Surg Oncol 1992; 18:604–606
73. Gough A, Clapperton M, Rolando N, et al: Randomized placebo-controlled trial of granulocyte-colony stimulating factor in diabetic foot infection. Lancet 1997; 350:855–859
74. De Lalla F, Pellizzer G, Strazzabosco M, et al: Randomized prospective controlled trial of recombinant granulocyte colony-stimulating factor as adjunctive therapy for limb- threatening diabetic foot infection. Antimicrob Agents Chemother 2001; 45: 1094–1098

Drugs, Wound Healing and Cutaneous Ulcers 16

Contents

16.1 Overview

This chapter deals with the association between medications and the wound healing process.

Schematically, three major categories of medications may be considered:
- Drugs that directly ulcerate the skin (whether by injection, topical use, or systemic administration)
- Drugs that interfere with the natural wound healing process
- Drugs that affect skin quality in general

This classification into three categories is somewhat artificial, and in many cases there is an overlap between the various types of effects listed above for a given drug. For example, it is reasonable to assume that each medication that directly causes ulcers (e.g., a drug that induces systemic lupus erythematosus), interferes with the healing of existing ulcers as well.

Drugs such as calcium blockers, which may cause leg edema, may serve as another example. Edema, in itself, has a generally adverse effect on the skin. As a result, the skin is more vulnerable, and even trivial trauma can result in ulceration. At the same time, since the skin's overall quality is adversely affected, it is reasonable to assume that its ability to heal is diminished, even for pre-existing ulcers. Nevertheless, for the sake of simplicity, in this chapter we restrict ourselves to the three-category classification.

A major issue presented is the category of medications that directly cause ulceration. In some cases, the drug causes ulceration following its injection into the skin at the injection site. In addition, ulceration may develop following cutaneous application of certain topical preparations.

Certain drugs administered systemically may cause ulceration directly, through various mechanisms such as the induction of vasculitis, the causing or aggravating of existing diseases, or by affecting coagulation. In some instances the mechanism leading to ulceration is not known with certainty.

16.2 Ulceration at the Injection Site

Some drugs are known to cause ulceration when injected into the skin.

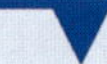

Drugs may be injected for various reasons:
- For therapeutic purposes (see Table 16.1)
- Accidental injections
- Drug abuse
- Self-inflicted (factitious) ulcers

(Drugs causing ulceration through accidental injections, drug abuse, and self-inflicted ulcers are detailed in Table 16.2).

16.2.1 Injections for Therapeutic Purposes – Subcutaneous or Intramuscular

Ulceration of the skin may occur at the injection site following subcutaneous or intramus-

Table 16.1. Ulceration at the injection site – injections for therapeutic purposes

Subcutaneous or intramuscular injections	Extravasation
Aseptic necrosis (*embolia cutis medicamentosa*) Phenylbutazone Local anesthetics Corticosteroids	Doxorubicin hydrochloride (Adriamycin) *cis*-Platinum 5-Fluorouracil Vinblastine Vincristine
Formation of sterile abscess Paraldehyde Clindamycin Intralesional BCG Prophylactic plague vaccination	Actinomycin D Daunorubicin
Induction of destructive vasculitis Pentazocine Interferon α, β, and γ	
Vasospastic effect Cocaine Ergotamine Interferon injections	
Granulomatous reaction Silicone injections	
Other medications Sclerosing agents Papaverin injections Heparin	

Table 16.2. Injected drugs – ulceration at the injection site

Accidental injections	Drug abuse	Self-inflicted ulcers[a]
Phenytoin	Cocaine	Phenol
Diazepam	Heroin	Sodium hydroxide
Dopamine	Pentazocine	Kerosene
Methylphenidate		Talc
Penicillin		Fillers of analgesic tablets
Terbutaline sulfate		Oily substances such as paraffin

[a] Numerous materials have been documented, including those listed here.

cular injections, as described below. Ulceration may be due to a variety of mechanisms:

■ **Aseptic Necrosis (*embolia cutis medicamentosa*).** Aseptic necrosis is a relatively rare, adverse effect of injected drugs. It has been documented following i.m. injections of phenylbutazone type analgesics and following injections containing local anesthetics or corticosteroids [1–4].

Soon after the injection, pain (which may be very intense) occurs, followed by skin necrosis of varying degrees in the affected area. The necrosis, in this case, is thought to be the result of an arterial occlusion, which could result from either embolus of the injected drug or direct compression of the artery by the injected material adjacent to the affected vessel [2, 5].

■ **Sterile Abscesses.** Intramuscular injections of paraldehyde or clindamycin have been reported to result in the formation of sterile abscesses with subsequent ulceration [1, 6]. A patient treated with multiple intramuscular injections is at a greater risk of developing this complication [6].

Sterile abscesses have also been reported following injections containing other materials, such as prophylactic plague vaccination [7].

Note that improper injection technique may result in local infection, sometimes accompanied by abscess formation and ulceration. However, this being the case, the abscess is not sterile and this phenomenon is not related to the injected drug.

■ **Induction of Destructive Vasculitis.** Injections of pentazocine [8] have induced obliterative vasculitis with subsequent ulceration. Note that pentazocine, apart from being used for genuine therapeutic indications, is commonly used by drug abusers.

Certain immunomodulators injected i.m., such as interferon α, β, and γ, have also been described as causing necrotizing vasculitis [9]. Note that recently, the most common drugs documented as causing ulceration following i.m. or s.c. injections are cytokines such as interferon α, β, or γ, used as immunomodulators [9–14]. With the increasing use of these substances, there are increasing numbers of reports of cutaneous ulceration following their use.

A biopsy of the ulcer may reveal necrotizing vasculitis [9]. However, this particular pathology is not necessarily seen in many other cases of ulceration following s.c. or i.m. injections of immunomodulators. Other suggested possible mechanisms of ulceration in these cases are vasospastic effects of the drug or direct toxic effects of the drug on the endothelium, with its subsequent formation of fibrin thrombi in deep dermal vessels [11, 14]. Note that certain immunomodulators such as interferon β-1b may result in non-injection site ulceration as well [13].

■ **Vasospastic Effect.** As mentioned above, a vasospastic effect has been suggested as a possible mechanism for the induction of ulceration following interferon injections [14]. Note that digital blocks with adrenaline (epinephrine) are known to result in vasospasm, which may result in severe ischemia [15, 16]. Local anesthetic containing adrenaline should therefore not be used in acral areas such as the fingers, toes, penis, and nose, which may be particularly affected by these preparations [17]. However, some researchers have pointed out that there have been no documented reports of ischemic necrosis of a digit from the appropriate use of local anesthetics containing adrenaline [18].

On the other hand, ulceration in drug abusers may be induced by the vasospastic effects of certain drugs such as cocaine (discussed below). Ergotamine preparations (which may, on occasion, be given as intramuscular injections) are discussed in Sect. 16.4.3.

■ **Granulomatous Reaction.** Silicone injections may induce granulomatous reactions. Typical reactions to silicone injections may manifest as classic signs of inflammation such as erythema, edema, and local sensitivity. However, more severe reactions with subcutaneous atrophy, fibrosis, and ulceration have been documented [19, 20]. Currently, the FDA has not approved liquid silicone injections for any purpose.

■ **Other Medications.** Ulceration has been documented following injections of sclerosants for telangiectasia [21]. Penile ulcerations have been documented following injections of papaverine [22]. In the latter case, there is no clear explanation for the development of ulceration. The authors suggest that it may be attributed to a combination of vascular trauma (due to the needle) and the low pH of the papaverine solution.

Heparin, given subcutaneously, may also cause ulceration. This issue is discussed below in Sect. 16.4.4.

16.2.2 Injection for Therapeutic Purposes – Extravasation

Extravasation injury is defined as leakage of pharmacologic solutions into the skin and subcutaneous tissue during intravenous administration. It is not an uncommon event; the reported incidence is 11% in children and 22% in adults treated with intravenous drugs [23, 24]. Doxorubicin hydrochloride (Adriamycin) is the most 'notorious' extravasated drug [25–29] in terms of skin ulceration. Other cytotoxic drugs, such as *cis*-platinum, 5-fluorouracil, vinblastine, vincristine, actinomycin D, and daunorubicin, are reported as causing ulceration when extravasated [1, 30–33]. Extravasation of contrast medium may also result in cutaneous ulceration [34].

The clinical course of a typical extravasation injury has been documented mainly with regard to extravasated doxorubicin [35, 36]. Extravasation is initially followed by the appearance of swelling and redness in the area of injury, accompanied by pain. Induration at the extravasation site may develop into an ulcer within a period of weeks or months.

The extent of ulceration depends on the:
- Type of offending drug
- Amount of extravasated material
- Site of extravasation: more severe reactions tend to develop on the dorsum of the hand and in the area of the antecubital fossa [1].

16.2.3 Accidental Injections

Accidental intra-arterial injections of various drugs, including phenytoin, diazepam, dopamine, methylphenidate, and penicillin, have been documented as resulting in digital gangrene or cutaneous ulceration at the site of injection [37–43]. An accidental finger stab with a needle used for administration of terbutaline sulphate (a β-adrenergic drug) has been documented as causing local necrosis [44].

16.2.4 Drug Abuse

Cutaneous ulcers within injection sites of cocaine and heroin have been documented [45–47] (Fig. 16.1). Pentazocine ulcers are com-

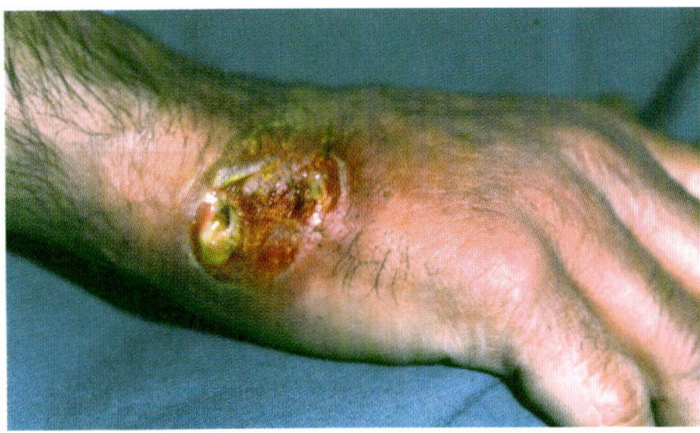

Fig. 16.1. A cutaneous ulcer in a drug addict following an injection of heroin

mon among drug abusers [48]. Drugs such as heroin may be adulterated with fillers containing other drugs (e.g., quinine, barbiturates, mannitol) or certain chemicals, including dextrose, cocaine, caffeine, procaine, talc, baking soda, starch, battery acid, butacaine, and nicotine [48].

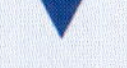

There are several pathophysiological mechanisms by which ulcers occur [49]:
- The drug itself, e.g., vasospastic properties of cocaine [46]
- Irritant or caustic effects of adulterants or excipients
- The use of contaminated needles with consequent infection

Kirchenbaum and Midenberg [49] reported the following incidence of ulceration at injection sites in the lower extremities of 56 drug abusers: dorsal venous arch of the foot (68%), greater saphenous vein (14%), veins in the digits (10%), and the spaces between the toes (7%). **'Puffy foot syndrome'** was described in patients who repeatedly used their limbs for drug injections, resulting in the blockage of lymphatics and the distortion of the venous return, with an increased risk of ulceration [49].

16.2.5 Self-Inflicted Ulcers

In most cases, self-inflicted ulcers are caused by continuous scratching, rubbing, or cutting of the skin. Once an ulcer appears, the continual 'fiddling' with it by the patient interferes with its healing.

Sometimes, self-inflicted ulcers are deliberately induced by injecting certain materials, including drugs, into the skin. Some injected drugs may be identified, since they are incorporated in specific vehicles. Jackson et al. [50] reported factitious ulcers caused by injections of certain pulverized tablet materials, originating from analgesic tablets or pentazocine hydrochloride tablets. Numerous materials such as phenol [48], sodium hydroxide [51], and kerosene [52] have been documented as being used for self-mutilation.

A lesion caused by the injection of an offending material may initially appear in the form of a nodule, or an abscess, which subsequently undergoes ulceration. In these cases, histology may contribute to a diagnostic identification of the ulcer's cause. The lesion may show (but not always) giant cells or epitheloid cells.

The unique characteristics of specific materials may also be reflected in the histology. For example, oil-containing substances are identified by the 'Swiss-cheese pattern' (as seen in paraffinoma), with numerous ovoid spaces of varying size, filled with the oily substance [53].

Using polarized light, one may identify the presence of inorganic birefringent materials. Some of these, such as talc, which is used as a filler in certain analgesic tablets, may be injected into the skin.

Substances that are doubly refractile on polarizing examination include:
- Nylon sutures
- Wood
- Talc
- Starch powder
- Silica
- Beryllium

Other substances may be identified by chemical or spectrophotometric methods [54].

Jackson et al. [50] introduced the electron-probe microanalysis method to determine accurately the presence and chemical nature of foreign material. This technique can identify certain pulverized tablet materials such as microcrystalline cellulose (found in pentazocine hydrochloride tablets) or talc (used as a filler in certain analgesic tablets), which may be injected into the skin and subcutaneous tissue.

16.3 Direct Cutaneous Exposure

The long-term use of suppositories containing ergotamine is reported to have caused perianal ulcers [55, 56]. Certain drugs, such as povidone-iodine [57], may induce ulceration by causing severe contact dermatitis (see Chap. 4).

In addition to the comments presented earlier regarding drug abuse, Tirney and Stadelmann [58] documented extensive facial necrosis, resulting from ischemia and subsequent infection, following the intranasal impaction of 'crack' cocaine.

16.4 Systemic Drugs that Directly Induce Ulceration

16.4.1 Causing or Aggravating Certain Diseases

Some drugs tend to cause or aggravate certain diseases in which cutaneous ulcers may be a feature (Table. 16.3). The classical example of such a disease is systemic lupus erythematosus (SLE). The most common drugs related etiologically to SLE are hydralazine, procainamide, β-blockers, phenytoin, and isoniazid [59]. These drugs, among many others, may result in SLE-like syndromes that are indistinguishable from SLE. In some cases, ulceration may develop, similar to that seen in SLE. Certain other medications may exacerbate pre-existing SLE: griseofulvin, sulfonamides, testosterone, and estrogens [60].

Despite the abundance of information in the literature regarding medications that cause SLE or SLE-like syndromes, there are no accurate statistical data regarding the development of cutaneous ulcers following treatment with such

Table 16.3. Systemic drugs that directly induce ulceration

Cause or aggravate certain diseases	Induce vasculitis
SLE • Hydralazyne	• Clyndamycin • Non-steroidal anti-inflammatory drugs • Propylthiouracil • Diltiazem • Oral contraceptives • Levamisole • Minocycline • Hydralazine • Warfarin
Lichen planus • Hydroxyurea • Methyldopa • Propanolol • Lithium carbonate	**Affect coagulability** • Warfarin • Heparin • Low-molecular-weight-heparin
Pyoderma gangrenosum • Granulocyte colony-stimulating factor • Isotretinoine • Montelukast sodium • Ibuprofen	**By unidentified mechanisms** • Hydroxyurea • Methotrexate • Bleomycin

medications, and the information available is limited to isolated case reports. Drug-induced SLE associated with the development of ulcers has been documented following the ingestion of hydralazine [59, 61, 62]. In some cases, histology shows that the hydralazine itself apparently induces vasculitis [62]. However, it should be noted that other conditions associated with SLE, such as Raynaud's phenomenon or the anti-phospholipid syndrome, may cause ulceration as well (see Chap. 4).

There are several other systemic diseases in which ulceration may occur following the use of certain drugs. The anti-phospholipid syndrome has been reported following the use of chloro-promazine, procaine-amide, quinidine, hydralazine, phenytoin, and interferon [63]. Dermatomyositis may also be precipitated by several drugs, including penicillamine, NSAIDs, or carbamazepine [60]. Nevertheless, for the above cases there are no data relating to the induction of ulceration by drugs in these diseases.

The association between drugs, scleroderma and cutaneous ulcers is discussed in Sect. 16.6.2.

Finally, certain ulcerative cutaneous processes may be induced by certain drugs: Lichen planus of the ulcerative type has been associated with the use of hydroxyurea [68], methyldopa [65], propanolol [66], and lithium carbonate [67]; pyoderma gangrenosum has been documented in association with the use of granulocyte colony-stimulating factor, isotretinoin, montelukast sodium (Singulair®), and ibuprofen [68–71]. In addition, sulpiride has been documented as a possible inducer of pyoderma gangrenosum-like eruption [72].

6.4.2 Induction of Vasculitis

Drugs that most commonly cause leukocytoclasic vasculitis are penicillin, sulfonamides, thiazides, allopurinol, and non-steroidal anti-inflammatory agents [73]. However, specific documentation as to drug-induced leukocytoclasic vasculitis manifested by ulceration is rather infrequent. Certain medications have been reported to induce vasculitis with subsequent formation of cutaneous ulcers. These in-

clude clindamycin [74], NSAIDs [75], propylthiouracil [76], diltiazem [77], oral contraceptives [78], levamisole [79], and minocycline [80]. However, in some of these reports the association between the drug and vasculitis may be questionable, and other factors may be involved.

Hydralazine, as discussed above, has been reported to induce SLE-reactions with vasculitis [62]. Vasculitis has also been documented in several cases of warfarin administration [81–83]. There are no accurate and well-established epidemiological reports regarding medications that tend to induce vasculitis presenting as cutaneous ulcers. As mentioned earlier in this chapter, certain drugs may induce a local vasculitic response when injected s.c. or i.m.

16.4.3 Vasospasm

Certain medications mentioned-above have been reported as having a vasospastic effect when administered by injection. Ergotamine preparations (usually given orally) have also been documented as resulting in severe vasospasm with subsequent ulceration [84–87]. Most of the existing reports have documented ischemic events of the lower extremities.

16.4.4 Drugs Affecting Coagulability

Skin necrosis may be induced by drugs that affect coagulability, such as warfarin or heparin. As noted below, the exact mechanism by which these drugs induce ulceration has not yet been fully established.

■ **Warfarin-induced Skin Necrosis.** The phenomenon appears in 0.01%–0.1% of patients treated with warfarin or its derivatives [88]. In most cases, warfarin necrosis usually appears within 3–6 days following ingestion of the drug, but it can also appear within the first two weeks. This process tends to develop in areas containing relatively high amounts of subcutaneous fat, such as buttocks, thighs, and breasts. This preference is attributed to the reduced vascularity of adipose tissue. However, other areas may also be affected. The initial cutaneous finding is an erythematous area, usually poorly demarcated, which gradually darkens to blue-black and progresses towards a well-demarcated area of necrosis. Hemorrhagic blisters may develop prior to the onset of ulceration [17, 89, 90]. Most of the affected patients are adult women with a tendency to obesity, the female-to-male ratio being 9:1 [88]. In most cases there is only a single lesion, but in one third of patients multiple lesions have been documented [88].

The initial mechanism of warfarin-induced ulceration involves a hypercoagulable state [88, 90]. The histological findings support this assumption: The early pathologic changes are microvascular damage with fibrin deposits in the postcapillary venules and small veins. Later, areas of hemorrhage and diffuse necrosis are seen in the dermis and subcutaneous tissue [91, 92]. However, in some cases, evidence of vasculitis has been documented following warfarin administration [86, 87]. One may conclude that there is probably more than one mechanism of ulceration.

Predisposing factors to warfarin necrosis are protein C deficiency or protein S deficiency [89, 93–99]. These associations further support the assumption that the mechanism causing warfarin necrosis is basically mediated via processes affecting coagulability.

■ **Heparin-Induced Necrosis.** Skin necrosis usually develops within 6–8 days following subcutaneous injection of heparin, but it can also appear after two weeks [100, 101]. In most cases the ulceration appears right at the injection site. Rarely, other sites may also be involved. Lesions of heparin necrosis have been reported to occur on the nose, hand, forearm, ankle, and thigh [101]. The clinical and histologic findings are indistinguishable from those of warfarin necrosis [101–103], which implies that similar mechanisms are responsible for necrosis. There are several reports of necrosis following the use of low-molecular-weight-heparin [104–107].

6.4.5 Drugs Causing Bullae

As mentioned in Chap. 4, even a superficial erosion (due to trauma, or bullous disease) may become an ulcer following bacterial infection. The probability of this occurring is much higher when there is an underlying problem such as diabetes mellitus or prolonged glucocorticoid therapy (as is the case with many patients suffering from bullous diseases). Numerous drugs may induce bullae; a detailed discussion, however, is beyond the scope of this chapter.

16.4.6 Unidentified Mechanisms

Apart from the groups of drugs presented above, certain drugs may result in cutaneous ulcers by mechanisms that are not currently fully understood. Hydroxyurea is a relatively frequent inducer of cutaneous ulcers [108–114]. It is reasonable to assume that hydroxyurea ulceration is not attributed to its anti-neoplastic effect, since other anti-neoplastic medications from the same group are not known to cause skin ulcers.

Similarly, methotrexate is known to induce the formation of mucosal and, less commonly, skin ulcers[115, 116]. Kaplan et al. [117] documented erosion of psoriatic plaques following chronic methotrexate administration.

Bleomycin-induced digital gangrene has been reported following i.m. injection [118]. In this report, the exact mechanism was not clarified, although the authors suggested that the drug may have induced Raynaud's phenomenon.

16.5 Interference with Normal Mechanisms of Wound Healing

In most cases, drugs belonging to this group do not cause ulceration directly. These drugs may interfere with the healthy physiological mechanisms of wound healing, and their use may significantly impede the healing of existing ulcers. Glucocorticoids are the most notorious drugs of this group, in respect to their influence on heal-

Table 16.4. Drugs that Interfere healing

Glucocorticoids

Non-steroidal anti-inflammatory drugs

**Anti-neoplastic
and immunosuppressive drugs**

Others

- colchicine
- penicillamine

ing. Other drugs that may interfere with healing are presented in Table 16.4.

Note that the use of some drugs in the presence of certain diseases such as diabetes mellitus or venous insufficiency may significantly increase the risk of developing cutaneous ulcers.

Generally speaking, it is difficult to predict the extent to which the medications discussed below impede the healing of chronic cutaneous ulcers. In the few cases described, when research studies were planned in order to examine the detrimental effect of drugs on healing, they focused on *acute* surgical wounds only.

16.5.1 Glucocorticoids

The detrimental effect of glucocorticoids on wound healing has been recognized and documented for many years [119]. Not surprisingly, the same qualities, namely anti-inflammatory, immunosuppressive, and anti-proliferative, that impart the therapeutic value of glucocorticoids in certain diseases are those that interfere with the normal course of wound repair.

Glucocorticoids influence and interfere with various aspects of wound healing. Laboratory research studies have documented decreased production of cytokines and growth factors, suppression of inflammatory response and mobilization of white cells, and the stabilization of lysosomal membranes in white blood cells, thereby decreasing phagocytic activity [120–122]. Host defense mechanisms become less efficient, resulting in an increased susceptibility to various infections.

Reduced proliferation of epidermal cells and fibroblasts occurs, associated with impaired angiogenesis [123–126]; wound contraction is impaired and reduced synthesis of proteins and collagen further delays the normal course of wound healing and closure of cutaneous ulcers [127, 128].

Research studies have shown that if glucocorticoids are administered within the first three days following injury, the effect on wound healing is much more significant than if they are administered more than three days after the trauma [129, 130]. Therefore, one may conclude that the detrimental effect of glucocorticoids is related mainly to their anti-inflammatory effects in the initial stages of injury.

In traumatic wounds in adults, it appears that low-dosage glucocorticoids (less than 10 mg prednisone per day) do not have a discernible effect on wound healing. Moderate dosages of 10–30 mg prednisone per day result in a mild mechanical impairment of wound strength. A dosage of 40 mg prednisone or more per day has a direct inhibitory effect on wound healing [121]. To the best of our knowledge, the data presented above have not been confirmed or re-evaluated in recent years by up-dated research studies.

The above conclusions may be reached only as regards acute traumatic wounds. When dealing with chronic cutaneous ulcers, it is difficult to assess the effects of glucocorticoids, and there is no definite information on this subject in the literature. Note that prolonged glucocorticoid therapy results in skin atrophy, with specific consequent ramifications on the process of wound healing (see below).

Through clinical experience we do know that even low doses of steroids, when taken for long periods, can result in such cutaneous damage as atrophy of the skin. It is reasonable to assume that those same mechanisms would interfere with wound healing and skin repair.

The obvious conclusion that can be drawn from the above information is that every effort should be made to discontinue glucocorticoid therapy (or at least reduce the dosage) in patients with chronic cutaneous ulcers.

Two further comments should be made here:

- To some extent, vitamin A may counteract the effects of glucocorticoids on wound healing. This issue is discussed in more detail in Chap. 19.
- The question as to whether topical growth factors may prevent some of the glucocorticoid effects on wound healing is still unanswered. Controlled research studies are needed.

16.5.2 Non-Steroidal Anti-Inflammatory Drugs

Medications such as aspirin and ibuprofen have been shown to impair collagen production and to lower the tensile strength of healing wounds [131, 132]. Whether the effect of non-steroidal anti-inflammatory drugs (NSAID) on the healing of cutaneous wounds is similar to their effect on gastric mucosa requires further investigation.

The extent to which the healing of cutaneous ulcers is hampered by NSAID is questionable. However, for patients with cutaneous ulcers, one should consider avoiding the use of NSAID and using alternative analgesic drugs. At present, there are no data regarding whether the use of advanced forms of NSAID may have a certain advantage with respect to their effect on healing.

16.5.3 Anti-Neoplastic and Immunosuppressive Drugs

Observations that anti-neoplastic and immunosuppressive drugs interfere with the normal course of wound healing, with respect to surgical wounds, are well documented in the literature [133]. Animal experiments have demonstrated that the extent of these detrimental effects depends on the specific medication used. Severe impairment of healing was observed following the use of actinomycin D, bleomycin, or BCNU, whereas the effect caused by vincristine, cyclophosphamide, or 5FU was relatively mild [134].

At present, the mechanism by which anti-neoplastic drugs exert their effects on the healing of cutaneous ulcers is not fully understood. Some of these effects may be attributed to nutritional deficiencies and the catabolic effects associated with these drugs [135–137]. In any case, the identification and correction of nutritional deficiencies may prevent the negative consequences of anti-neoplastic treatment on healing of wounds and chronic ulcers of the skin.

The issue of extravasation injury following intravenous injections of anti-neoplastic drugs is discussed above.

16.5.4 Other Drugs that Interfere with Healing

Colchicine has been shown to delay the normal course of wound healing. This effect may be due to its inhibitory effect on tubulin-dependent cell functions, including interference with fibroblasts, secretion of collagen precursors, and the inhibition of wound contraction [121, 138, 139]. Another medication that has been detected as a possible inhibitor of wound contraction and cutaneous healing is penicillamine [121, 139].

16.6 Drugs that Adversely Affect Skin Quality

16.6.1 Leg Edema

Calcium channel blockers, especially nifedipine, may cause edema of the legs [140–142]. Edema adversely affects the quality of the skin [143, 144], which can result in the formation of leg ulcers and the aggravation of pre-existing ulcers. The effect of calcium channel blockers is highly significant in patients who suffer from venous stasis or lymph vessel disease. In the presence of cutaneous ulcers, whenever possible, one should consider discontinuing these

Table 16.5. Drugs that adversely affect skin quality

Formation of leg edema[a]

Dihydropyridine calcium antagonists
- Nifedipine
- Amlodipine
- Felodipine
- Isradipine
- Nicardipine

Drugs causing skin atrophy or scleroderma-like reactions[b]

- glucocorticoids
- penicillamine
- bleomycin
- appetite suppressants
- pentazocine
- bromocriptine

a. The use of non-dihydropyridine calcium antagonists (i.e., verapamil and diltiazem) has also been reported to induce leg edema [147].
b. Exposure to various agents (e.g., polyvinyl chloride, epoxy resins, organic solvents, and pesticides) is also associated with sclerodrema or scleroderma-like changes [150, 151].

drugs. Luca and Romero [145] reported improvement of leg ulcers following the discontinuation of nifedipine. The phenomenon of drug-induced leg edema is commonly associated with the dihydropyridine calcium antagonists (nifedipine, felodipine, isradipine, nicardipine, nisoldipine) (see Table 16.5) [146]. However, it may occur following the use of non-dihydropyridine calcium antagonists (i.e., verapamil and diltiazem) as well [147]. The edema formation is caused, most probably, by arteriolar dilatation (which is greater than venous dilatation) and increased transcapillary pressure gradients [146].

16.6.2 Skin Atrophy or Scleroderma-Like Reactions

The effects of glucocorticoids on wound healing have been discussed above. As noted, glucocorticoid usage, whether systemic or topical, has been known for many years to cause skin

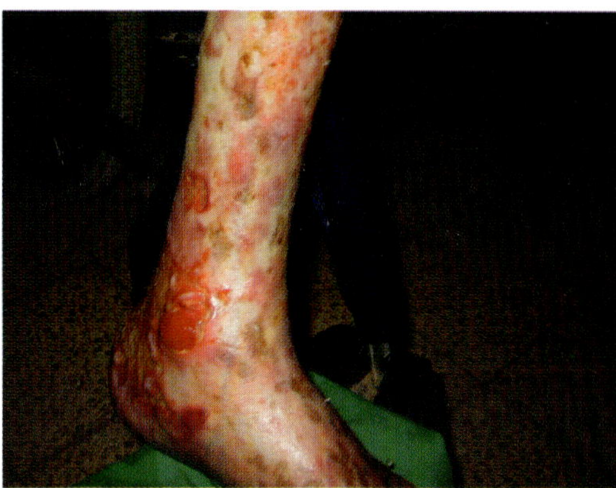

Fig. 16.2. Cutaneous ulcers on sclerodermoid skin

atrophy [148]. Atrophic skin is poorly vascularized and very vulnerable, and its ability to heal wounds is reduced.

Prolonged penicillamine therapy may also result in cutaneous atrophy [149].

Scleroderma-like reactions (Fig. 16.2) which affect the quality of the skin may develop following the use of certain medications including pentazocine, bleomycin, appetite suppressants, and bromocriptine [150–152]. Exposure to various agents (e.g., polyvinyl chloride, epoxy resins, organic solvents, and pesticides) is also associated with scleroderma or scleroderma-like changes [150, 151]. There are no clear data in the literature regarding the formation of ulcers under these circumstances.

References

1. Bork K: Ulcers and necroses; atrophies. In: Cutaneous Side Effects of Drugs, 1st edn. Philadelphia: WB Saunders. 1988; pp 360–369
2. Kohler LD, Schwedler S, Worret WI: Embolia cutis medicamentosa. Int J Dermatol 1997; 36:197
3. Kunzi T, Ramstein C, Pirovino M: Circumscribed skin necrosis following intramuscular injection (embolia cutis medicamentosa). Schweiz Rundsch Med Prax 1995; 84:640–643
4. Muller-Vahl H: Aseptic tissue necrosis: a severe complication after intramuscular injections. Dtsch Med Wochenschr 1984; 109:786–792
5. Gammel JA: Arterial embolism, an unusual complication following the intramuscular administration of bismuth. JAMA 1927; 88:998

6. Fiscina S: Injections followed by a sterile abscess. Mil Med 1986; 151:452

7. Smith AL, Khan F, De Mello W: Sterile abscess formation following plague vaccination. J R Army Med Corps 1997; 143:116–117

8. Cosman A, Feliciano WC, Wolff M: Pentazocine ulcers. Plast Reconst Surg 1977; 59:255–259

9. Krainick U, Kantarjian H, Broussard S, et al: Local cutaneous necrotizing lesions associated with interferon injections. J Interferon Cytokine Res 1998; 18:823–827

10. Webster GF, Knobler RL, Lublin FD, et al: Cutaneous ulcerations and pustular psoriasis flare caused by recombinant interferon β injections in patients with multiple sclerosis. J Am Acad Dermatol 1996; 34:365–367

11. Weinberg JM: Cutaneous necrosis associated with recombinant interferon injection. J Am Acad Dermatol 1998; 39:807–808

12. Oeda E, Shinohara K: Cutaneous necrosis caused by injection of α-interferon in a patient with chronic myelogenous leukemia. Am J Hematol 1993; 44:213–214

13. Gaines AR, Varricchio F: Interferon β-lb injection site reactions and necroses. Mult Scler 1998; 4:70–73

14. Weinberg JM, Wolfe JT, Sood S, et al: Cutaneous necrosis associated with recombinant interferon injection. Report of three cases with interferon beta-1b and review of the literature. Acta Derm Venereol (Stockh) 1997; 77:146–148

15. Hinterberger JW, Kintzi HE: Phentolamine reversal of epinephrine-induced digital vasospasm. How to save an ischemic finger. Arch Fam Med 1994; 3:193–195

16. Maguire WM, Reisdorff EJ, Smith D, Weigenstein JG: Epinephrine-induced vasospasm reversed by phentolamine digital block. Am J Emerg Med 1990; 8:46–47

17. Bork K: Necrosis and ulcers. In: Cutaneous Side Effects of Drugs. 1st edn. Philadelphia: W.B Saunders. 1988; pp 220–230

18. Sylaidis P, Logan A: Digital blocks with adrenaline. An old dogma refuted. J Hand Surg [Br] 1998; 23:17–19

19. Rae V, Pardo RJ, Blackwelder PL, et al: Leg ulcers following subcutaneous injection of a liquid silicone preparation. Arch Dermatol 1989; 125:670–673

20. Mastruserio DN, Pesqueira MJ, Cobb MW: Severe granulomatous reaction and facial ulceration occurring after subcutaneous silicone injection. J Am Acad Dermatol 1996; 34:849–852

21. Bihari I, Magyar E: Reasons for ulceration after injection treatment of telangiectasia. Dermatol Surg 2001; 27:133–136

22. Borgstrom E: Penile ulcer as complication in self-induced papaverine erections. Urology 1988; 32:416–417

23. Brown AS, Hoelzer DJ, Piercy SA: Skin necrosis from extravasation of intravenous fluids in children. Plast Reconstr Surg 1979; 64:145–150

24. Riyami A: Complications of intravenous infusions. J Ir Med Assoc 1968; 61:23–25

25. Disa JJ, Chang RR, Mucci SJ, et at: Prevention of Adriamycin induced full-thickness skin loss using hyaluronidase infiltration. Plast Reconstr Surg 1998; 101:370–374

26. Barden GA: Venous extravasation of doxorubicin HCI with secondary skin ulceration. South Med J 1980; 73:1543–1544

27. Mehta P, Najar N: Skin ulceration due to faulty adriamycin administration. Clin Pediatr (Phila) 1978; 17:663–664

28. Luedke DW, Kennedy PS, Rietschel RL: Histopathogenesis of skin and subcutaneous injury induced by Adriamycin. Plast Reconstr Surg 1979; 63:463–465

29. Bowers DG Jr, Lynch JB: Adriamycin extravasation. Plast Reconstr Surg 1978; 61:86–92

30. Bertelli G: Prevention and management of extravasation of cytotoxic drugs. Drug Saf 1995; 12:245–255

31. Boman NL, Tron VA, Bally MB, et al: Vincristine induced dermal toxicity is significantly reduced when the drug is given in liposomes. Cancer Chemother Pharmacol 1996; 37:351–355

32. Blair WF, Kilpatrick WC Jr, Saiki JH, Alter EJ: Extravasation of chemotherapeutic agents. Clin Orthop 1980; 151:228–230

33. Bairey O, Bishara J, Stahl B, et al: Severe tissue necrosis after cisplatin extravasation at low concentration: possible "immediate recall phenomenon". J Natl Cancer Inst 1997; 89:1233–1234

34. Elam EA, Dorr RT, Lagel KE, Pond GD: Cutaneous ulceration due to contrast extravasation. Experimental assessment of injury and potential antidotes. Invest Radiol 1991; 26:13–16

35. Heckler FR: Current thoughts on extravasation injuries. Clin Plast Surg 1989; 16:557–563

36. Rudolph R, Stein RS, Pattillo RA: Skin ulcers due to Adriamycin. Cancer 1976; 3:1087–1094

37. Sintenie JB, Tuinebreijer WE, Kreis RW, et al: Digital gangrene after accidental intra-arterial injection of phenytoin (epanutin). Eur J Surg 1992; 158:315–316

38. Joist A, Tibesku CO, Neuber M, et al: Gangrene of the fingers caused by accidental intra-arterial injection of diazepazn. Dtsch Med Wochenschr 1999; 124:755–758

39. Steib A, Jeanpierre C, Mole JP, et al: Tissue necrosis after accidental perivenous injection of dopamine. Ann Fr Anesth Reanim 1984; 3:328–329

40. De Myttenaere S, Heifetz M, Shilansky H, et al: Different treatments used in a case of gangrene due to accidental intra-arterial injection of methylphenidate (rilatine). Anesth Analg (Paris) 1977; 34:405–410

41. Schanzer H, Gribetz I, Jacobson JH: Accidental intra-arterial injection of penicillin G. A preventable catastrophe. JAMA 1979; 242:1289–1290

42. Schanzer H, Jacobson JH: Tissue damage caused by the intramuscular injection of long-acting penicillin. Pediatrics 1985; 75:741–744

43. Wynne JM, Williams GL, Ellman BA: Accidental intra-arterial injection. Arch Dis Child 1978; 53: 396–400
44. Yasin M, Vishne TH, Hendel D: Local necrosis of finger following stab with needle used to pump terbutaline sulfate (bricalin). Harefuah 2001; 140: 398–399
45. Bertoncini RL, Silveira PG, Ceola L, et at: Vascular complications in intravenous drug addicts. Rev Assoc Med Bras 1992; 38: 204–208
46. Abidin MR, Gillinov MA, Topol BM, et al: Injection of illicit drugs into the granulation tissue of chronic ulcers. Ann Plast Surg 1990; 24: 268–270
47. Dunne JH, Johnson WC: Necrotizing skin lesions in heroin addicts. Arch Dermatol 1972; 105: 544–547
48. Fellner MJ, Ledesma GN: Leg ulcers secondary to drug reactions. Clin Dermatol 1990; 8: 144–149
49. Kirchenbaum SE, Midenberg ML: Pedal and lower extremity complications of substance abuse. J Am Podiatry Assoc 1982; 72: 380–387
50. Jackson RM, Tucker SB, Abraham JL, et al: Factitial cutaneous ulcers and nodules: the use of electron-probe microanalysis in diagnosis. J Am Acad Dermatol 1984; 11: 1065–1069
51. Gschnait F, Brenner W, Berger E, et al: An unusual case of repeated self-mutilation. Wien Kim Wochenschr 1981; 93: 127–131
52. Qaryoute SM: Skin ulceration induced by kerosene injection. Ann Plast Surg 1984; 12: 361–363
53. Shapiro PE: Non infectious granulomas. In: Elder D, Elenitas R, Jaworsky C, Johnson B (eds) Lever's Histopathology of the Skin, 8th edn. Philadelphia: Lippincott-Raven. 1997; pp 317–340
54. Ackerman AB: Nodular and diffuse dermatitis. In: Histologic Diagnosis of Inflammatory Skin Diseases: An Algoritmic Method Based on Pattern Analysis. 1st edn. Baltimore Philadelphia: Lea & Febiger. 1978; pp 385– 495
55. Brandt O, Abeck D, Breitbart E, et al: Perianal ergotismus gangraenosus. Hautarzt 1997; 48: 199–202
56. Baptista AP, Mariano A, Machado A: Peranal ulcers caused by ergotamine-containing suppositories. Acta Med Port 1992; 5: 39–41
57. Mochida K, Hisa T, Yasunaga C, et al: Skin ulcerations due to povidone-iodine. Contact Dermatitis 1995; 33: 61–62
58. Tierney BP, Stadelmann WK: Necrotizing infection of the face secondary to intranasal impaction of "-crack" cocaine. Ann Plast Surg 1999; 43: 640–643
59. Bork K: Drug-induced Lupus Erythemtosus. In: Bork K: Cutaneous Side Effects of Drugs. 1st edn. Philadelphia: WB Saunders. 1988; pp 181–184
60. Breathnach SM, Hintner H: Patterns of clinical disease. Types of clinical reaction. In: Breathnach SM, Hintner H: Adverse Drug Reactions and the Skin. 1st edn. Oxford: Blackwell Scientific Publications. 1992; pp 41–136
61. Kissin MW, Williamson RC: Hydrallazine-induced SLE- like syndrome presenting as a leg ulcer. Br Med J 1979; 2: 1330
62. Bernstein RM, Egerton-Vernon J, Webster J: Hydralazine-induced cutaneous vasculitis. Br Med J 1980; 280: 156–157
63. Gibson GE, Su WP, Pittelkow MR: Antiphospholipid syndrome and the skin. J Am Acad Dermatol 1997; 36: 970–982
64. Renfro L, Kamino H, Raphael B, et al: Ulcerative lichen planus-like dermatitis associated with hydroxyurea. J Am Acad Dermatol 1991; 24: 143–145
65. Burry JN: Ulcerative lichenoid eruption from methyldopa (letter). Arch Dermatol 1976; 112: 880
66. Massa MC, Jason SM, Gradini R, et at: Lichenoid drug eruption secondary to propranolol. Cutis 1991; 48: 41–43
67. Srebrnik A, Bar-Nathan EA, Ilie B, et al: Vaginal ulcerations due to lithium carbonate therapy. Cutis 1991; 48: 65–66
68. Ross HJ, Moy LA, Kaplan R, et al: Bullous pyoderma gangrenosum after granulocyte colony-stimulating factor treatment. Cancer 1991; 68: 441–443
69. Gangaram HB, Tan LP, Gan AT, et al: Pyoderma gangrenosum following treatment with isotretinoine. Br J Dermatol 1997; 136: 636–637
70. Cohen AD, Grossman N, Halevy S: Pyoderma gangrenosum induced by montelukast sodium – confirmation by interferon-γ (IFN-γ) release test. In: 32nd Annual European society for dermatology research (ESDR) meeting. Geneva: September, 2002
71. Cohen AD, Cagnano E, Halevy S: Ibuprofen-induced pyoderma gangrenosum. J Am Acad Dermatol (in press)
72. Srebrnik A, Shachar E, Brenner S: Suspected induction of a pyoderma gangrenosum-like eruption due to sulpiride treatment. Cutis 2001; 67: 253–256
73. Soter NA: Cutaneous necrotizing venulitis. Freedberg IM, Eisen AZ, Wolff K, Austen KF, Goldsmith LA, Katz SI, Fitzpatrick TB (eds) In: Fitzpatrick's Dermatology in General Medicine. 5th edn. New-York: McGraw-Hill. 1999; pp 2044–2053
74. Lambert WC, Kolber LR, Proper SA: Leukocytoclastic angiitis induced by clindamycin. Cutis 1982; 30: 615–619
75. Veraguth AJ, Hauselmann HJ, Hunziker T, Gerber NJ: Vasculitic skin lesions caused by nonsteroidal anti-inflammatory agents. Schweiz Med Wochenschr 1992; 122: 923–929
76. Houston BD, Crouch ME, Brick JE, et al: Apparent vasculitis associated with propylthiouracil use. Arthritis Rheum 1979; 22: 925–928
77. Carmichael AJ, Paul CJ: Vasculitic leg ulcers associated with diltiazem. Br Med J 1988; 297: 562
78. Mosovich B, Biton A, Avinoach I: Vasculitis with cutaneous necrosis induced by oral contraceptive. Harefuah 1991; 120: 451–453
79. Menni S, Pistritto G, Gianotti R, et al: Ear lobe bilateral necrosis by levamisole-induced occlusive vasculitis in a pediatric patient. Pediatr Dermatol 1997; 14: 477–479

80. Schrodt BJ, Kulp-Shorten CL, Callen JP: Necrotizing vasculitis of the skin and uterine cervix associated with minocycline therapy for acne vulgaris. South Med J 1999; 92:502–504

81. Altmeyer P, Welke S, Renger A, et al: Zur pathogenese der sogenannten Cumarin-Nekrose. Aktuel Dermatol 1976; 2:65–68

82. Slutzki S, Bogokowsky H, Gilboa Y, et al: Coumadin induced skin necrosis. Int J Dermatol 1984; 23:117–119

83. Tanay A, Yust I, Brenner S, et al: Dermal vasculitis due to coumadin hypersensitivity. Dermatologica 1982; 165:178–185

84. Stoebner PE, Gaspard C, Meynadier J, et al: Tongue necrosis provoked by ergotamine tartrate and disclosing a giant cell arteritis. Eur J Dermatol 1999; 9:652–653

85. Zavaleta EG, Fernandez BB, Grove MK, et al: St. Anthony's fire (ergotamine induced leg ischemia) – a case report and review of the literature. Angiology 2001; 52:349–356

86. Bongard O, Bounameaux H: Severe iatrogenic ergotism: incidence and clinical importance. Vasa 1991; 20:153–156

87. Payne B, Sasse B, Franzen D, et al: Manifold manifestations of ergotism. Schweiz Med Wochenschr 2000; 130:1152–1156

88. DeFranzo AJ, Marasco P, Argenta LC: Warfarin-induced necrosis of the skin. Ann Plast Surg 1995; 34:203–208

89. Chan YC, Valenti D, Mansfield AO, et al: Warfarin induced skin necrosis. Br J Surg 2000; 87:266–272

90. Ad-El DD, Meirovitz A, Weinberg A, et al: Warfarin skin necrosis: local and systemic factors. Br J Plast Surg 2000; 53:624–626

91. Cole MS, Minifee PK, Wolma FJ: Coumarin necrosis – a review of the literature. Surgery 1988; 103:271–277

92. Faraci PA, Deterling RA Jr, Stein AM, et al: Warfarin induced necrosis of the skin. Surg Gynecol Obstet 1978; 146:695–700

93. Makris M, Bardhan G, Preston FE: Warfarin induced skin necrosis associated with activated protein C resistance. Thromb Haemost 1996; 75:523–524

94. McGehee WG, Klotz TA, Epstein DJ, et al: Coumarin necrosis associated with hereditary protein C deficiency. Ann Int Med 1984; 101:59–60

95. Broekmans AW: Hereditary protein C deficiency. Haemostasis 1985; 15:233–240

96. Comp P, Elrod J, Karzenski S: Warfarin-induced skin necrosis. Semin Thromb Hemost 1990; 16:293–298

97. Rose VL, Kwaan HC, Williamson K, et al: Protein C antigen deficiency and warfarin necrosis. Am J Clin Pathol 1986; 86:653–655

98. Ng T, Tillyer ML: Warfarin-induced skin necrosis associated with Factor V Leiden and protein S deficiency. Clin Lab Haematol 2001; 23:261–264

99. Broekmans AW, Bertina RM, Loeliger EA, et al: Protein C and the development of skin necrosis during anticoagulant therapy (letter). Thromb Haemost 1983; 49:251

100. Breathnach SM, Hintner H: Anticoagulants, fibrinolytic agents and antiplatlet drugs. In: Adverse Drug Reactions and the Skin, 1st edn. Oxford: Bleckwell Scientific Publications. 1992; pp 247–253

101. Gold JA, Watters AK, O'Brien E: Coumadin versus heparin necrosis. J Am Acad Dermatol 1987; 16:148–150

102. White PW, Sadd JR, Nensel RE: Thrombotic complications of heparin therapy: including six cases of heparin- induced necrosis. Ann Surg 1979; 190:595–608

103. Levine LE, Bernstein JE, Soltani K, et al: Heparin-induced cutaneous necrosis unrelated to injection sites: a sign of potentially lethal complications. Arch Dermatol 1983; 119:400–403

104. Santamaria A, Romani J, Souto JC, et al: Skin necrosis at the injection site induced by low-molecular-weight heparin: case report and review. Dermatology 1998; 196:264–265

105. Balestra B, Quadri P, Dermarmels-Biasiutti F, et al: Low-molecular-weight heparin-induced thrombocytopenia and skin necrosis distant from injection sites. Eur J Haematol 1994; 53:61–63

106. Montserrat I, Lopez D, Zuazu-Jausoro I, et al: Low-molecular-weight subcutaneous heparin-induced skin necrosis. Blood Coag Fibrinol 1990; 1:751–752

107. Drew PJ, Smith MJ, Milling MA: Heparin-induced skin necrosis and low molecular weight heparins. Ann R Coll Surg Engl 1999; 81:266–269

108. Sirieix ME, Debure C, Baudot N, et al: Leg ulcers and hydroxyurea: Forty-one cases. Arch Dermatol 1999; 135:818–820

109. Velez A, Garcia-Aranda JM, Moreno JC: Hydroxyurea-induced leg ulcers: is macroerythrocytosis a pathogenic factor? J Eur Acad Dermatol Venereol 1999; 12:243–244

110. Best PJ, Daoud MS, Pittelkow MR, et al: Hydroxyurea-induced leg ulceration in 14 patients. Ann Intern Med 1998; 128:29–32

111. Weinlich G, Fritsch P: Leg ulcers in patients treated with hydroxyurea for myeloproliferative disorders: what is the trigger? Br J Dermatol 1999; 141:171–172

112. Ravandi-Kashani F, Cortes J, Cohen P, et al: Cutaneous ulcers associated with hydroxyurea therapy in myeloproliferative disorders. Leuk Lymphoma 1999; 35:109–118

113. Demircay Z, Comert A, Adiguzel C: Leg ulcers and hydroxyurea: report of three cases with essential thrombocythemia. Int J Dermatol 2002; 41:872–874

114. Cohen AD, Hallel-Halevy D, Hatskelzon L, et al: Longitudinal melanonychia associated with hydroxyurea therapy in a patient with essential thrombocytosis. J Eur Acad Dermatol Venereol 1999; 13:137–139

115. Lawrence CM, Dahl MG: Two patterns of skin ulceration induced by methotrexate in patients with psoriasis .J Am Acad Dermatol 1984; 11:1059–1065

116. Ben-Amitai D, Hodak E, David M: Cutaneous ulceration: an unusual sign of methotrexate toxicity – first report in a patient without psoriasis. Ann Pharmacother 1998; 32:651–653

117. Kaplan DL, Olsen EA: Erosion of psoriatic plaques after chronic methotraxate administration. Int J Dermatol 1988; 27:59–62

118. Surville-Barland J, Caumes E, Ankri A, et al: Bleomycin-induced digital gangrene. Eur J Dermatol 1998; 8:221

119. Green JP: Steroid therapy and wound healing in surgical patients. Br J Surg 1965; 52:523–525

120. Anstead GM: Steroids, retinoids, and wound healing. Adv Wound Care 1998; 11:277–285

121. Pollack SV: Wound healing: A review. 4. Systemic medications affecting wound healing. J Dermatol Surg Oncol 1982; 8:667–672

122. Mogford JE, Mustoe TA: Experimental models of wound healing. In: Falanga V (ed) Cutaneous Wound Healing. London: Martin Dunitz. 2001; pp 109–122

123. Lenco W, McKnight M, MacDonald AS: Effects of cortisone acetate, methylprednisolone, and medroxyprogesterone on wound contracture and epithelization in rabbits. Ann Surg 1975; 181:67–73

124. Durant S, Duval D, Homo-Delarche F: Factors involved in the control of fibroblast proliferation by glucocorticoids: a review. Endocr Rev 1986; 7:254–269

125. Hashimoto I, Nakanishi H, Shono Y, et al: Angiostatic effects of corticosteroid on wound healing of the rabbit ear. J Med Invest 2002; 49:61–66

126. Chedid M, Hoyle JR, Csaky KG, et al: Glucocorticoids inhibit keratinocyte growth factor production in primary dermal fibroblasts. Endocrinology 1996; 137:2232–2237

127. Stadelmann WK, Digenis AG, Tobin GR: Impediments to wound healing. Am J Surg 1998; 176 [Suppl 2A]: 39S–47S

128. Autio P, Oikarinen A, Melkko J, et al: Systemic glucocorticoids decrease the synthesis of type I and type III collagen in human skin in vivo, whereas isotretinoin treatment has little effect. Br J Dermatol 1994; 131:660–663

129. Edwards LC, Dunphy JE: Wound healing. 2. Injury and abnormal repair. N Engl J Med 1958; 259:275–285

130. Sandberg N: Time relationship between administration of cortisone and wound healing in rats. Acta Chir Scand 1964; 127:446–455

131. Kulick MI, Smith S, Hadler K: Oral ibuprofen: evaluation of its effect on peritendinous and the breaking strength of a tenorrhaphy. J Hand Surg [Am] 1986; 11:110–120

132. Lee KH: Studies on the mechanism of action of salicylates. 3. Effect of vitamin A on the 'wound healing retardation action of aspirin. J Pharm Sci 1968; 57:1238–1240

133. Falcone RE, Nappi JF: Chemotherapy and wound healing. Surg Clin North Am 1984; 64:779–794

134. Cohen SC, Gabelnick HL, Johnson RK, Goldin A: Effects of antineoplastic agents on wound healing in mice. Surgery 1975; 78:238–244

135. McGrath P: Reflections on nutritional issues associated with cancer therapy. Cancer Pract 2002; 10:94–101

136. Capra S, Ferguson M, Ried K: Cancer: impact of nutrition intervention outcome – nutrition issues for patients. Nutrition 2001; 17:769–772

137. Donaldson SS, Lenon RA: Alterations of nutritional status: impact of chemotherapy and radiation therapy. Cancer 1979; 43 [Suppl]: 2036–2052

138. Alster Y, Varssano D, Loewenstein A, Lazar M: Delay of corneal wound healing in patients treated with colchicine. Ophthalmology 1997; 104:118–119

139. Joseph HL, Anderson GL, Barker JH, et al: Inhibition of wound contraction with colchicine and D-penicillamine. J Surg Res 1996; 61:197–200

140. Williams GH: Hypertensive vascular diseases. In: Fauci As, Braunwald E, Isselbacher KJ, Wilson JD, Martin JB, Kasper DL, Hauser SL, Longo DL (eds) Harrison's Principles of Internal Medicine,14th edn. New York: McGraw-Hill. 1998; pp 1380–1394

141. Parfitt K (ed) Nifedipine. In: Martindale – The complete drug reference, 32nd edn. London: Pharmaceutical Press. 1999; pp 916–922

142. Lewis JG: Adverse reactions to calcium antagonists. Drugs 1983; 25:196–222

143. Pierard-Franchimont C, Letawe C, Fumal I, et al: Gravitational syndrome and tensile properties of skin in the elderly. Dermatology 1998; 197:317–320

144. Casley-Smith JR, Casley-Smith JR: Pathology of oedema- Effect of oedema. In: Casley-Smith JR, Casley-Smith JR (eds) Modern Treatment for Lymphoedema, 5th revised edn. Adelaide: The Lymphoedema Association of Australia. 1997; pp 60–73

145. Luca S, Romeo S: Edema and skin ulcers of the lower limbs as a collateral effect of nifedipine. A clinical case report. Minerva Cardioangiol 1999; 47:219–222

146. Weir MR: Dihydropyridine calcium antagonists. In: Izzo JL, Black HR (eds) Hypertension Primer. The Essentials of High Blood Pressure, 2nd edn. Dallas: American Heart Association (Lippincott Williams & Wilkins). 1999; pp 379–381

147. Levine TB, Sica DA: Non-dihydropyridine calcium antagonists. In: Izzo JL, Black HR (eds) Hypertension Primer. The Essentials of High Blood Pressure. 2nd edn. Dallas: American Heart Association (Lippincott Williams & Wilkins). 1999; pp 382–384

148. Valencia IC, Kerdel FA: Topical glucocorticoides. In: Freedberg IM, Eisen AZ, Wolff K, Austen KF, Goldsmith LA, Katz SI (eds) Fitzpatrick's Dermatology in General Medicine, 6th edn. New York: McGraw-Hill. 2003; pp 2324–2328

149. Lever WF, Schaumburg-Lever G: Eruptions due to drugs. In: Histopathology of the Skin, 7th edn. Philadelphia: J.B. Lippincott. 1990; pp 284–297

150. Rowell NR, Goodfield MJD: The 'connective tissue diseases'. In: Champion RH, Burton JL, Burns DA, Breathnach SM (eds) Rook/Wilkinson/Ebling Textbook of Dermatology, 6th edn. Oxford: Blackwell Scientific Publications. 1998; pp 2437–2575

151. Tu JH, Eisen AZ: Scleroderma. In: Freedberg IM, Eisen AZ, Wolff K, Austen KF, Goldsmith LA, Katz SI, Fitzpatrick TB (eds) Fitzpatrick's Dermatology in General Medicine, 5th edn. New York: McGraw-Hill. 1999; pp 2023–2033

152. Leshin B, Piette WW, Caplan RM: Morphea after bromocriptine therapy. Int J Dermatol 1989; 28: 177–179

Alternative Topical Preparations

17

> and with a knife cut from his thigh
> the sharp-piercing arrow,
> and from the wound washed the
> black blood with warm water, and
> upon it cast a bitter root, when he
> had rubbed it between his hands, a
> root that slayeth pain, which stayed
> all his pangs; and the wound waxed
> dry, and the blood ceased.
>
> (Homer; *The Iliad XI: 845*)

Contents

17.1 Overview

This chapter discusses the efficacy and value of certain alternative topical preparations. We cannot cover all the preparations used topically for the management of cutaneous wounds and ulcers. Since the dawn of mankind thousands of such substances have been used.

The topical agents reviewed below are, in fact, traditional home remedies, such as honey or herbal extracts. Recently there has been increased interest in determining the precise mode of action of these old remedies and their value in a controlled, scientific manner.

However, there is a dearth of controlled studies of this kind, i.e., comparing alternative medications with placebo. Lacking just as much are studies comparing the beneficial effects of these alternative medications with those of advanced treatment modalities such as growth factors or composite grafts.

Many of these topical treatment modalities cannot be evaluated on the basis of 'evidence-based medicine'. We therefore suggest in most cases that cutaneous ulcers be treated in accordance with the scheme presented in Chap. 20. Where possible, the advanced treatment modalities should be preferred, since their therapeutic value is well documented.

In which cases may one prefer to use one of the topical preparations presented in this chapter (or, additional topical preparations, discussed in the following chapter)?
- When the physician has special experience with the specific substance

> ▬ When, in spite of continued efforts and a variety of accepted therapeutic measures, the treated ulcer is 'stuck' and fails to show any improvement.

Most of these alternative topical preparations will at least provide useful coverage of the ulcer surface. The use of alternative topical preparations is subject to regulations determined by medical/legal authorities of each country.

In most cases, adverse effects of these preparations have rarely been documented. This is in contrast to certain 'accepted' preparations whose usage, especially over relatively long periods, may have some undesirable effects; (e.g., toxicity of certain antibacterial preparations). Nevertheless, these alternative measures have been studied less intensively than have accepted treatment modalities, and physicians are less aware of their potential adverse effects.

In some cases there is definite improvement of cutaneous ulcers following the use of alternative topical preparations. Keep in mind that there are many mechanisms of wound repair that we still do not understand, so these treatment modalities may, sometimes unexpectedly, produce good results.

Cost-effectiveness is another aspect to consider when using alternative topical preparations. In most cases they are less expensive than currently accepted treatments. Honey or aloe vera preparations may be used for long periods without straining the patient's budget, compared with certain advanced modes of therapy, which are usually more expensive.

Nevertheless, alternative measures are better used after accepted treatment modalities have been used and found not to have helped. For the initial treatment, it is advisable to use accepted topical preparations or debridement techniques whose efficacy has been well documented and supported by evidence-based medicine.

In some cases, the success of a treatment is, in fact, due not to the active ingredient of the preparation, but rather to the vehicle in which the medication is formulated. Thus, a secreting ulcer tends to improve when repeatedly wetted with liquid preparations, and an ulcer covered by a dry black crust may improve following the application of preparations incorporated in a fatty vehicle, more or less regardless of the active ingredient in the preparation. On the other hand, treating a secreting wound with fatty preparations is likely to aggravate the ulcer.

Not all subtypes of certain old, traditional remedies are similar or identical. For example, there are various kinds of honey that may each have different pharmacological properties. Similarly, plant extracts such as aloe vera may vary in their pharmacological effects, depending on the specific subtype of the plant, the season of the year the plant was picked, the method of extraction, or the manufacturing process. This should be considered when discussing their clinical effects.

Finally, there is a trend in the pharmaceutical industry to combine alternative preparations with advanced ones. For example, aloe vera extract may be combined with a hydrogel preparation. Hopefully, the value of such combinations will be examined in the coming years.

17.2 Herbal and Traditional Home Remedies

Traditional remedies have been in use for hundreds or even thousands of years. Not all extracts produced from a given plant can be considered uniform and identical in their pharmacological effects. Each plant may have a wide variety of subtypes, and each subtype may possess different biological properties. Factors such as the season of the year in which the plant was picked or the method of extraction may affect the pharmacological properties of a herbal extract. Moreover, as stated earlier, the effect of a preparation containing the plant extract may depend on other components, such as the vehicle (base) which contains the active ingredient, not just the active substance itself.

17.2.1 Aloe Vera

The aloe vera plant has yellow flowers and fleshy leaves arranged in a rosette pattern, from which the extract is obtained (Fig. 17.1). Subtypes of this plant may vary in their pharmacological properties.

Since the dawn of human history, the aloe vera plant has been known to possess medical properties. It was widely used in Mesopotamia and Ancient Egypt. Over the years it has been used for a whole host of medical applications, ranging from gastrointestinal disorders to conditions such as asthma and tuberculosis.

> The leaves of the aloe vera plant contain two major pharmacological components:
> - 1. A bitter yellow fluid can be extracted from specific areas of the inner leaf; this substance, referred to as 'juice' or 'latex', is known to have a laxative effect.
> - 2. A characteristic gel is obtained from the inner part of the aloe leaf; this gel has been used for centuries for skin afflictions and wounds.

■ **Mode of Action.** In contrast to other alternative medications, the effects of aloe vera extracts on wound healing have been examined rather closely. The picture is still not clear, but there are several possibilities. The main thrust of the research suggests that aloe vera possesses antibacterial properties [1–3], and that an extract from its leaves shows antiprostaglandin activity, with subsequent increase of dermal perfusion [3].

■ **Research.** The results of animal studies examining the beneficial effect of aloe vera on wound healing are inconclusive [4–8]. When used on humans, aloe vera has been shown to be of benefit in conditions such as radiation dermatitis [9–11]. Fresh gel of aloe vera leaves has also been shown to enhance healing of leg ulcers [12]. All these studies, however, were not well-controlled clinical trials.

There are few controlled studies of the effect of aloe vera on chronic cutaneous ulcers. In 1998, Thomas et al. [13] examined the effect of a hydrogel dressing derived from the aloe plant (acemannan hydrogel wound dressing) on pressure ulcers. The aloe-hydrogel preparation was found to be just as effective as a moist saline wound dressing used as a control.

17.2.2 Calendula

The plant *Calendula officinalis*, more commonly known as pot marigold, has been used for skin diseases since ancient times. It is used in the treatment of wounds, cutaneous ulcers, burns, and various rashes, including diaper dermatitis [14]. The extract is derived from the petals of the plant and may be prepared as an ointment or as a lotion.

There is evidence from animal studies that calendula extract may increase granulation tissue formation. *In vitro* studies have shown that it may have antimicrobial properties and an immune-modulating effect [15]. However, there are no controlled clinical research studies that unequivocally support its use for wounds or chronic cutaneous ulcers.

17.2.3 Other Herbal Extracts

There are other herbal extracts widely used in traditional and folk medicine for healing cuta-

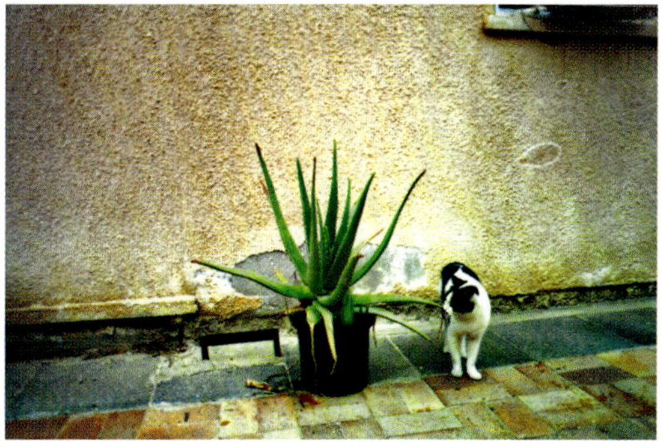

Fig. 17.1. An aloe vera plant, being closely examined

neous ulcers. These include substances such as sea buckthorn seed oil or tannin-containing herbs [15]. There are no data in the literature that support their value in wound healing.

17.2.4 Balsam of Peru

The source of balsam of Peru is *Myroxyolon pereirae (balsamum)*, a tree of mahogany-like wood, which grows in Central America, almost exclusively in El Salvador. When the tree bark is incised, an oily resin-like liquid with a characteristic aroma seeps out.

The main constituents of balsam of Peru are benzylesters of benzoic and cinnamic acid. It contains numerous other compounds, not all of which have been identified.

In folk medicine, balsam of Peru has been given orally for various diseases such as rheumatic pain or chronic cough. Topically, it has been used for certain skin diseases, mainly for wounds and burns.

Balsam of Peru has soothing properties that may alleviate pain. It is also said to have antibacterial properties. However, there is no scientific evidence of its beneficial effect on wounds and cutaneous ulcers.

Certainly, its pleasant, characteristic aroma makes it suitable for use on wounds with an unpleasant odor. However, it must be remembered that a foul-smell is often a sign of infection. This being the case, the preferred treatment may involve antibiotics or antibacterial substances.

Chemically similar allergens are included in other balsams and essential oils. Therefore, an allergic reaction to balsam of Peru (a standard component of patch testing), should be considered as an indication of the possibility of contact allergy to other fragrances and flavoring agents [16].

17.2.5 Clay

Natural clay is a worldwide folk remedy, used for various medical purposes. It may be used topically for wounds and cutaneous ulcers.

Montmorillonite is an active mineral used in alternative medicine; it derives its name from a deposit in Montmorillon, in southern France. It is the main constituent of 'bentonite', a powdered clay derived from deposits of weathered volcanic ash. The name 'bentonite' was derived from Fort Benton, Wyoming, where it was first identified.

Clay products may have a beneficial effect on wounds, as they can absorb fluids. Clay is also claimed to be able to absorb microorganisms and toxins. Its action is assumed to be purely physical, without any chemical reaction.

There is neither any information in the literature, nor are there any controlled studies on the use of clay in cutaneous ulcers.

17.3 Honey

17.3.1 General

Honey has held a unique significance in the treatment of wounds and ulcers throughout history. Honey was first used for healing purposes in Ancient Egypt, more than 4000 years ago [17, 18], and it has continued to be used ever since. However, note that the term 'honey' does not define a single substance. Honey is derived from many possible sources. Thus, its effect on the healing process may vary, depending on its specific origin and the type of processing it has undergone.

17.3.2 Mode of Action: Why Does Honey Have a Beneficial Effect?

Generally speaking, any type of honey may have certain beneficial properties when used on wounds or cutaneous ulcers. Honey is a relatively occlusive agent that can provide a protective coating against external infective agents. In addition, the use of honey prevents adhesion of the dressing material to the wound (adhesion damages the wound bed when the dressing is removed).

Apart from those possible advantages, there are reports of several unique properties of honey in its ability to enhance healing.

Some of these features are listed below, but further research is required to clarify the issue.
- Occlusive and hygroscopic effect
- Antimicrobial activity
- Enzymatic debridement
- Activation of the body's immune system

■ **Occlusive and Hygroscopic Effect.** Being a viscous compound, honey may help to maintain a moist environment within the ulcer, thereby providing ideal conditions for healing. Being a hyperosmotic compound, honey may help to absorb excessive fluids and secretions from the ulcer bed, which would otherwise tend to interfere with normal wound healing [19].

■ **Antimicrobial Activity.** Generally speaking, compounds of high osmolarity, such as honey or solutions containing high concentrations of sugars, inhibit bacterial growth [20, 21]. However, when used as dressings, because of gradual dilution, the antibacterial activity resulting from the hyperosmolarity is significantly reduced [22].

Some researchers have suggested that honey possesses intristic antibacterial properties unrelated to its hyperosmolarity [23, 24]. Jeddar et al. [25] documented a bactericidal effect of honey at a concentration of 40% on gram-positive and gram-negative bacteria; it was particularly effective against *Salmonella, Shigella,* and *Escherichia coli.* Cooper et al. [24] have shown that certain types of honey, manuka honey and a honey of a mixed pasture source, when diluted, were still effective against *Staphylococcus aureus* strains, beyond the effect that could be attributed only to hyperosmolarity. The antibacterial activity of pasture honey was attributed to the release of hydrogen peroxide, while in the case of manuka honey the effect may be attributed to a phytochemical component [24].

Eradication of methicillin-resistant *Staphylococcus aureus* from a hydroxyurea-induced leg ulcer has been reported [26].

Willix and Molan [27] demonstrated that even when diluted 10 times or more, honey inhibits the growth of common species of wound-infecting bacteria. The antibacterial effect has been attributed to hydrogen peroxide, produced within the honey dressing, although Molan [28] has emphasized that the concentration of hydrogen peroxide produced in a honey dressing is about 1 mmol/l, which is only 0.1% of the accepted concentration of hydrogen peroxide used medically (3% solution). Honey has also been shown to be effective against *Candida* strains [29].

■ **Enzymatic Debridement.** Honey contains enzymes, such as catalase [19]. These enzymes may contribute to healing by digesting necrotic material on the ulcer bed. Others have suggested that autolytic debridement, induced by honey, may be enhanced by the presence of hydrogen peroxide, since matrix metalloproteases are activated by oxidation [23].

■ **Activation of the Body's Immune System.** Honey may stimulate mitogenesis in B and T lymphocytes, activate neutrophils [30] and stimulate the release of tumor necrosis factor-α from monocytes [31].

17.3.3 Research

Much research, including *in vitro* studies, animal studies, and clinical studies, has been done to evaluate the effects of honey on wound healing. These studies are detailed in comprehensive monographs [23, 32]. Several controlled clinical studies have demonstrated a beneficial effect of honey on burn wounds [33–35]. However, there are few scientific studies on the use of honey in chronic cutaneous ulcers.

Efem et al. [36] described their clinical observations in 59 patients with long-standing wounds (including pressure ulcers, diabetic ulcers, and ulcers due to sickle cell disease and malignancy), most of which (80%) had not responded to conventional therapy. Honey was shown to be effective in debriding and cleansing unclean and foul-smelling ulcers and in inducing granulation and epithelialization. They summarized their findings by reporting a "remarkable improvement", although the article did not present exact data on the number of healed ulcers or changes in the surface area of the ulcers.

Similarly, Ndayisaba et al. [37] reported the beneficial effect of honey on 40 patients with wounds and cutaneous ulcers of mixed etiology.

17.3.4 Mode of Use

The frequency with which the dressing is changed depends on the extent of the oozing and secretion from the ulcer and may vary from once to three times a day. In general, it is not advisable to use honey on a heavily secreting ulcer, but rather some other treatment such as rinsing the ulcer with saline. Since honey attracts insects, it must be covered with a dressing.

Note that honey may be contaminated by various infective organisms such as yeasts, spore-forming bacteria, and *Paenibacillus larvae* [38– 41]. It would therefore be advisable to purchase honey products intended to be used for topical application, which have been sterilized by γ-irradiation and prepared by a reliable manufacturer.

17.3.5 Summary

At present, one cannot make a definite statement with respect to the use of honey in the management of cutaneous ulcers. The general comments at the beginning of the chapter regarding the use of alternative topical applications are equally applicable to honey. Further controlled studies on the role of honey in the treatment of cutaneous ulcers are required.

17.4 Conclusion

Recently, in parallel with the development of advanced treatment modalities for the management of cutaneous ulcers (such as composite grafting or growth factors), there have also been attempts to assess the value of alternative preparations and to identify their mode of action (if such exists) on the healing process. In an article reviewing the beneficial effects of honey, published in the *Journal of the Royal Society of Medicine* in 1989, Zumla et al. [19] stated, "The time has now come for conventional medicine to lift the blinds off this 'traditional remedy' and give it its due recognition." This can be applied not only to the use of honey, but to a wide range of alternative substances, some of which have been discussed in this chapter. More and more studies are currently being conducted using the principles of evidence-based medicine to evaluate various alternative treatments.

There are basically two situations in which one may consider using alternative substances: The first is when the physician is very familiar with the substance, has experience with it, and is well acquainted with its properties; the second situation is when a range of currently used treatments, including advanced treatment modalities, have been unsuccessful in achieving healing of an ulcer in a specific patient.

References

1. Shelton RM: Aloe vera. Its chemical and therapeutic properties. Int J Dermatol 1991; 30:679–683
2. Robson MC, Heggers JP, Hagstorm WJ: Myth, magic witchcraft, or fact? Aloe vera revisited. J Burn Care Rehabil 1982; 3:157–163
3. Klein AD, Penneys NS: Aloe vera. J Am Acad Dermatol 1988; 18:714–720
4. Watcher MA, Wheeland RG: The role of topical agents in the healing of full-thickness wounds. J Dermatol Surg Oncol 1989; 15:1188–1195
5. Rowe TD, Lovell BK, Parks LM: Further observations on the use of aloe vera leaf in the treatment of third degree x-ray reactions. J Am Pharm Assoc 1941; 30:266–269
6. Sjostrom B, Weatherly White RCA, Paton BC: Experimental studies in cold injury. J Surg Res 1964; 53:12–16
7. Rodriguez-Bigas M, Cruz NI, Suarez A: Comparative evaluation of aloe vera in the management of burn wounds in guinea pigs. Plast Reconstr Surg 1988; 81:386–389
8. Kaufman T, Kalderon N, Ullmann Y, et al: Aloe vera gel hindered wound healing of experimental second-degree burns: a quantitative controlled study. J Burn Care Rehabil 1988; 9:156–159

9. Collins CE, Collins C: Roentgen dermatitis treated with fresh whole leaf of aloe vera. Am J Roentgenol 1935; 33: 396–397

10. Loveman AB: Leaf of aloe vera in treatment of roentgen ray ulcers. Arch Dermatol Syph 1937; 36: 838–843

11. Mandeville FB: Aloe vera in the treatment of radiation ulcers of mucous membranes. Radiology 1939; 32: 598–599

12. Zawahry ME, Hegazy MR, Helal M: Use of aloe in treating leg ulcers and dermatoses. Int J Dermatol 1973; 12: 68–73

13. Thomas DR, Goode PS, LaMaster K, et al: Acemannan hydrogel dressing versus saline dressing for pressure ulcers. Adv Wound Care 1998; 11: 273–276

14. Brown DJ, Dattner AM: Phytotherapeutic approaches to common dermatologic conditions. Arch Dermatol 1998; 134: 1401–1404

15. Bedi MK, Shenefelt PD: Herbal therapy in dermatology. Arch Dermatol 2002; 138: 232–242

16. Rietchel RL, Fowler JF: Medication from plants. In: Rietchel RL, Fowler JF (eds) Fisher's Contact Dermatitis, 4th edn. Philadelphia: Williams & Wilkins. 1995; pp 171–183

17. The Swnw (Egypt). In: Majno G: The Healing Hand. Man and Wound in the Ancient World, 2nd edn. Cambridge, Massachusetts: Harvard University Press. 1975; pp 69– 139

18. Caldwell MD: Topical wound therapy – An historical perspective. J Trauma 1990; 30: S116–S122

19. Zumla A, Lulat A: Honey – a remedy rediscovered. J R Soc Med 1989; 82: 384–385

20. Chirife J, Scarmato G, Herszage L: Scientific basis for use of granulated sugar in treatment of infected wounds. Lancet 1982; 1: 560–561

21. Seal DV, Middleton K: Healing of cavity wounds with sugar. Lancet 1991; 338: 571–572

22. Chirife J, Herszage L, Joseph A, et al: *In vitro* study of bacterial growth inhibition in concentrated sugar solutions: microbiological basis for use of sugar in treating infected wounds. Antimicrob Agents Chemother 1983; 23: 766–773

23. Molan PC: Potential of honey in the treatment of wounds and burns. Am J Clin Dermatol 2001; 2: 13–19

24. Cooper RA, Molan PC, Harding KG: Antibacterial activity of honey against strains of Staphylococcus aureus from infected wounds. J R Soc Med 1999; 92: 283–285

25. Jeddar A, Kharsany A, Ramsaroop UG, et al: The antibacterial action of honey. An *in vitro* study. S Afr Med J 1985; 67: 257–258

26. Natarajan S, Williamson D, Grey J, et al: Healing of an MRSA-colonized, hydroxyurea-induced leg ulcer with honey. J Dermatolog Treat 2001; 12: 33–36

27. Willix DJ, Molan PC, Harfoot CG: A comparison of the sensitivity of wound infecting species of bacteria to the antibacterial activity of manuka honey and other honey. J Appl Bacteriol 1992; 73: 388–394

28. Molan PC: The antibacterial activity of honey. Variation in the potency of the antibacterial activity. Bee World 1992; 73: 59–76

29. Obaseiki-Ebor EE, Afonya TC: *In vitro* evaluation of the anti-candidiasis activity of honey distillate (HY-1) compared with that of some antimycotic agents. J Pharm Pharmacol 1984; 34: 283–284

30. Abuharfeil N, Al-Oran R, Abo-Shehada M: The effect of bee honey on the proliferative activity of human B- and T-lymphocytes and the activity of phagocytes. Food Agric Immunol 1999; 11: 169–177

31. Tonks A, Cooper RA, Price AJ, et al: Stimulation of TNF-α release in monocytes by honey. Cytokine 2001; 14: 240–242

32. Molan PC: A brief review of honey as a clinical dressing. Primary Intention 1998; 6: 148–159

33. Subrahmanyam M: Topical application of honey in treatment of burns. Br J Surg 1991; 78: 497–498

34. Subrahmanyam M: Honey-impregnated gauze versus polyurethane films (Opsite) in the treatment of burns-a prospective randomized study. Br J Plast Surg 1993; 46: 322–323

35. Subrahmanyam M: A prospective randomized clinical and histological study of superficial burn wound healing with honey and silver sulfadiazine. Burns 1998; 24: 157–161

36. Efem SE: Clinical observations on the wound healing properties of honey. Br J Surg 1988; 75: 679–681

37. Ndayisaba G, Bazira L, Habonimana E: Treatment of wounds with honey. 40 cases. Presse Med 1992; 21: 1516–1518

38. Snowdon JA, Cliver DO: Microorganisms in honey. Int J Food Microbiol 1996; 31: 1–26

39. Nevas M, Hielm S, Lindstrom M, et al: High prevalence of Clostridium botulinum types A and B in honey samples detected by polymerase chain reaction. Int J Food Microbiol 2002; 72: 45–52

40. Tanzi MG, Gabay MP: Association between honey consumption and infant botulism. Farmacotherapy 2002; 22: 1479–1483

41. Lauro FM, Favaretto M, Covolo L, et al: Rapid detection of Paenibacillus larvae from honey and hive samples with a novel nested PCR protocol. Int J Food Microbiol 2003; 81: 195–201

Additional Topical Preparations

18

Contents

18.1 Overview

This chapter discusses the efficacy and value of several additional preparations. Some of those presented below can be considered to be 'preparations of early modern dermatology', such as topical zinc. Others are developments of recent years, such as hyaluronic acid, and are included here since they do not belong to a specific family of preparations intended for healing wounds. The use of the topical preparations presented below is subject to the regulations determined by medical/legal authorities of each country.

18.2 Vitamins and Trace Elements

18.2.1 Topical Vitamin A and Derivatives

Few studies have been published regarding the use of topical preparations containing vitamin A for experimental wounds or cutaneous ulcers [1–4]. However, there have not been sufficient data to substantiate the beneficial effect of these preparations unequivocally.

In Chap. 19, note is made of the fact that there is some evidence, albeit inconclusive, that systemic vitamin A may be beneficial in patients with cutaneous ulcers who are being treated with glucocorticoids for some other reason. Thus, vitamin A may counteract some of the inhibitory effects of glucocorticoids on wound healing.

It has been suggested, however, that vitamin A may not only counteract the inhibitory effects of glucocorticoids, but also neutralize the desired anti-inflammatory effects of glucocorticoids – those very anti-inflammatory effects for which the steroids were prescribed [5]. In view of this, there may be a place for considering the use of topical vitamin A in patients with cutaneous ulcers who are also receiving glucocorticoids. Indeed, in 1969 Hunt [6] showed that a topical preparation of vitamin A (containing 7500 I.U. vitamin A ester per milliliter of anhydrous ointment base) may have some beneficial effect on wound healing in animals as well as in patients receiving glucocorticoid therapy.

■ **Cod Liver Ointment.** Pursuant to studies from the 1930s [3, 4], Terkelsen et al. [7] showed that topical applications of cod liver ointment may enhance the healing of traumatic wounds in hairless mice. Note that cod liver, apart from containing vitamin A, contains relatively high amounts of various types of fatty acids. Hence, it would be difficult to assess the contribution of each component to the healing effect.

■ **Topical Retinoic Acid.** Retinoic acid was shown to impair epithelialization and to inhibit wound healing in an animal model. At the same time, retinoic acid enhanced formation of granulation tissue [8]. Similar observations regarding the topical use of retinoic acid have been documented in the past [9, 10]. Kligman and Popp [11] reported that topical retinoic acid cream (0.05–0.1%) accelerated the closure of punch wounds in four patients with photo-damaged skin.

Recently, short-contact topical retinoic acid therapy has been documented as having a beneficial effect on chronic wounds [12]. In five patients with chronic leg ulcers, topical retinoic acid solution 0.05% was applied to the wound bed for a maximum of 10 min, and then rinsed off with normal saline. The procedure was repeated once daily, for a period of four weeks. There was improvement in terms of granulation tissue and collagen formation, although actual healing or a reduction in size of the ulcers was not documented. From those studies, which involved very small patient numbers, no conclusions can be derived with regard to the value of retinoic acid in the treatment of chronic ulcers. In view of the above, it may be worthwhile to examine the effect of topical retinoic acid on ulcers with 'unhealthy' granulation tissue on their surface.

Reports have also documented the beneficial effect of pretreating photo-damaged skin with retinoic acid prior to procedures such as chemical peeling or dermabrasion. The reported benefit is seen in the form of more rapid healing and better cosmetic results [13, 14]. Conclusions cannot be drawn regarding the use of this substance in chronic cutaneous ulcers based only on these studies.

To a certain degree, retinoic acid has an irritating effect on normal skin [15, 16]. It is unclear whether it causes irritation to granulation tissue or to newly formed epithelial tissue. Therefore, until there is clear scientific evidence of the value of retinoic acid in the treatment of cutaneous ulcers, its routine clinical use is not recommended for this purpose.

18.2.2 Topical Zinc

Topical preparations containing zinc are 'classical' substances applied to wounds (Fig. 18.1). The assumption that zinc may have a beneficial effect on wound healing is discussed in Chap.

19. Several mechanisms have been suggested for the beneficial effect of zinc in general. They include possible modulation of various cytokines [17–20], a possible effect on Langerhans' cells [21], and perhaps the induction of an increase in mitotic activity [22]. These same mechanisms may play a role when zinc is applied topically. However, since the beneficial effect of topical zinc remains questionable, it would be too early and perhaps pretentious to presume its mechanism of action.

The beneficial effect of topical zinc is usually discussed without any reference to zinc levels in the serum. Even when there is no clinical evidence of zinc deficiency, and its level in the serum is within the normal range, it is not known whether there is an increased demand for certain ingredients, including zinc, within tissues in an ulcer.

One should distinguish between the effect of the zinc itself on the healing process and the formulation and the vehicle in which it is incorporated. Zinc oxide paste bandage, for example, being a paste, may absorb exudates and improve healing of secreting ulcers, independent of the biochemical or biologic properties of the zinc.

■ 'Unna Boot'. Unna zinc-gelatin boot, commonly known as 'Unna's boot', used to be an ac-

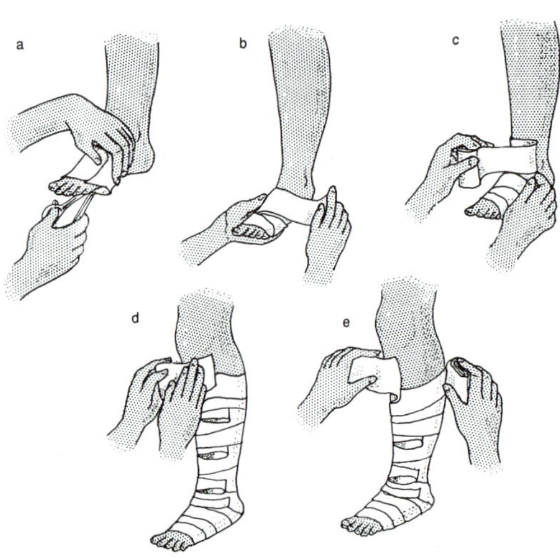

Fig. 18.1. Application of medicated paste bandage

cepted treatment in early modern dermatology for stasis dermatitis and venous ulceration and is still used even today. The topical preparation consisted of zinc oxide, calamine, gelatin, and glycerin, in proportions that varied from manufacturer to manufacturer. It was used together with leg raising to reduce edema. The zinc-gelatin preparation was usually applied to a stockinette bandage encasing the entire extremity, over which a firm bandage was then applied (Fig. 18.2). The bandage was left on for several days, depending on the amount of oozing [23, 24].

More advanced forms consisted of medicated bandages that had been impregnated with zinc oxide and were applied layer upon layer, as a spiral bandage encircling the extremity. In both cases the moist surface was molded with the hands and allowed to harden to form a rigid case or 'boot' [24].

■ **Zinc Oxide Preparations.** The common formulation of zinc in topical preparations is zinc oxide, widely used in powders, shaking lotions, creams, and pastes. It has covering and protective properties and a cooling effect. It is also said to be slightly astringent and to have anti-bacterial properties [25, 26]. Some of its beneficial effect may be attributable to the induction of debridement. In addition, zinc oxide preparations have been shown to be capable of debriding necrotic pressure ulcers [26, 27].

Stromberg and Agren [28] documented the effect of topical zinc oxide in the management of venous ulcers and ulcers caused by peripheral arterial disease, whereby sterile compresses impregnated with zinc oxide were compared with plain sterile compresses. Improvement was found in 83% of the patients treated with zinc oxide but in only 42% of the control group. Agren [29] also documented the beneficial effect of zinc oxide on wound healing.

Other researchers [30, 31] were not able to demonstrate enhanced healing following the topical use of zinc. Brandrup et al. [31] compared zinc oxide dressings with hydrocolloid dressings in the treatment of leg ulcers and found no significant difference between the two.

■ **Conclusion.** The precise role of topical zinc in wound healing remains unclear. Controlled studies are required to confirm its beneficial effect. Thus, for the present, it is probably advisable to favor the more advanced, accepted therapeutic modalities. Perhaps if conventional treatment for the ulcer is not successful, zinc-containing preparations may be considered.

Recently, combinations of zinc with hydrogel dressings were shown to induce a certain degree of autolytic debridement of dermal burns in an animal model [26, 32]. Perhaps combinations of zinc with advanced dressing modalities may be implemented in the near future to enhance wound healing.

18.3 Scarlet Red

Scarlet red is an aniline dye which has been used in the treatment of wounds and ulcers since the beginning of the past century. The most common formulation of scarlet red is an ointment containing lanolin, olive oil, and petrolatum. Researchers have found at least four chemically different dyestuffs marketed as 'scarlet red' [33]. Although the effect of each one of the substances should be evaluated separately, we will review below the properties of this compound in general.

The majority of reports do not indicate that scarlet red has anti-bacterial or antiseptic qualities [33], although there are several conflicting reports in this regard [34]. It is also possible that when scarlet red is incorporated into certain preparations, other ingredients of the same preparation may have some antiseptic effect.

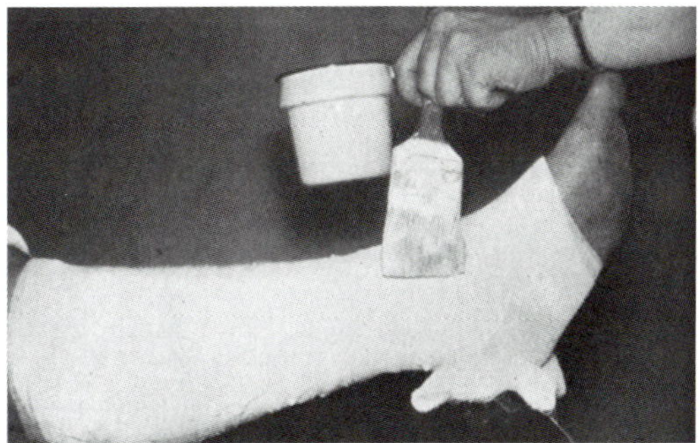

Fig. 18.2. Zinc-gelatin dressing (from [24])

The main mechanism by which scarlet red is considered to exert its effect on healing is mitogenic activity. Early trials demonstrated that subcutaneous injections of scarlet red resulted in increased mitosis of the germinal layer of the epidermis, hair follicles, and sweat glands [35]. These were followed by other studies that demonstrated epidermal proliferation and enhancement of epithelialization [35–39]. The reason for the enhancement of mitogenic activity has not yet been clarified.

Scarlet red has been compared with biobrane, a synthetic collagen dressing, in two controlled studies of the management of donor-site wounds. Prasad et al. [40] conducted a prospective study with 21 burn patients in which it was found that biobrane-treated wounds took longer to heal and had a higher incidence of infection, compared with wounds treated with scarlet red. On the other hand, biobrane was found to be more effective in reducing pain.

Zapata-Sirvent [41] compared biobrane with scarlet red in 31 patients with burns. Two graft donor sites of identical size were treated with either scarlet red or biobrane. They did not find a significant difference in healing times, and biobrane was again found to be more effective in reducing pain.

Cannon [42] emphasized that dressings containing scarlet red seemed to be most effective for donor-site wounds when applied over bloody coagulum; he suggested that blood on the surface of the wound not be removed before applying the dressing.

18.4 Hyaluronic Acid Derivatives

Hyaluronic acid is a major component of the extracellular matrix. Recently, the use of hyaluronic acid and certain derivatives on cutaneous ulcers has been examined. Observations based on tissue cultures and animal studies indicate that hyaluronic acid may induce processes such as angiogenesis, fibroblast and keratinocyte migration, and epithelial and endothelial proliferation [43–47].

Hyaluronan is a benzyl esterified hyaluronic acid derivative that has been shown, in a number of case reports and uncontrolled studies, to have beneficial effects on chronic cutaneous ulcers [48, 49]. Two of these reports are worthy of mention: Ortonne et al. [50] used hyaluronan in 50 patients with venous leg ulcers and demonstrated a significant reduction in wound size after three weeks of treatment, compared with a control group treated with dextranomer paste. Mekkes et al. [51] compared hyaluronan with hydrogel in ten patients with large non-healing ulcers, eight of which were due to venous insufficiency and two to vasculitis. The ulcers treated with hyaluronan healed faster than the control lesions.

Hyaluricht® is zinc hyaluronate. It was used on 315 patients with diabetic ulcers, in a controlled randomized study [52]. Forty (93%) of 43 ulcers in the treatment group were healed (Hyaluricht® plus conventional therapy), compared with 23 (82%) of 28 in the control group (conventional therapy).

18.5 Biafine®

Biafine® is a water-based emulsion used for radiation dermatitis, burns, wounds, and cutaneous ulcers. Its aqueous phase contains demineralized water, alginate of sodium salts, and triethanolamine. The oily phase is composed of paraffin liquid, ethylene glycol stearic acid, propylene glycol, paraffin wax, squalene, avocado oil, cetyl palmitate, and fragrance [53].

■ **Mode of Action.** The influence of Biafine on wound-healing processes has not been identified. Its water content may provide good hydration to the wound environment. As an emulsion, it may serve as an emollient that moisturizes the treated area. However, it may be asked whether Biafine, in itself, has unique intrinsic properties apart from its emollient and hydration effects, which may be provided by oily substances and ointments, or water-based preparations, respectively.

Biafine® is chemotactic for macrophages and it reduces the secretion of IL-6 and increases the IL-1/IL-6 ratio [54]. The current assumption is that, by resulting in inflammatory cell migration and cytokine release, Biafine enhances granulation tissue formation.

■ **Mode of Use.** According to the manufacturer's instructions, Biafine® should be applied as a relatively thick layer, three to five times a day. Each time it is applied, any remnants from the previous application should first be removed by gentle irrigation.

■ **Indications.** As described above, Biafine® may be considered for use in radiation dermatitis, burns, wounds, and cutaneous ulcers. To the best of our knowledge, there have been no controlled studies on the use of Biafine® for cutaneous ulcers. Several studies have shown that it is of benefit in minimizing or preventing radiation-induced dermatitis in women undergoing breast irradiation [53–55].

References

1. Prutkin L: Wound healing and vitamin A acid. Acta Derm Venereal 1972; 52:489–492
2. Tumberello J: Using vitamin A+D Ointment for wounds. Oncol Nurs Forum 1995; 22:989
3. Brandaleone H: The effect of the direct application of cod liver upon the healing of ulcers of the feet in patients with diabetes mellitus. Ann Surg 1938; 108:141–152
4. Steel JP: The cod-liver oil treatment of wounds. Lancet 1935; 2:290–292
5. Anstead GM: Steroids, retinoids, and wound healing. Adv Wound Care 1998; 11:277–285
6. Hunt TK, Ehrlich HP, Garcia JA, et al: Effects of vitamin A on reversing the inhibitory effect of cortisone on healing of open wounds in animals and man. Ann Surg 1969; 170:633–641
7. Terkelsen LH, Eskild-Jensen A, Kjeldsen H, et al: Topical application of cod liver oil ointment accelerates wound healing: an experimental study in wounds in the ears of hairless mice. Scand J Plast Reconstr Hand Surg 2000; 34:15–20
8. Watcher MA, Wheeland RG: The role of topical agents in the healing of full-thickness wounds. J Dermatol Surg Oncol 1989; 15:1188–1195
9. Lee KH, Tong TG: Mechanism of action of retinyl compounds on wound healing. 2. Effect of active retinyl derivatives on granuloma formation. J Pharm Sci 1970; 59:1195–1197
10. Hung VC, Lee JY, Zitelli JA, et al: Topical tretinoin and epithelial wound healing. Arch Dermatol 1989; 125:65–69
11. Popp C, Kligman AM, Stoudemayer TJ: Pretreatment of photoaged forearm skin with topical tretinoin accelerates healing of full-thickness wounds. Br J Dermatol 1995; 132:46–53
12. Paquette D, Badiavas E, Falanga V: Short-contact topical tretinoin therapy to stimulate granulation tissue in chronic wounds. J Am Acad Dermatol 2001; 45:382–386
13. Hevia O, Nemeth AJ, Taylor JR: Tretinoin accelerates healing after trichloroacetic acid chemical peel. Arch Dermatol 1991; 127:678–682
14. Mandy SH: Tretinoin in the preoperative and postoperative management of dermabrasion. J Am Acad Dermatol 1986; 15 [Suppl]:878–879, 888–889
15. Griffiths CE, Kang S, Ellis CN, et al: Two concentrations of topical tretinoin (retinoic acid) cause similar improvement of photoaging but different degrees of irritation. A double-blind, vehicle-controlled comparison of 0.1% and 0.025% tretinoin creams. Arch Dermatol 1995; 131:1037–1044
16. Griffiths CE, Voorhees JJ: Topical retinoic acid for photoaging: clinical response and underlying mechanisms. Skin Pharmacol 1993; 6 [Suppl 1]:70–77
17. Driessen C, Hirv K, Kirchner H, et al: Zinc regulates cytokine induction by superantigens and lipopolysaccharide. Immunology 1995; 84:272–277
18. Driessen C, Hirv K, Rink L, et al: Induction of cytokines by zinc ions in human peripheral blood mononuclear cells and separated monocytes. Lymphokine Cytokine Res 1994; 13:15–20
19. Tarnow P, Agren M, Steenfos H, et al: Topical zinc oxide treatment increases endogenous gene expression of insulin-like growth factor 1 in granulation from porcine wounds. Scand J Plast Reconstr Surg Hand Surg 1994; 28:255–259
20. Watanabe S, Wang XE, Hirose M, et al: Insulin-like growth factor 1 plays a role in gastric wound healing: evidence using a zinc derivative, polaprezinc, and an *in vitro* rabbit wound repair model. Aliment Pharmacol Ther 1998; 12:1131–1138
21. Kohn S, Kohn D, Schiller D: Effect of zinc supplementation on epidermal Langerhans' cells of elderly patients with decubital ulcers. J Dermatol 2000; 27:258–263
22. Jin L, Murakami TH, Janjua NA, et al: The effects of zinc oxide diethyldithiocarbamate on the mitotic index of epidermal basal cells of mouse skin. Acta Med Okayama 1994; 48:231–236
23. Solomon LM: Eczema. In: Moschella SL, Hurley HJ (eds) Dermatology, 2nd edn. Philadelphia: WB Saunders. 1985; pp 354–388
24. Sulzberger MB, Wolf J: Eczematous Dermatoses. In: Sulzberger MB, Wolf J: Dermatologic Therapy in General Practice, 2nd edn. Illinois: Year Book Publishers. 1942; pp 88–124
25. Ryan TJ: Wound healing and current dermatologic dressings. Clin Dermatol 1990; 8:21–29
26. Keefer KA, Iocono JA, Ehrlich HP: Zinc-containing wound dressings encourage autolytic debridement of dermal burns. Wounds 1998; 10:54–58

27. Agren MS, Stromberg HE: Topical treatment of pressure ulcers. A randomized comparative trial of Varidase and zinc oxide. Scand J Plast Reconstr Surg 1985; 19:97–100

28. Stromberg HE, Agren MS: Topical zinc oxide treatment improves arterial and venous leg ulcers. Br J Dermatol 1984; 111:461–468

29. Agren MS: Zinc in wound repair. Arch Dermatol 1999; 135:1273–1274

30. Williams KJ, Meltzer R, Brown RA, et al: The effect of topically applied zinc on the healing of open wounds. J Surg Res 1979; 27:62–67

31. Brandrup F, Menne T, Agren MS, et al: A randomized trial of two occlusive dressings in the treatment of leg ulcers. Acta Derm Venereol (Stockh) 1990; 70:231–235

32. Davis SC, Mertz PM, Bilevich ED, et al: Early debridement of second-degree burn wounds enhances the rate of epithelization – an animal model to evaluate burn wound therapies. J Burn Care Rehabil 1996; 17:558–561

33. Fodor PB: Scarlet red. Ann Plast Surg 1980; 4:45–47

34. Parfitt K (ed) Disinfectants and preservatives. In: Martindale – The complete drug reference, 32nd edn. London: Pharmaceutical Press. 1999; pp 1097–1127

35. Fischer B: Die experimentelle Erzeugung atypischer Epithelwucherungen und die Entstehung bösartiger Geschwülste. Münch Med Wochenschr 1906; 42:2041–2047

36. Davis JS: The effect of scarlet red in various combinations upon the epithelization of granulating surfaces. Ann Surg 1910; 51:40–51

37. Davis JS: A further note on the clinical use of scarlet red and its component amido-azotolud in stimulating the epitheliation of granulated surfaces. Ann Surg 1911; 53:702–719

38. Bettman AG: A simpler technic for promoting epithelialization and protecting skin grafts. JAMA 1931; 97:1879–1881

39. Fisher LB, Maibach HI: The effect of occlusive and semipermeable dressings on the mitotic activity of normal and wounded human epidermis. Br J Dermatol 1972; 86:593–600

40. Prasad JK, Feller I, Thomson PD: A prospective controlled trial of Biobrane versus scarlet red on skin graft donor areas. J Burn Care Rehabil 1987; 8:384–386

41. Zapata-Sirvent R, Hansbrough JF, Carroll W, et al: Comparison of Biobrane and scarlet red dressings for treatment of donor site wounds. Arch Surg 1985; 120:743–745

42. Cannon B: Scarlet red. Plast Reconstr Surg 1983; 72:116

43. West DC, Hampson IN, Arnold F, et al: Angiogenesis induced by degradation products of hyaluronic acid. Science 1985; 228:1324–1326

44. Deed R, Rooney P, Kumar P, et al: Early response gene signalling is induced by angiogenic oligosaccharides of hyaluronan in endothelial cells. Inhibition by non-angiogenic, high-molecular-weight hyaluronan. Int J Cancer 1997; 10:251–256

45. Doillon CJ, Silver FH: Collagen based wound dressing: effects of hyaluronic acid and fibronectin on wound healing. Biomaterials 1986; 7:3–8

46. Iocono JA, Ehrlich HP, Keefer KA, et al: Hyaluronan induces scarless repair in mouse limb organ culture. J Pediatr Surg 1998; 33:564–567

47. Ellis IR, Schor SL: Differential effects of TGF-beta 1 on hyaluronan synthesis by fetal and adult skin fibroblasts: Implications for cell migration and wound healing. Exp Cell Res 1996; 228:326–333

48. Hollander DA, Schmandra T, Windolf J: A new approach to the treatment of recalcitrant wounds: A case report demonstrating the use of a hyaluronan esters fleece. Wounds 2000; 12:111–117

49. Wollina U, Karamfilov T: Treatment of recalcitrant ulcers in pyoderma gangrenosum with mycophenolate mofetil and autologous keratinocyte transplantation on a hyaluronic acid matrix. J Eur Acad Dermatol Venereol 2000; 14:187–190

50. Ortonne JP: Comparative study of the activity of hyaluronic acid and dextranomer in the treatment of leg ulcers of venous origin. Ann Dermatol Venereol 2001; [Suppl]:13–16

51. Mekkes JR, Nahuys M: Induction of granulation tissue formation in chronic wounds by hyaluronic acid. Wounds 2001; 13:159–164

52. Koev D, Tankova T, Dakovska G: Hyaluricht in the treatment of diabetic foot ulcers. Diabetic Foot Study Group of the EASD. Balatonfured, Hungary. September, 2002

53. Szumacher E, Wighton A, Franssen E, et al: Phase II study assessing the effectiveness of Biafine cream as a prophylactic agent for radiation-induced acute skin toxicity to the breast in women undergoing radiotherapy with concomitant CMF chemotherapy. Int J Radiat Oncol Biol Phys 2001; 51:81–86

54. Coulomb B, Friteau L, Dubertret L: Biafine applied on human epidermal wounds is chemotactic for macrophages and increases the IL-1/ IL-6 ratio. Skin Pharmacol 1997; 10:281–287

55. Fisher J, Scott C, Stevens R, et al: Randomized phase-III study comparing best supportive care to Biafine as a prophylactic agent for radiation-induced skin toxicity for women undergoing breast irradiation: Radiation Therapy Oncology Group (RTOG) 97–13. Int J Radiat Oncol Biol Phys 2000; 48:1307–1310

Nutrition and Cutaneous Ulcers

19

Contents

ulceration is secondary to a systemic disease which, in itself, may also result in physiological stress.

During physiological stress, energy requirements are significantly increased [1–4], as is the demand for components such as protein, vitamins, and trace elements [1–8]. Several decades ago, Levenson conducted several research studies on wounds associated with significant bodily injury [9–11]. The body's capacity for repair is impaired in cases of widespread burns, sepsis, or multi-organ trauma.

However, cutaneous ulcers are not necessarily associated with acute stress. Many chronic ulcers develop slowly. In these cases, appropriate nutrition is also of importance. The repair process requires energy and nutritional elements for tissue repair and replacement.

Note that states of nutritional deficiency are not always obvious. Some of these states may develop unnoticed if the diet is inadequate, or due to the administration of anti-neoplastic drugs. It is still not clear whether interference with wound repair can occur even before certain types of nutritional deficiency have manifested themselves clinically.

19.1 Overview

Various nutritional deficiency states can have a profound impact on the mechanisms of wound healing. Those that have to be considered in patients with cutaneous ulcers, such as protein, carbohydrate, and lipid deficiency, will be discussed below. The various vitamin and trace element deficiencies will also be covered. It is important to remember that the presence of a skin wound or a cutaneous ulcer can be associated with a state of stress, i.e., severe trauma that has caused the wounding. At times, skin

19.2 Malnutrition

Malnutrition is clinically associated with a high incidence of skin ulcers, impaired healing, and wound complications [12–17]. Apart from adversely affecting mechanisms of wound healing, malnutrition also damages basic functions such as cell-mediated immunity, phagocytosis, and the bactericidal effect of macrophages [18, 19].

Malnourished patients usually present with combined protein/energy deficiency states. Several studies have examined the significance of each component separately; most have documented the clinical consequences of protein depletion. A few studies, presented below, have examined the association between healing and low caloric intake or inadequate intake of lipids.

However, it is unusual for patients to present with an isolated protein or essential-fatty-acid deficiency. Malnutrition usually involves a combination of these as well as caloric deficiency. Thus, most animal studies that have investigated the consequences of isolated deficiency states do not have practical clinical significance. These isolated states of deficiency are seen only rarely, in patients treated with total parenteral nutrition, in which a specific component has been accidentally omitted.

19.2.1 Assessment of Nutritional Status

A basic assessment of nutritional status is required in patients with chronic ulcers of the skin. This is especially significant in populations which are prone to inadequate nutrition, e.g., nursing-home residents with pressure ulcers.

Nutritional evaluation, with respect to history taking, physical examination, and laboratory assessment is reviewed in most textbooks of internal medicine. Hence, this section should serve as a reminder for the general parameters to be evaluated regarding protein-calorie malnutrition.

The very basic indicators of nutritional status are weight and height. Patients at high risk for involuntary weight loss should be weighed once or twice weekly. It must be taken into account that the presence of edema may lead to false conclusions as to nutritional status [20, 21].

Additional parameters for more thorough nutritional assessment may be measured, such as the triceps skin-fold thickness and upper-mid-arm circumference [21]. These should be assessed with respect to standard values, according to age and gender.

In laboratory assessments, the albumin level can serve as an indicator of nutritional status.

However, it is not a fully accurate parameter, since certain conditions may rapidly affect its plasma concentration. Dehydration leads to an increase in the concentration of various plasma components, thereby masking the presence of low albumin. Shifts of fluids from intravascular to extravascular spaces (following surgery or burns) may also alter albumin levels in the plasma [21].

On the other hand, neither the synthesis nor the catabolism of albumin is subject to sudden changes, since its half-life is approximately 20 days. Measurement of proteins with a shorter half-life (e.g., prealbumin [transthyretin] and transferrin) may provide a better estimation as to the protein status. The half-life of prealbumin is only 2 days and it responds quickly to deficient protein states (and refeeding), which makes it a more sensitive indicator for this purpose [20, 22, 23].

A screening method was suggested for detecting malnourishment in patients with chronic obstructive pulmonary disease [24], in which the nutritional evaluation included measurement of weight and height, serum albumin and prealbumin, total lymphocyte count, triceps skin-fold thickness, mid-arm muscle circumference, and information on unintentional weight loss. It would be advisable to implement similar screening methods for the identification of malnutrition in high-risk patients with cutaneous ulcers as well.

19.2.2 Protein Depletion

Protein depletion can prolong the inflammatory phase of chronic cutaneous ulcers. It affects a variety of basic wound healing functions such as proliferation of fibroblasts, collagen synthesis, angiogenesis, and wound remodeling [25–27]. Most studies in human beings have examined the correlation between low protein intake and pressure ulcers. Nevertheless, it is reasonable to assume that protein depletion may also affect cutaneous ulcers of other etiologies by similar mechanisms.

Several studies have demonstrated that hospitalized patients with pressure ulcers are prone to suffer from malnutrition with protein depletion [28, 29]. The serum albumin concentration may reflect nutritional status; a level less than 3.3 g/dl is associated with increased risk for the formation of pressure ulcers [17].

Berlowitz et al. [30] also reported a correlation between impaired nutritional status (intake of less than 50 g protein per day) and the formation of cutaneous ulcers within six weeks. In this context it should be noted that low albumin concentrations facilitate the development of lower-extremity edema, which further impairs repair of leg ulcers.

Breslow et al. [31] have shown that high protein diets may improve the healing of pressure ulcers in malnourished nursing-home patients. The current recommended amount of protein intake for patients suffering from pressure ulcers is 1.25–1.50 g/kg per day [32]. Some suggest intake of up to 3.0 g/kg protein per day [33]. The administered amount should be adjusted to the patient's general condition, the patient's weight, the presence of other diseases, the presence of infection, and the severity of ulcers.

19.2.3 Supplementation of Amino Acids

Several studies have been conducted to identify specific amino acids that have a significant effect on wound repair mechanisms. However, since amino acids produce a complex alignment of interactive mechanisms, they should all be regarded as significant to the healing process. The provision of essential amino acids according to the recommended daily allowance (RDA) to patients with chronic ulcers is mandatory.

At present, there are no established guidelines as to whether specific amino acids should be provided beyond the recommended daily allowance, and if so, at what dose. Two amino acids have been suggested as playing a central role in wound healing:

■ **Methionine.** Methionine is converted to cysteine, which serves as a cofactor in enzymatic systems required for collagen synthesis. The addition of methionine and cysteine has been shown to enhance collagen formation and fibroblast proliferation [34]. The addition of methionine to the diet of protein-depleted animals has been shown to reverse some of the detrimental effects protein deficiency has on healing [25].

■ **Arginine.** Arginine deficiency may impair wound healing by its effect on T-cells and macrophages [35]. While some researchers have indicated that supplementation with arginine may enhance immune functions and healing of wounds [36], the results of other studies have been contradictory [37, 38]. At present, the above data are not sufficient to establish a policy regarding the administration of arginine in patients with cutaneous ulcers who are not protein deficient.

Moreover, recent evidence has been accumulating as to the various effects of nitric oxide (NO) on wound healing. Current data suggest that a certain increase in NO production may be beneficial to normal healing [39]. Hence, the fact that L-arginine is the sole substrate for nitric oxide synthesis suggests that the value of arginine supplementation for patients with chronic ulcers should be re-examined.

19.2.4 Caloric- and Lipid-Deficient States

The provision of adequate energy is required for the basic functions of healing, such as cellular proliferation and tissue regeneration. In rats, reduced granulation tissue formation and decreased matrix protein deposition has been observed when the caloric intake was only 50% of the required amount [40].

The results of a multi-center study of 672 severely ill elderly patients, conducted by Bourdel-Marchasson et al. [41], showed that daily supplements of 200 kcal to a regular diet of 1880 kcal/day significantly reduced the incidence of pressure ulcers. The currently recommended calorie intake for patients suffering from pressure ulcers is approximately 30–35 kcal/kg per day [32]. A higher amount, of 40 kcal/kg per day has been given to patients with stage IV pressure ulcers with a beneficial effect [31].

Fats, as well as being providers of energy, are constituents of phospholipids and help build cell membranes. Thus, their presence is essential for cellular proliferation. A deficiency in essential fatty acids has been shown to impair wound healing in rats [42, 43]. Total parenteral nutrition (TPN) with inadequate provision of lipids may result in the depletion of essential fatty acids. This condition has been seen to cause impaired wound healing in infants during prolonged fat-free parenteral alimentation [44, 45].

Other functions of essential fatty acids require further investigation. For example, arachidonic acid is a precursor for prostaglandins, which may have a variety of effects on the wound-healing process. Prostaglandins participate in the early inflammatory phase of wound healing as well as in its more advanced phases [46–48]. Note that an omega-3 fatty-acid-enriched diet, albeit beneficial in terms of the cardiovascular aspect, may impede the normal processes of wound healing [49].

19.2.5 Practical Conclusions

- Physicians should be alert as to the nutritional status of patients with cutaneous ulcers, or of patients who are prone to develop cutaneous ulcers (e.g., bed-ridden patients). Malnutrition should be evaluated clinically. Measurement of serum levels of proteins such as albumin and prealbumin may be of assistance.
- Patients should receive enough proteins, carbohydrates, and lipids in their diet so as to meet the respective RDAs.
- In medical conditions associated with physiological stress, appropriate nutrition should be provided according to the accepted medical guidelines. In general, the amount administered should be adjusted to the patient's general condition,

weight, presence of other diseases, presence of infection, and severity of ulcers. For patients with pressure ulcers, a protein intake of at least 1.5 g/kg per day should be provided.
- There is no conclusive evidence to date showing that supplementation of specific elements (e.g., specific amino acids or fatty acids) contributes to the wound-healing process.

19.2.6 Maintaining Appropriate Hydration

Nursing-home residents with pressure ulcers, who are prone to inadequate nutritional status, are also at increased risk of suffering from inadequate hydration. It is important to maintain proper hydration in these patients (see Chap. 7).

19.2.7 Specific Types of Ulcers Directly Associated with Malnutrition

Two types of ulcers are directly associated with malnutrition:
- Noma (cancrum oris, necrotizing ulcerative gingivitis)
- Tropical ulcer (tropical sloughing phagedena)

In both cases, the exact mechanisms leading to ulceration have not been identified, but opportunistic infection may play a major role.

19.3 Vitamins

Because of the vast scope of this subject, the discussion here will be limited to the association between wound healing and vitamins A, C, and E. These vitamins function as anti-oxidants and are generally associated with wound healing. One question is whether these anti-oxidant compounds reduce the damage caused by oxygen radicals, with subsequent enhanced healing. Another possibility is that the beneficial effect of each vitamin described below is due to its unique properties and not necessarily to its anti-oxidant activity.

In any event, whenever there is clinical evidence of deficiency of one of these vitamins (or any other vitamin or nutritional element) it should be rectified. The clinical signs of vitamin deficiency are detailed in Table 19.1. The question of whether, in some deficiency states, interference with wound repair may occur even before the clinical manifestations of deficiency are evident remains unanswered. The discussion below will also relate to the issue of whether supplementing one or more of these vitamins may enhance healing of cutaneous ulcers, even if there is no clinical evidence of a deficiency state (Table 19.2).

Table 19.1. Clinical manifestations of deficiency

Vitamin/ Mineral	Cutaneous manifestations	Other manifestations
Vitamin A	Dry skin; fine scaling; follicular hyperkeratosis ('phrynoderma')	Ocular lesions: xerophthalmia; keratomalacia; night blindness General: diarrhea, apathy, hindered growth in children
Vitamin C	Dry, rough skin; follicular hyperkeratosis. In severe deficiency: perifollicular purpuric macules and papules; coiled hair shafts	Fatigue, weakness, malaise In severe deficiency: gastrointestinal bleeding; jaundice; generalized edema; dyspnea; congestive heart failure; hypotension and shock; convulsions Oral: swollen bleeding gums; loose teeth
Vitamin E	No clear data regarding cutaneous manifestations yet documented	Peripheral neuropathy; arreflexia; decreased vibration or position sensation; skeletal myopathy In severe deficiency: ataxic gait; ophtalmoplegia; pigmented retinopathy
Zinc	Dry rough skin; eczematous and erosive eruptions located around the body orifices (mouth and genitalia) or acral; seborrheic-dermatitis like eruptions; alopecia (sometimes generalized; angular stomatitis	Diarrhea; decreased appetite; hypoguesia; glossitis; mental disturbances; lethargy
Iron	Pallor (in presence of anemia); Pruritus; koilonychia (spoon-shaped nails); chilosis; hair loss	Features of anemia, if present Oral: glossitis; sore tongue with atrophic filiform papillae In severe deficiency: dysphagia

A deficiency of one of the above vitamins or trace elements may induce poor wound healing.

Table 19.2. Supplementation of vitamins to consider[a] in patients with cutaneous ulcers for whom no nutritional deficiencies have been identified

Vitamin	Medical conditions
Vitamin A	Glucocorticoid treatment
	Treatment with antineoplastic drugs
	During/following radiation therapy
Vitamin E	Following laser injury[b]
	During/following radiotherapy[b]

[a] Cannot be regarded as evidence-based medicine.
[b] Based on animal studies only.

19.3.1 Vitamin A

In the 1940s, Brandaleone et al. [50] documented the detrimental effect of vitamin A deficiency on wound healing in the skin of rats. A similar animal experiment conducted by Freiman et al. [51] in 1970 confirmed these observations. Vitamin A deficiency was shown to inhibit epithelialization, reduce collagen synthesis, and induce increased susceptibility to infective agents [52, 53].

In light of the above, there is universal agreement that vitamin A should be provided when found to be deficient, and that replacement therapy can improve the body's ability to repair wounds and cutaneous ulcers. Another important question, discussed below, is whether vitamin A supplementation should be recommended for patients with an ulcer that does not heal well, in whom there is no clinical evidence of vitamin A deficiency.

19.3.1.1 Cutaneous Ulcers Without Clinical or Laboratory Evidence of Vitamin A Deficiency

Currently, there is no clinical evidence to support the routine administration of vitamin A in patients with cutaneous ulcers who are *not* vitamin A deficient. It should be kept in mind that high doses of vitamin A may lead to toxicity, which may, in turn, have a detrimental effect on wound repair [54]. However, vitamin A deficiency is a relatively common condition. Clinical deficiency of vitamin A may evolve relatively rapidly under traumatic stress or severe illness [5, 55]. As mentioned above, the question as to whether, in some deficiency states, interference with wound repair may occur even before the clinical manifestations of deficiency are evident, is still unanswered.

19.3.1.2 When to Consider Supplementation of Vitamin A

In view of the above, physicians treating chronic cutaneous ulcers, should consider administration of vitamin A under the following conditions:

- Vitamin A deficiency
- Patients receiving glucocorticoids
- Patients receiving chemotherapy or radiation therapy

Note that items 2 and 3 are suggestions that cannot be regarded, for the time being, as evidence-based. More studies are needed to establish the beneficial effect of vitamin A in these cases.

■ **Vitamin A Deficiency.** In view of the above, improved wound repair can be expected if vitamin A deficiency is corrected. The physical characteristics of vitamin A deficiency should be identified, as detailed in Table 19.1 [56–58]. These include dry skin with fine scaling and follicular hyperkeratosis and pathognomonic ocular lesions (e.g., xerophthalmia, keratomalacia). In most cases, vitamin A deficiency is usually accompanied by a deficiency of other nutrients.

Diagnosis is confirmed by measuring the level of vitamin A in the blood, although this is not considered a reliable indicator of the status of body stores of vitamin A. An ophthalmologic examination may be required to assess the severity of the condition. Measurement of body stores is done either by liver biopsy or by isotopic dilution, using vitamin A's isotope [54]. A good clinical response to oral vitamin A can help to confirm the diagnosis. When a deficiency state is diagnosed, vitamin A should be administered in accordance with the degree of severity.

■ **Patients Receiving Glucocorticoids.** Eherlich [59] and Hunt et al. [60] reported in 1968 and 1969, respectively, that orally administered vitamin A may partially antagonize the inhibitory effects of steroid therapy on wound healing. The mechanism of this effect is still unclear. Vitamin A has been shown to increase cell-mediated immune response, release growth factors, enhance fibroblast differentiation, and increase collagen synthesis [10, 11, 61].

When addressing the effects of vitamin A on the wound repair process, it may be important to distinguish between its effect on acute wounds and that on chronic cutaneous ulcers. To date it is not clear whether its main effect is on the initial inflammatory response to wounding, the healing of chronic ulcers, or both.

Levenson and Demetriou [10] have suggested that vitamin A may alter fibroblast gene expression, thereby increasing fibroblast activity and the proliferation rate. Other researchers have suggested that glucocorticoids stabilize lysosomal membranes (with subsequent reduction of macrophage and phagocytic activity), whereas vitamin A tends to decrease the stability of lysosomal membranes [55, 62]. It should be also noted, however, that some studies have not shown a beneficial effect of systemic retinoids (other than vitamin A) in counteracting the effect of steroid therapy in wound healing [63–65].

Some researchers have suggested that a dose of 25,000 IU/day of vitamin A, given for a few weeks, would benefit patients under glucocorticoid therapy [66, 67]. However, it should be kept in mind that the RDA of vitamin A is 5000 IU (1000 µg) for men, and 4000 IU (800 µg) for women [2]. An excess intake of vitamin A can be toxic: Normal adults ingesting 50,000 IU/day of vitamin A for several months may develop chronic vitamin A intoxication. Extreme care should also be taken not to exceed the safety level in pregnant women.

Anstead [63] has pointed out that a high systemic dose of vitamin A may actually reverse the *desired* anti-inflammatory effects of steroid therapy, thereby aggravating the disease for which the patient is being treated with glucocorticoids. In these cases, topical application of vitamin A derivatives might be considered.

Since there are no clear published guidelines on this issue, it seems, for the time being, at least, that vitamin A in doses slightly more than the RDA should be recommended – excluding pregnant women. A diet containing foodstuffs rich in vitamin A such as carrots, may also be recommended.

■ **Patients Receiving Chemotherapy or Radiation Therapy.** The results of animal experiments suggest that, similar to its effect on wound healing in cases of steroid therapy, vitamin A may counteract the effect of anti-neoplastic drugs such as cyclophosphamide or 5-fluorouracil [68, 69]. It may also have a beneficial effect following radiation therapy [70, 71].

19.3.1.5 Vitamin A: Practical Conclusions

– A physician should always be aware of the possibility of vitamin A deficiency in patients with cutaneous ulcers. Appropriate intervention should be carried out in such cases.

– Excessive intake of vitamin A (in the form of vitamin pills) should be avoided.

– Supplementation of vitamin A in patients with cutaneous ulcers during steroid treatment, chemotherapy, or radiation therapy may be considered.

– Ensure that patients with cutaneous ulcers receive at least the RDA of vitamin A. A diet of foodstuffs containing higher amounts of vitamin A may be recommended.

19.3.2 Vitamin C

Vitamin C (ascorbic acid) is an essential cofactor in the hydroxylation of proline and lysine residues in the process of collagen synthesis. Vitamin C deficiency impedes the normal course of wound repair mainly by interfering with collagen synthesis and its cross-linking. Collagen formed in vitamin C deficiency states is under-hydroxylated, relatively unstable, and subject to collagenolysis [40, 72, 73].

Vitamin C is also required for an appropriately functioning immune system, including neutrophil function and efficient phagocytosis. The addition of vitamin C to cultures of neutrophils and macrophages has been shown to increase their motility and capacity for phagocytosis [74, 75].

Vitamin C deficiency is associated with a higher incidence of wound infection [40]. The histology of skin specimens in scurvy patients demonstrates a reduced amount of collagen, reduced angiogenesis, and the presence of perifollicular hemorrhages [76].

19.3.2.1 Administration of Vitamin C in Non-Deficient Patients with Chronic Ulcers of the Skin

Silverstein et al. [77] studied 20 guinea pigs and concluded that increased vitamin C intake before and after a surgical procedure may induce faster recovery of skin integrity and increase wound strength. However, based on this report alone, it would be inappropriate to make recommendations for patients with chronic cutaneous ulcers.

There is no conclusive evidence that vitamin C supplementation is beneficial for patients with chronic cutaneous ulcers who have normal vitamin C levels [10, 78]. Still, severe traumatic stress or illness may result in the depletion of vitamin C. For a severely ill patient, it may be worthwhile to increase the dose of vitamin C to 1–2 g/day for a short period, until signs of recovery are seen [62].

19.3.2.2 Vitamin C Deficiency

■ **Clinical Manifestations.** The clinical manifestations of vitamin C deficiency were described in full by Hirschmann and Raugi [73] in the *Journal of the American Academy of Dermatology* in 1999, as well as by Lind in his original descriptions of scurvy [79]. These manifestations are diverse and affect many systems. Constitutional symptoms of vitamin C deficiency are fatigue, weakness, and malaise. These usually recede following vitamin C supplementation. Severe deficiency may be manifested by gastrointestinal bleeding, jaundice, and generalized edema, dyspnea with high-output congestive heart failure, and hypotension with subsequent shock and convulsions [73, 79].

Typical cutaneous manifestations are dry and rough skin with follicular hyperkeratosis, presenting mainly on the buttocks and legs. In the advanced disease, perifollicular purpuric macules and papules can be seen. The latter are attributed to increased fragility of blood vessel walls and are seen primarily on the legs, due to increased hydrostatic pressure. Petechiae may be seen in other areas such as the eyelids [80]. Fractured and coiled hair shafts ("corkscrew hair") are seen over the body.

The oral manifestations are characteristic and may direct the physician to the correct diagnosis. They include swollen, red gums that may gradually become necrotic, with loose teeth.

■ **Treatment.** If scurvy is suspected, therapy should be initiated immediately after a sample of blood is drawn. In adults, the current recommendation for scurvy in *Harrison's Principles of Internal Medicine* is 200 mg/day of vitamin C orally. This usually relieves symptoms of scurvy within a few days [54]. Others recommend higher doses of 500–1000 mg/day. In infants and children, vitamin C should be given i.v. or p.o. at a dose of 25–50 mg/24 h, given as a single dose [81].

Note that vitamin C deficiency is frequently accompanied by other nutritional deficiencies and by concurrent opportunistic infections.

19.3.2.3 Vitamin C: Practical Conclusions

- Provision of vitamin C to patients who are vitamin C deficient, especially to those who suffer from cutaneous ulcers or wounds, is extremely important.
- Make sure that the patient is receiving the RDA of vitamin C, i.e., approximately 60 mg/ day for adults [2].
- At present, there is no evidence that high doses of vitamin C are beneficial for patients with cutaneous ulcers who are not vitamin C deficient. However, it is reasonable to consider administering higher doses of vitamin C to patients suffering from severe traumatic stress.

19.3.3 Vitamin E

Vitamin E is the accepted term for a group of compounds that possess similar biological activities. Tocopherols are the most common representatives of this group, of which α-tocopherol is the most active.

Vitamin E, as an antioxidant, is considered to neutralize oxygen free radicals and prevent tissue damage. Supplementation of the vitamin has been claimed to have a beneficial effect on coronary heart disease, but this claim has not yet been fully confirmed scientifically [82–86]. In view of the above, it seems to be a reasonable step to assess the effect of vitamin E on wound healing.

However, to date there are no data confirming either the value of vitamin E in chronic cutaneous ulcers or a beneficial effect of high-dose vitamin E supplementation on wound repair. If there were any beneficial effect, it could well be on wounds that stem from radiation or laser therapy. Radiation tissue injury involves an overproduction of free radicals; thus, the antioxidant effect of vitamin E may be beneficial in these cases.

Animal studies have been conducted using models of laser or radiation skin injury. In these studies a degree of beneficial effect of vitamin E was demonstrated [87, 88]. However, a beneficial effect of vitamin E on chronic ulcers or traumatic injury has not yet been demonstrated in human beings. Furthermore, some investigators have suggested that high levels of vitamin E may even impair wound repair, as is seen with glucocorticoids [89]. In any case, the dietary intake of vitamin E is usually adequate. In summary, at this stage there is no clinical evidence in support of supplementary vitamin E therapy in patients with chronic ulcers.

Vitamin E deficiency states are extremely rare. They may develop as a result of gastrointestinal diseases with prolonged malabsorption (such as celiac or cystic fibrosis) or in rare familial forms.

The deficiency is usually manifested clinically as neurologic and ophthalmologic deficits, as detailed in Table 19.1 [54, 90–92]. When vitamin E deficiency is suspected, the serum level of α-tocopherol should be determined.

19.4 Trace Elements

We shall discuss here the association between zinc and iron, wound repair, and cutaneous ulcers. The clinical signs of zinc and iron deficiency are shown in Table 19.1.

19.4.1 Zinc

Zinc is an essential trace element. To date, researchers have identified more than 70 metalloenzymes that require zinc for their function. Some of these enzymes play a key role in the synthesis of nucleic acids and proteins [93, 94]. Physiologic levels of zinc are needed for the maintenance of immune functions [95–99] as well as dermal and epidermal functions [100– 102].

Early observations that zinc depletion tends to impede wound repair [102–104] led investigators to the assumption that zinc supplementation may be beneficial for cutaneous healing mechanisms in general, and not necessarily in states of zinc deficiency only.

In the following discussion, we will distinguish between two different conditions:

- Cutaneous ulcers in patients with normal levels of zinc
- Cutaneous ulcers in patients with zinc deficiency

19.4.1.1 Normal Levels

Suggested mechanisms by which zinc supplementation may exert its beneficial effect on wound healing – even when serum and body zinc levels are normal – include:

- Modulation of cytokines: Several studies have shown that zinc may affect the production of various cytokines by mononuclear cells [96, 105, 106]. Zinc oxide has also been shown to increase the endogenous expression of growth factors, such as insulin-like growth factor I, in granulation tissue [107, 108].
- Effect on Langerhans' cells: Kohn et al. have suggested that zinc may enhance the migrating capacity of Langerhans' cells, thereby positively affecting immune mechanisms and tissue repair [109].
- Induction of increase of mitotic activity [110], with subsequent enhanced epithelial migration and improved endothelial repair [108, 111–113].

Although several studies have demonstrated enhanced wound repair following zinc supplementation [102, 114, 115], other researchers have reported contrasting results [116, 117].

Currently, there is no clinical evidence supporting the administration of zinc in patients with chronic ulcers of the skin if they are not zinc deficient [118, 119]. This issue requires fur-

ther clarification, and more research studies should be conducted before a consensus policy can be determined.

Note that a high level of zinc may be detrimental to cutaneous physiologic functions and normal processes of wound repair [120, 121]. In cases where zinc deficiency is not suspected, the RDA of zinc should be maintained.

19.4.1.2 Zinc Deficiency

Zinc deficiency interferes with normal processes of wound healing, including delayed epithelialization, reduced proliferation of fibroblasts, and reduced collagen synthesis [100–102, 121]. Zinc-deficient patients are more susceptible to various infections [119]. Therefore, in patients with cutaneous ulcers and clinical or laboratory evidence of zinc deficiency, there is no doubt that oral zinc should be provided, in order to replenish bodily stores.

A normal plasma level of zinc lies between 70 and 100 µg/dl [122]. The plasma level of zinc provides some indication of bodily stores but is not necessarily accurate, especially in mild deficiency. Despite a certain degree of deficiency of zinc in bodily stores, its level in the serum may still be normal [54, 123–125].

Serum zinc levels show a diurnal variation, and the level tends to decrease two hours after a meal. The plasma level of zinc may fall due to its redistribution from plasma to tissues in certain conditions such as infection or malignancy. Even when deficient, zinc may be released from bodily tissues into the blood. Only when the degree of deficiency becomes critical, a rapid onset of both biochemical and clinical signs becomes evident [123–125].

Some of the clinical signs of mild zinc deficiency (see below) may be somewhat 'vague', such as a mild decrease in appetite or mild weakness. The extent of interference with wound repair processes in such circumstances is not known. The question of whether, in such patients, serum zinc levels may indeed reflect this state is unresolved.

Serum alkaline phosphatase is a zinc-dependent enzyme, and its activity may provide some indication as to zinc status. The value of tests such as leukocyte and erythrocyte zinc values still has to be validated [122–126].

■ **Clinical Manifestations of Zinc Deficiency.** Zinc deficiency affects cellular division and differentiation. As a result, clinical manifestations appear in those tissues that have a high level of cellular turnover, such as skin or gastrointestinal mucosa [54]. The cutaneous manifestations of acquired deficiency are presented in Table 19.1 [54, 127–130].

■ **Recommended Dietary Allowance.** The RDA for adult men and women is 15 mg and 12 mg/day, respectively [2]. Zinc supplements can be administered as $ZnSo_4$ (given orally) or as $ZnCl_2$ (administered intravenously). The amount of zinc given is determined by both the level of deficiency and the type of preparation. Note that the amount of elemental zinc contained in preparations varies. For example, a capsule of 220 mg $ZnSo_4 \cdot 7H_2O$, contains approximately 55 mg Zn^{2+} [127].

Mild zinc deficiency may be treated with 220 mg zinc sulfate given orally, once daily. In severe deficiency states, a dose of 220 mg may be given two or three times per day. However, this dosage should be given for a short period only, to avoid toxicity [127].

Practical conclusions are as follows:
- It may be advisable to check zinc levels in patients with cutaneous ulcers. However, the value of routine serum zinc tests has not yet been proven.
- Make sure that patients with cutaneous ulcers do not show any clinical signs of zinc deficiency.
- If there is evidence of zinc deficiency, it should be corrected.
- Currently, there is no clinical evidence to suggest that zinc supplementation is beneficial to patients with chronic ulcers of the skin if they are not zinc deficient.

19.4.2 Iron

Significant iron deficiency impairs the process of wound repair. A significantly low iron level causes anemia and reduced oxygen delivery to tissues. However, an important question is whether iron deficiency that is not severe enough to cause anemia also impairs normal wound repair processes. The answer to this question is most likely positive.

Iron plays a major role in cellular respiration, cellular proliferation, and differentiation, as well as in gene expression [131]. Impairment of host defense mechanisms may be a result of the effect of iron deficiency on lymphocyte proliferation [132, 133]. In addition, iron is a cofactor in the hydroxylation of proline and lysine in the process of collagen synthesis [134], so it may affect wound repair processes in this way as well.

In general, it appears that a low iron level tends to have an adverse effect on dermal and epidermal functions. This effect is seen in cases of hair loss due to iron deficiency, which improves with the restoration of normal bodily iron levels. Additional clinical signs of iron deficiency are listed in Table 19.1 [135, 136].

Practical conclusions regarding iron deficiency are:
- It is advisable to check serum iron levels, as well as transferrin iron-binding capacity and ferritin, in all patients with chronic cutaneous ulcers, even if the hemoglobin concentration is normal.
- Iron deficiency should be corrected.
- In any case, serum iron below the normal level demands a thorough work-up to identify the cause.

19.4.3 Other Vitamins and Trace Elements

Other vitamins and other trace elements have not been discussed here. Some may yet have an unidentified role as cofactors or components of enzymes that are important in the mechanisms of wound repair. It should be noted, however, that deficiencies in certain elements cannot necessarily be identified and may be sub-clinical in nature. In many cases, measurements of various vitamin levels in the blood or serum cannot be regarded as a reliable indicator of deficiency states.

As presented below, multivitamin supplementation may well be considered in patients with chronic cutaneous ulcers. In general it is easier, in such cases, to correct mild 'suboptimal' deficiency states by prescribing multivitamin supplementation than to diagnose them.

19.4.4 Vitamin and Trace Element Supplementation in Patients with Cutaneous Ulcers

Recent evidence has shown that an optimal amount of all vitamins is not fully provided by the diet of many people, even in developed countries and especially among the elderly. There is a high prevalence of suboptimal vitamin and mineral levels, which are nevertheless above the level of a classic deficiency syndrome and are not manifested clinically. This pertains to the vitamins and minerals that have been specifically detailed in this chapter (vitamins A, C, and E, zinc, and iron) as well as to a wide range of other vitamins and trace elements. Such suboptimal states are considered to be risk factors for chronic illnesses such as cardiovascular diseases and cancer [137, 138].

Whether suboptimal levels of vitamins or trace elements may impede the healing of cutaneous ulcers has still not been established. Similarly, the mechanisms by which healing could be affected in these mild states of deficiency have not yet been identified. One of many possible mechanisms may be supported by the finding that vitamin and trace element supplementation reduces the incidence of infections in elderly patients [139–141]. Restoring optimal levels of vitamins and minerals in patients with cutaneous ulcers may therefore affect the immune system, with a subsequent beneficial effect on healing.

Considering that leg ulcers are much more prevalent in the elderly, it would be reasonable to advise these patients on how to improve their diet, and to consider prescribing vitamin and mineral supplements.

19.5 Summary

Summary comments on malnutrition and protein and on carbohydrate and lipid deficiency appear earlier in this chapter.

The following are general comments on the association between vitamins and trace elements and the presence of cutaneous ulcers:

- Blood tests such as serum iron and ferritin may assist in determining states of deficiency.
- When a state of deficiency is diagnosed, it should be corrected.
- All patients with cutaneous ulcers must receive the appropriate RDAs.
- Stress adds to the depletion of vitamins and trace elements. In these cases, possible deficiency states should be monitored and nutritional supplementation provided as required.
- Due to the risk of toxicity, in no event should excess supplementation be provided.
- In the absence of a confirmed deficiency of a particular vitamin or trace element, there is no proven benefit in administering high doses of these compounds for wound repair. However, the following reservations should be kept in mind: (a) There are specific situations, detailed above, in which it is reasonable to consider administration of specific vitamins, such as vitamin A to patients who are receiving glucocorticoids. (b) Vitamin and trace element supplementation may be considered for patients with cutaneous ulcers.

References

1. Lin E, Lowry SF, Calvano SE: The systemic response to injury. In: Schwartz SI, Shires GT, Spencer FC, et al (eds) Principles of Surgery, 7th edn. New York: McGraw-Hill. 1998; pp 3–52

2. Dwyer J: Nutritional requirements and dietary assessment. In: Braunwald E, Fauci AS, Kasper DL, Hauser SL, Longo DL, Jameson JL (eds) Harrison's Principles of Internal Medicine, 15th edn. New York: McGraw-Hill. 2001; pp 451–455

3. Frank GC: Nutritional requirements for patients with chronic wounds. In: McCulloch JM, Kloth LC, Feedar JA (eds) Wound Healing: Alternatives in Management, 2nd edn. Philadelphia: FA Davis. 1995; pp 87–108

4. Garner WL: Thermal berns. In: Achauer BM, Eriksson EE (eds) Plastic Surgery: Indications, Operations, and Outcomes. St. Louis: Mosby. 2000; pp 357–373

5. Rai K, Courtemanche AD: Vitamin A assay in burned patients. J Trauma 1975; 15 : 419–424

6. Berger MM, Shenkin A: Trace elements in trauma and burns. Curr Opin Clin Nutr Metab Care 1998; 1 : 513–517

7. Levenson SM, Seifter E: Dysnutrition, wound healing and resistance to infection. Clin Plast Surg 1977; 4 : 375–388

8. Gottschlich MM, Warden GD: Vitamin supplementation in the patient with burns. J Burn Care Rehabil 1990; 11 : 275–279

9. Levenson SM, Upjohn HL, Preston JA, et al: Effect of thermal burns on wound healing. Ann Surg 1957; 146 : 357–368

10. Levenson SM, Demetriou AA: Metabolic factors. In: Cohen IK, Diegelmann RF, Lindblad WJ (eds) Wound Healing: Biochemical and Clinical Aspects. Philadelphia: WB Saunders. 1992; pp 248–273

11. Albina JE: Nutrition and wound healing. J Parenteral Ent Nutr 1994; 18 : 367–376

12. Kay SP, Moreland JR, Schmitter E: Nutritional status and wound healing in lower extremity amputations. Clin Orthop 1987; 217 : 253–256

13. Dickhaut SC, DeLee JC, Page CP: Nutrition status: Importance in predicting wound healing after amputation. J Bone Joint Surg Am 1984; 66 : 71–75

14. Casey J, Flinn WR, Yao JS, et al: Correlation of immune and nutritional status with wound complications in patients undergoing vascular operations. Surgery 1983; 93 : 822–827

15. Allman RM, Goode PS, Patrick MM, et al: Pressure ulcer risk factors among hospitalized patients with activity limitation. JAMA 1995; 273 : 865–870

16. Thomas DR, Goode PS, Tarquine PH, et al: Hospital acquired pressure ulcers and risk of death. J Am Geriatr Soc 1996; 44 : 1435–1440

17. Pinchcofsky Devin GD, Kaminski MV Jr: Correlation of pressure sores and nutritional status. J Am Geriatr Soc 1986; 34 : 435–440

18. Daly JM, Reynolds J, Sigal RK, et al: Effect of dietary protein and amino acids on immune function. Crit Care Med 1990; 18 [Suppl] : S86–S93

19. Redmond HP, Shou J, Kelly CJ, et al: Immunosuppressive mechanisms in protein-calorie malnutrition. Surgery 1991; 110 : 311–317

20. Collins N: Assessment and treatment of involuntary weight loss and protein-calorie malnutrition. Adv skin Wound Care 2000; 13 [Suppl 1] : 4–10

21. Halsted CH: Nutrition and nutritional assessment. In: Braunwald E, Fauci AS, Kasper DL, Hauser SL, Longo DL, Jameson JL (eds) Harrison's Principles of Internal Medicine, 15th edn. New York: McGraw-Hill. 2001; pp 455–461

22. Mears E: Outcomes of continuous process improvement of a nutritional care program incorporating serum prealbumin measurements. Nutrition 1996; 12 : 479–484

23. Lopez-Hellin J, Baena-Fustegueras JA, Schwartz-Riera S, et al: Usefulness of short-lived proteins as nutritional indicators surgical patients. Clin Nutr 2002; 21 : 119–125

24. Thorsdottir I, Gunnarsdottir I, Eriksen B: Screening method evaluated by nutritional status measurements can be used to detect malnurishment in chronic obstructive pulmunary disease. J Am Diet Assoc 2001; 101 : 648–654

25. Ruberg RL: Role of nutrition in wound healing. Surg Clin North Am 1984; 64 : 705–714

26. Lindstedt E, Sandblom P: Wound healing in man: tensile strength of healing wounds in some patient groups. Ann Surg 1975; 181 : 842–846

27. Pollack SV: Wound healing: A review. III. Nutritional factors affecting wound healing. J Dermatol Surg Oncol 1979; 5 : 615–619

28. Thomas DR: The role of nutrition in prevention and healing of pressure ulcers. Clin Geriatr Med 1997; 13 : 497–511

29. Guenter P, Malyszek R, Bliss DZ, et al: Survey of nutritional status in newly hospitalized patients with stage III or stage IV pressure ulcers. Adv Skin Wound Care 2000; 13 : 164–168

30. Berlowitz DR, Wilking SV: Risk factors for pressure sores: a comparison of cross sectional and cohort-derived data. J Am Geriatr Soc 1989; 37 : 1043–1050

31. Breslow RA, Hallfrisch J, Guy DG, et al: The importance of dietary protein in healing pressure ulcers. J Am Geriatr Soc 1993; 41 : 357–362

32. Bergstrom N, Bennett MA, Carlson, et al: Treatment of pressure ulcers. Clinical practice guideline, no 15. AHCPR publication no. 95-0652. Rockville, Maryland: U.S. Department of Health and Human Services. Public Health Services, Agency for Health Care Policy and Research, December 1994

33. Phillips LG: Therapeutic options in management of pressure ulcers. In: Falanga V (ed) Cutaneous Wound Healing, 1st edn. London: Martin Dunitz. 2001; pp 343–356

34. Williamson MB, Fromm HJ: The incorporation of sulfur amino acids into the proteins of regenerating wound tissue. J Biol Chem 1955; 212 : 705–712

35. Barbul A, Lazarou SA, Efron DT, et al: Arginine enhances wound healing and lymphocyte immune responses in humans. Surgery 1990; 108: 331–337

36. Kirk SJ, Hurson M, Regan MC, et al: Arginine stimulates wound healing and immune function in elderly human beings. Surgery 1993; 114: 155–159

37. Sigal RK, Shou J, Daly JM: Parenteral arginine infusion in humans: nutrient substrate or pharmacologic agent? J Parenter Enteral Nutr 1992; 16: 423–428

38. Langkamp-Henken B, Herrlinger-Garcia KA, Stechmiller JK, et al: Arginine supplementation is well tolerated but does not enhance mitogen-induced lymphocyte proliferation in elderly nursing home residents with pressure ulcers. J Parenter Enteral Nutr 2000; 24: 280–287

39. Efron DT, Most D, Barbul A: Role of nitric oxide in wound healing. Curr Opin Clin Nutr Metab Care 2000; 3: 197–204

40. Barbul A, Purtill WA: Nutrition in wound healing. Clin Dermatol 1994; 12: 133–140

41. Bourdel-Marchasson I, Barateau M, Rondeau V, et al: A multi-center trial of the effects of oral nutritional supplementation in critically ill older inpatients. Nutrition 2000; 16: 1–5

42. Hulsey TK, O'Neill JA, Neblett WR, et al: Experimental wound healing in essential fatty acid deficiency. J Ped Surg 1980; 15: 505–508

43. Caffrey BB, Jonsson HT Jr: Role of essential fatty acids wound healing in rats. Prog Lipid Res 1981; 20: 641–647

44. Caldwell MD, Jonsson HT, Othersen HB Jr: Essential fatty acid deficiency in an infant receiving prolonged parent alimentation. J Pediatr 1972; 81: 894–898

45. Burney DP, Goodwin C, Caldwell MD, et al: Essential fatty acid deficiency and impaired wound healing in an infant with gastroschisis. Am Surg 1979; 45: 542

46. Kloth LC, McCulloch JM: The inflammatory response to wounding. In: McCulloch JM, Kloth LC, Feedar JA (eds) Wound Healing: Alternatives in Management, 2nd edn. Philadelphia: FA Davis. 1995; pp 3–15

47. Laulederkind SJ, Thompson-Jaeger S, Goorha S, et al: Both constitutive and inducible prostaglandin H synthase affect dermal wound healing in mice. Lab Invest 2002; 82: 919–927

48. Kohyama T, Liu X, Kim HJ et al: Prostacyclin analogs inhibit fibroblast migration. Am J Physiol Lung Cell Mol Physiol 2002; 283: L428–L432

49. Albina JE, Gladden P, Walsh WR: Detrimental effects of an omega 3 fatty acid-enriched diet on wound healing. J Parenter Enteral Nutr 1993; 17: 519–521

50. Brandaleone H, Papper E: The effect of the local and oral administration of cod liver oil on the rate of wound healing in vitamin A deficient and normal animals. Ann Surg 1941; 114: 791–798

51. Freiman M, Seifter E, Connerton C, et al: Vitamin A deficiency and surgical stress. Surg Forum 1970; 21: 81–82

52. Dreizen S: Nutrition and the immune response – A review. Int J Vit Nutr Res 1979; 49: 220–228

53. Jarrett A, Spearman RI: Vitamin A and the skin. Br J Dermatol 1970; 82: 197–199

54. Russell RM: Vitamin and trace mineral deficiency and excess. In: Braunwald E, Fauci AS, Kasper DL, Hauser SL, Longo DL, Jameson JL (eds) Harrison's Principles of Internal Medicine, 15th edn. New York: McGraw-Hill. 2001; pp 461–469

55. Hunt TK: Vitamin A and wound healing. J Am Acad Dermatol 1986; 15: 817–821

56. Soni BP, McLaren DS, Sherertz EF: Cutaneous changes in nutritional disease. In: Freedberg IM, Eisen AZ, Wolff K, Austen KF, Goldsmith LA, Katz SI, Fitzpatrick TB (eds) Fitzpatrick's Dermatology in General Medicine, 5th edn. New York: McGraw-Hill. 1999; pp 1725–1737

57. Bleasel NR, Stapleton KM, Lee MS, et al: Vitamin A deficiency phrynoderma: due to malabsorption and inadequate diet. J Am Acad Dermatol 1999; 41: 322–324

58. Goskowicz M, Eichenfield LF: Cutaneous findings of nutritional deficiencies in children. Curr Opin Pediatr 1993; 5: 441–445

59. Ehrlich HP, Hunt TK: Effects of cortisone and vitamin A on wound healing. Ann Surg 1968; 167: 324–328

60. Hunt TK, Ehrlich HP, Garcia JA, et al: Effect of vitamin A on reversing the inhibitory effect of cortisone on healing of open wounds in animals and man. Ann Surg 1969; 170: 633–641

61. Barbul A, Thysen B, Rettura G, et al: White cell involvement in the inflammatory, wound healing, and immune actions of vitamin A. J Parenter Enternal Nutr 1978; 2: 129–138

62. Rackett SC, Rothe MJ, Grant-Kels JM: Diet and dermatology. The role of dietary manipulation in the prevention and treatment of cutaneous disorders. J Am Acad Dermatol 1993; 29: 447–461

63. Anstead GM: Steroids, retinoids, and wound healing. Adv Wound Care 1998; 11: 277–285

64. Salmela K: the effect of methylprednisolone and vitamin A on wound healing. II. Acta Chir Scand 1981; 147: 313–315

65. Oikarinen A, Vuorio E, Vuorio T: Comparison of the effects of dexamethasone and 13-cis-retinoic acid on connective tissue biosynthesis in human skin fibroblasts. Arch Dermatol Res 1989; 281: 273–278

66. Pollack SV: Wound healing: A review. IV. Systemic medications affecting wound healing. J Dermatol Surg Oncol 1982; 8: 667–672

67. Cohen BE, Cohen IK: Vitamin A: Adjuvant and steroid antagonist in the immune response. J Immunol 1973; 111: 1376–1380

68. Weinzweig J, Levenson SM, Rettura G, et al: Supplemental vitamin A prevents the tumor-induced defect in wound healing. Ann Surg 1990; 211:269–276

69. de Waard JW, Wobbes T, van der Linden CJ, et al: Retinol may promote fluorouracil-suppressed healing of experimental intestinal anastomoses. Arch Surg 1995; 130:959–965

70. Levenson SM, Gruber CA, Rettura G, et al: Supplemental vitamin A prevents the acute radiation induced defect in wound healing. Ann Surg 1984; 200:494–512

71. Winsey K, Simon RJ, Levenson SM, et al: Effect of supplemental vitamin A on colon anastomotic healing in rats given preoperative irradiation. Am J Surg 1987; 153:153–156

72. Englard S, Seifter S: The biochemical functions of ascorbic acid. Annu Rev Nutr 1986; 6:365–406

73. Hirschmann JV, Raugi GJ: Adult scurvy. J Am Acad Dermatol 1999; 41:895–906

74. Thomas WR, Holt PG: Vitamin C and immunity: An assessment of the evidence. Clin Exp Immunol 1978; 32:370–379

75. Anderson R, Oosthuizen R, Maritz R, et al: The effects of increasing weekly doses of ascorbate on certain cellular and humoral immune functions in normal volunteers. Am J Clin Nutr 1980; 33:71–76

76. Crandon JH, Lund CC, Dill DB: Experimental human scurvy. N Engl J Med 1940; 223:353–369

77. Silverstein RJ, Landsman AS: The effects of a moderate and high dose of vitamin C on wound healing in a controlled guinea pig model. J Foot Ankle Surg 1999; 38:333–338

78. ter Riet G, Kessels AG, Knipschild PG: Randomized clinical trial of ascorbic acid in the treatment of pressure ulcers. J Clin Epidemiol 1995; 48:1453–1460

79. Stewart CP, Guthrie D: Lind's treatise on scurvy: A bicentenary volume containing a reprint of the first edition of 'A Treatise on Scurvy by James Lind, MD', with additional notes. Edinburgh: Edinburgh University Press. 1953; pp 145–148

80. Hood J, Hodges RE: Ocular lesions in scurvy. Am J Clin Nutr 1969; 22:559–567

81. Levin RH, Zenk KE: Medication Table. In: Rudolph AM, Hoffman JIE, Rudolph CD (eds) Rudolph's Pediatrics, 20th edn. Englewood Cliffs: Prentice Hall. 1996; pp 2170–2210

82. Rimm EB, Stampfer MJ, Ascherio A, et al: Vitamin E consumption and the risk of coronary disease in men. N Engl J Med 1993; 328:1450–1456

83. Stampfer MJ, Hennekens CH, Manson JE, et al: Vitamin E consumption and the risk of coronary disease in women. N Engl J Med 1993; 328:1444–1449

84. Pruthi S, Allison TG, Hensrud DD: Vitamin E supplementation in the prevention of coronary disease. Mayo Clin Proc 2001; 76:1131–1136

85. Blumberg JB: An update: vitamin E supplementation and heart disease. Nutr Clin Care 2002; 5:50–55

86. MRC/BHF Heart Protection Study of antioxidant vitamin supplementation in 20,536 high-risk individuals: a randomized placebo-controlled trial. Lancet 2002; 360:23–33

87. Simon GA, Schmid P, Reifenrath WG, et al: Wound healing after laser injury to skin – the effect of occlusion and vitamin E. J Pharm Sci 1994; 83:1101–1106

88. Taren DL, Chvapil M, Weber CW: Increasing the breaking strength of wounds exposed to preoperative irradiation using vitamin E supplementation. Int J Vitam Nutr Res 1987; 57:133–137

89. Ehrlich HP, Tarver H, Hunt TK: Inhibitory effects of vitamin E on collagen synthesis and wound repair. Ann Surg 1972; 175:235–240

90. Burck U, Goebel H, Kuhlendahl HD, et al: Neuromyopathy and vitamin E deficiency in man. Neuropediatrics 1981; 12:267–278

91. Jackson CE, Amato AA, Barohn RJ: Isolated vitamin E deficiency. Muscle Nerve 1996; 19:1161–1165

92. Martinello F, Fardin P, Ottina M, et al: Supplemental therapy in isolated vitamin E deficiency improves the peripheral neuropathy and prevents the progressing of ataxia. J Neurol Sci 1998; 156:177–179

93. Lansdown AB: Zinc in the healing wound. Lancet 1996; 347:706–707

94. Nedler KN: The biochemistry and physiology of zinc metabolism. In: Goldsmith CA (ed) Biochemistry and Physiology of the Skin. Oxford: Oxford University Press. 1983; pp 1082–1101

95. Keen CL, Gershwin ME: Zinc deficiency and immune function. Annu Rev Nutr 1990; 10:415–431

96. Driessen C, Hirv K, Rink L, et al: Induction of cytokines by zinc ions in human peripheral blood mononuclear cells and separated monocytes. Lymphokine Cytokine Res 1994; 13:15–20

97. Salas M, Kirchner H: Induction of Interferon-γ human leukocyte cultures stimulated by Zn^{2+}. Clin Immunol Immunpathol 1987; 45:139–142

98. Shankar AH, Prasad AS: Zinc and immune function: The biological basis of altered resistance to infection. Am J Clin Nutr 1998; 68 [Suppl]: 447S–463S

99. Dardenne M: Zinc and immune function. Eur J Clin Nutr 2002; 56 [Suppl]: S20–S23

100. Solomons NW, Cousins RJ. Zinc. In: Solomons NW, Rosenberg IH (eds) Current topics in nutrition and disease, vol 12. Absorption and malabsorption of mineral nutrients. New York: Alan R Liss. 1984; pp 126–179

101. Pories WJ, Strain WH: The functional role of zinc in epidermal tissues. In: Mills CF (ed) Trace element metabolism in animals. Edinburgh and London: E. and S. Livingstone. 1970; pp 75–77

102. Agren MS: Studies on zinc in wound healing. Acta Derm Venereol (Stockh) 1990; 154:1–36

103. Pories WJ, Henzel JH, Rob CG, et al: Acceleration of healing with zinc sulfate. Ann Surg 1967; 165:432–436

104. Seymour CS: Trace metal disorders. In: Warrel DJ, Ledingham JG, Warrel DA (eds) Oxford Textbook of Medicine. Oxford: Oxford University Press. 1996; pp 1423–1424

105. Ibs KH, Rink L: Zinc-altered immune function. J Nutr 2003; 133 [5 Suppl 1]:1452S–1456S

106. Driessen C, Hirv K, Kirchner H, et al: Zinc regulates cytokine induction by superantigens and lipopolysaccharide. Immunol 1995; 84:272–277

107. Tarnow P, Agren M, Steenfos H, et al: Topical zinc oxide treatment increases endogenous gene expression of insulin-like growth factor 1 in granulation tissue from porcine wounds. Scand J Plast Reconstr Surg Hand Surg 1994; 28:255–259

108. Watanabe S, Wang XE, Hirose M, et al: Insulin-like growth factor 1 plays a role in gastric wound healing: evidence using a zinc derivative, polaprezinc, and an in vitro rabbit wound repair model. Aliment Pharmacol Ther 1998; 12:1131–1138

109. Kohn S, Kohn D, Schiller D: Effect of zinc supplementation on epidermal Langerhans' cells of elderly patients with decubital ulcers. J Dermatol 2000; 27:258–263

110. Jin L, Murakami TH, Janjua NA, et al: The effects of zinc oxide diethyldithiocarbamate on the mitotic index of epidermal basal cells of mouse skin. Acta Medica Okayama 1994; 48:231–236

111. Agren MS: Zinc in wound repair. Arch Dermatol 1999; 135:1273–1274

112. Agren MS: Zinc oxide increases degradation of collagen in necrotic wound tissue [letter]. Br J Dermatol 1993; 129:221

113. McClain C, Morris P, Hennig B: Zinc and endothelial function. Nutrition 1995; 11:117–120

114. Hallbook T, Lanner E: Serum zinc and healing of venous leg ulcers. Lancet 1972; 2:780–782

115. Husain SL: Oral zinc sulphate in leg ulcers. Lancet 1969; 1:1069–1071

116. Phillips A, Davidson M, Greaves MW: Venous leg ulceration: evaluation of zinc treatment, serum zinc and rate of healing. Clin Exp Dermatol 1977; 2:395–399

117. Sandstead HH, Henriksen LK, Greger JL, et al: Zinc nutriture in the elderly in relation to taste acuity, immune response, and wound healing. Am J Clin Nutr 1982; 36 [Suppl]:1046–1059

118. Wilkinson EA, Hawke CI: Does oral zinc aid the healing of chronic leg ulcers? A systematic literature review. Arch Dermatol 1998; 134:1556–1560

119. Wilkinson EAJ, Hawke CI: Oral zinc for arterial and venous leg ulcers (Cochrane Review). In: The Cochrane Library, Issue 4, 2000. Oxford: Update Software

120. Goode P, Allman R: The prevention and management of pressure ulcers. Med Clin North Am 1989; 73:1511–1524

121. Reed BR, Clark RA: Cutaneous tissue repair: practical implications of current knowledge. II. J Am Acad Dermatol 1985; 13:919–941

122. Nieves DS, Goldsmith LA: Cutaneous changes in nutritional disease. In: Freedberg IM, Eisen AZ, Wolff K, Austen KF, Goldsmith LA, Katz SI (eds) Fitzpatrick's Dermatology in General Medicine, 6th edn. New York: McGraw-Hill. 2003; pp 1139–1411

123. King JC: Assessment of zinc status. J Nutr 1990; 11:1474–1479

124. Wood RJ: Assessment of marginal zinc status in humans. J Nutr 2000; 130:1350S–1354S

125. Aggett PJ: The assessment of Zinc Status: a personal view. Proc Nutr Soc 1991; 50:9–17

126. Naber TH, van den Hamer CJ, Baadenhuysen H, et al: The value of methods to determine zinc deficiency in patients with Crohn's disease. Scand J Gastroenterol 1998; 33:514–523

127. Nelder KH: Acrodermatitis enteropathica and other zinc-deficiency disorders. In: Freedberg IM, Eisen AZ, Wolff K, Austen KF, Goldsmith LA, Katz SI, Fitzpatrick TB (eds) Fitzpatrick's Dermatology in General Medicine, 5th edn. New York: McGraw-Hill. 1999; pp 1738–1744

128. Prasad AS: Zinc deficiency in women, infants and children. J Am Coll Nutr 1996; 15:113–120

129. Krasovec M, Frenk E: Acrodermatitis enteropathica secondary to Crohn's disease. Dermatology 1996; 193:361–363

130. Prasad AS: Clinical manifestations of zinc deficiency. Annu Rev Nutr 1985; 5:341–363

131. Boldt DH: New perspectives on iron: an introduction. Am J Med Sci 1999; 318:207–212

132. Kuvibidila SR, Porretta C, Baliga BS: Iron deficiency alters the progression of mitogen treated murine splenic lymphocytes through the cell cycle. J Nutr 2001; 131:2028–2033

133. Brock JH, Mulero V: Cellular and molecular aspects of iron and immune function. Proc Nutr Soc 2000; 59:537–540

134. Iocono JA, Ehrlich HP, Gottrup F, et al: The biology of healing. In: Leaper DJ, Harding KG (eds) Wounds: Biology and Management. Oxford: Oxford University Press. 1998; pp 10–22

135. Hillman RS: Iron deficiency and other hypoproliferative anemias. In: Fauci AS, Braunwald E, Isselbacher KJ, Wilson JD, Martin JB, Kasper DL, Hauser SL, Longo DL (eds) Harrison's Principles of Internal Medicine, 14th edn. New York: McGraw-Hill 1999; pp 638–645

136. Black MM, Gawkrodger DJ, Seymour CA, Weismann K: Metabolic and nutritional disorders. In: Champion RH, Burton JL, Burns DA, Beathnach SM (eds) Rook/Wilkinson/Ebling Textbook of Dermatology, 6th edn. Oxford: Blackwell Scientific Publications 1998; pp 2577–2677

137. Fairfield KM, Fletcher RH: Vitamins for chronic disease prevention in adults. Scientific review. JAMA 2002; 287:3116–3126

138. Fletcher RH, Fairfield KM: Vitamins for chronic diseases prevention in adults. Clinical applications. JAMA 2002; 287:3127–3129

139. Chandra RK: Effect of vitamin and trace-element supplementation on immune responses and infection in elderly subjects. Lancet 1992; 340:1124–1127

140. Girodon F, Galan P, Monget AL, et al: Impact of trace elements and vitamin supplementation on immunity and infections in institutionalized elderly patients: a randomized controlled trial. Arch Intern Med 1999; 159:748–754

141. Chandra RK: Vitamin supplementation in elderly persons. JAMA 2003; 289:173–174

Therapeutic Approach to Cutaneous Ulcers According to Appearance

20

Contents

20.1 Overview

The currently accepted classification of cutaneous ulcers, based on their clinical appearance, refers to 'yellow', 'black', and 'red' ulcers. To the best of our knowledge, that general scheme was originally presented as a clinical aid by Hellgren and Vincent [1]. Later, this concept was adopted by pharmaceutical companies. Since then, the three-color classification has become the accepted method in the evaluation of chronic cutaneous ulcers and acute traumatic wounds [2–7]. A similar classifiation, based on the ulcer color and its morphological characteristics, has been recently introduced by Thomas [8].

As described in Chap. 1, the treatment of a cutaneous ulcer is governed by three considerations: (a) etiology, (b) clinical appearance, and (c) adjuvant therapy. The present chapter focuses on the appearance of ulcers. We present below flow charts (see Figs. 20.6, 20.8, 20.11) suggesting the therapeutic approach to cutaneous ulcers depending on their appearance.

> The three 'classical' clinical types of wounds or cutaneous ulcers, according to color, are:
> - Clean 'red' wounds
> - Secreting 'yellow' wounds
> - Dry 'black' wounds
>
> We shall expand here on the above classification and describe an additional type of ulcer, referred to as a 'sloughy' ulcer.

This chapter discusses the therapeutic options of chronic ulcers. Most of the following is applicable also to acute wounds. However, in acute wounds, there is a larger array of surgical options (e.g. skin flaps), not discussed in this book.

The approach introduced in this chapter, regarding the drying out of secretions or the moisturizing/softening of dry crusts is based on the very fundamentals of dermatologic therapy. However, the decision as to which type of product to use is not always clear cut and is subject to the clinical experience of the physician. We present our suggestions below.

Note that the main goal in the management of yellow, black, or sloughy ulcers is to 'convert' them into ulcers that are clean and red.

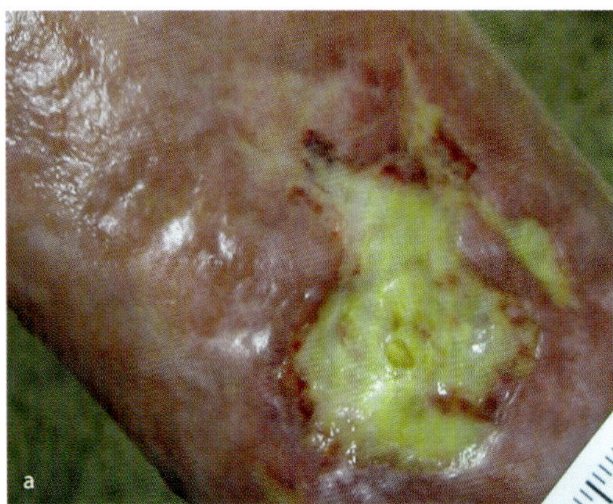

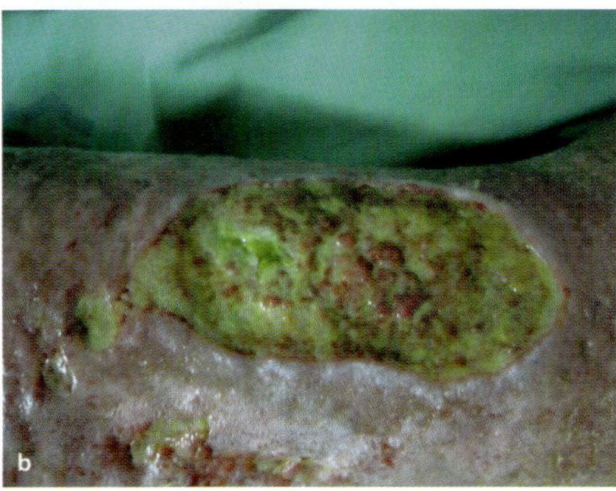

Fig 20.1 a, b. 'Yellow' ulcers

20.2 Secreting 'Yellow' Ulcers

It is the presence of a purulent or seropurulent discharge that imparts a characteristic yellowish appearance to these ulcers (Fig. 20.1 a, b). The secretions may vary from thin and relatively clear to heavy and thick.

When secretions are seen on the ulcer bed, they can be removed by irrigation with saline, which should be done as gently as possible. However, the purpose is not only to treat obvious secretions, but also to prevent their ongoing formation within the ulcer bed. We shall distinguish between an ulcer with profuse and/or purulent secretion and an ulcer with mild secretion (Fig. 20.2).

20.2.1 Ulcers with Profuse and/or Purulent Secretion

The primary objective here is to dry the ulcer. Traditionally, the simplest way of doing this is by repeated wetting. This can be done by gentle saline irrigation, several times a day. Alternatively, a wet dressings may be equally effective. This is done by applying a damp sterile cloth soaked in saline or Ringer's lactate solution, a few times a day, each time for 10–20 min (see Fig. 20.3).

In these cases, the added water cannot bind to the skin and it evaporates. In so doing, it 'pulls' water from the outer layers of the ulcer bed. We are not aware at present of any scientifically based research to explain this phenomenon, but as much as it seems paradoxical, repeated wetting or frequent washing does have a drying effect. Apart from its drying effect, frequent saline washing mechanically removes bacteria from the ulcer's surface.

The effectiveness of this technique depends on its being carried out correctly. For example, if the damp cloth/gauze is covered by a plastic wrap, evaporation will not be possible and the ulcer will not dry. Similarly, if, instead of using one layer of gauze or a thin cloth, one applies several layers of gauze which are repeatedly wet with a large amount of saline, a drying effect will not be achieved. On the contrary, excessive wetting may result in maceration and significant damage to the tissue.

Antiseptic solutions, such as potassium permanganate or chlorine-based solutions, may be used instead of saline to achieve some degree of antibacterial effect. Antibiotic solutions may also be considered, taking into account the controversy that surrounds this issue (see Chap. 10).

20.2.2 Ulcers with Mild to Moderate Secretion

Possible treatment for a mildly secreting ulcer is a hydrophilic dressing to absorb secretions. Preparations containing dextranomer granules, charcoal dressings, or alginate dressings may be used.

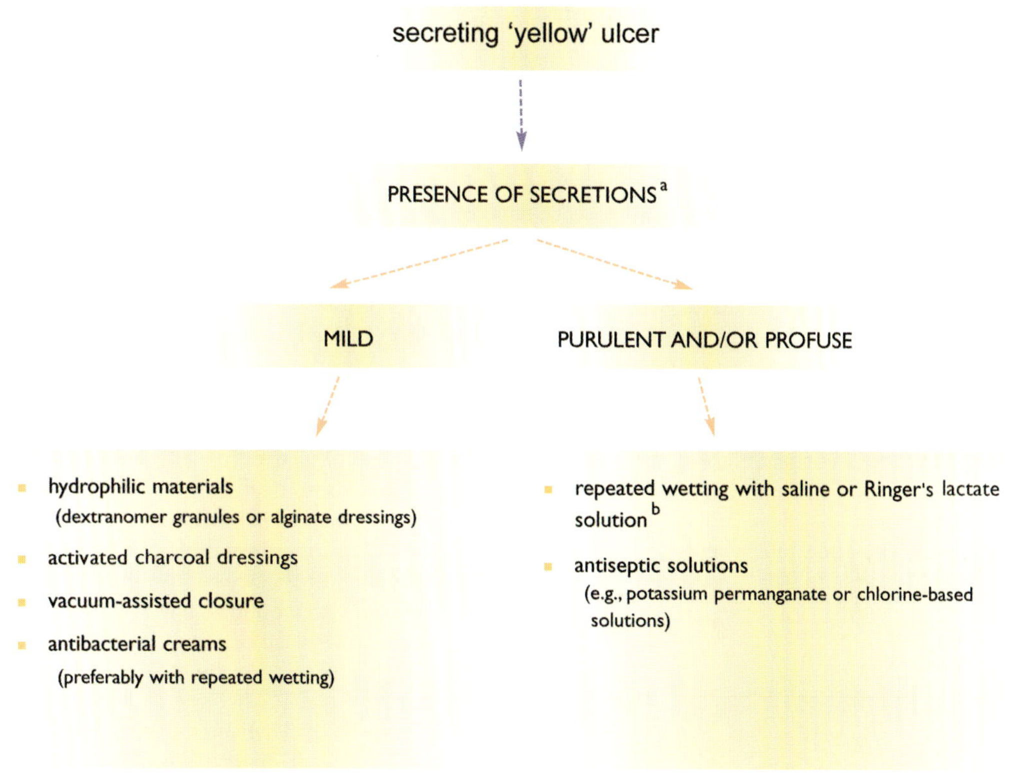

secreting 'yellow' ulcer

↓

PRESENCE OF SECRETIONS[a]

MILD

PURULENT AND/OR PROFUSE

MILD:
- hydrophilic materials
  (dextranomer granules or alginate dressings)
- activated charcoal dressings
- vacuum-assisted closure
- antibacterial creams
  (preferably with repeated wetting)

PURULENT AND/OR PROFUSE:
- repeated wetting with saline or Ringer's lactate solution[b]
- antiseptic solutions
  (e.g., potassium permanganate or chlorine-based solutions)

[a] When dealing with secreting ulcers, occlusive dressings should not be used.

[b] Wetting may be combined with the use of absorptive/hydrophilic dressings, depending on the patients' needs and their daily activities. However, absorptive dressings should not be used for covering such an ulcer for prolonged periods of time.

Fig. 20.2. Therapeutic approach to a secreting ulcer

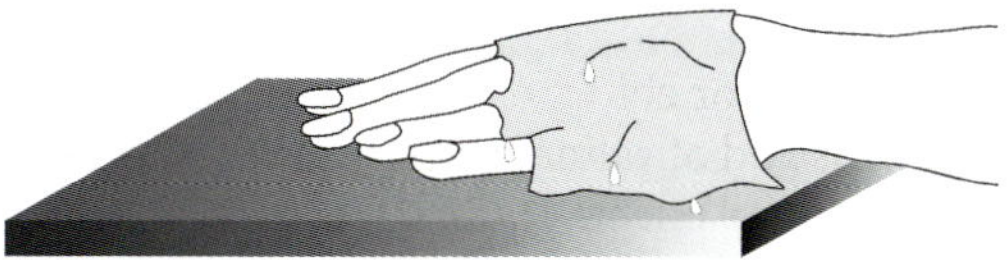

Fig. 20.3. Wetting a secreting lesion with a damp cotton cloth

Another reasonable form of treatment is to use a dressing that exerts topical negative pressure (vacuum-assisted closure®). This assists in absorbing fluid and debris from the ulcer bed with subsequent reduction of wound edema. In addition, it may draw the ulcer's edges towards its center, thereby enhancing wound contraction. (Note: All the methods described above are discussed in Chap. 8. The issue of negative topical pressure in presented in the Addendum to this chapter.)

It is reasonable to assume that, in many cases, the presence of secretions may represent a mild degree of bacterial infection that interferes with the processes of wound healing, even though there may be no clear signs of clinical infection (i.e., cellulitis or erysipelas). Therefore, if the amount of secretion is not very excessive, one may consider applying an antibacterial cream such as silver-sulfadiazine onto the ulcer. It may have some drying effect and can be combined with wetting at every dressing removal. In any case, an ointment should never be applied to a secreting wound.

20.2.3 Additional Comments

When treating secreting ulcers, the physician has to ascertain that there is no wound infection, i.e., cellulitis or erysipelas, that requires systemic antibiotics. It is also generally accepted that the presence of thick purulent secretions on an ulcer bed should be regarded as evidence of infection [9–13]. In such cases, occlusive dressings should be avoided.

A large amount of relatively thin and clear secretion from an ulcer is not necessarily the result of infection, but may represent edematous extracapillary fluid, which is released through the ulcer. Further investigation will determine the cause of the edema and its appropriate treatment.

Whenever a 'yellow' ulcer becomes clean and red, treatment should be re-evaluated.

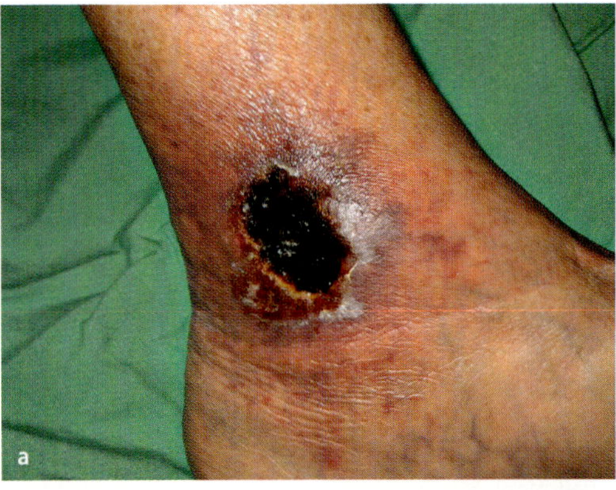

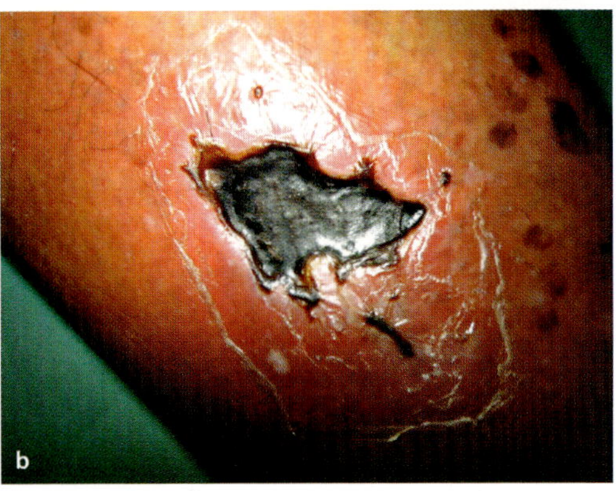

Fig. 20.4 a, b. Black ulcers

20.3 Dry 'Black' Ulcers

A dry ulcer is covered by black necrotic material, i.e., eschar composed mainly of devitalized tissues or an 'eschar-like' crust (Fig. 20.4 a, b). The accepted approach 40–50 years ago, was to allow wounds to dry out, enabling them to form a crust, as part of what was considered then to be a healthy process of wound healing. Winter et al. [14], followed by Hinman and Maibach [15], demonstrated the importance of moist healing on wounds and cutaneous ulcers.

It is now understood that creating a moist environment enables the black crust to gradually separate from the ulcer bed, thereby creating better conditions for healing. A suitable degree of moisture within an ulcer's environment creates a desirable biologic medium that provides optimal conditions for the processes of healing. It enables a more efficient metabolic activity, cellular interaction, and growth-factor activities that cannot occur within a dry environment.

■ **Ointments and Hydrogel Preparations.** In most cases, application of an ointment may be beneficial. The occlusive fatty layer above the ulcer prevents water evaporation; thus, the tissues become saturated with water. When the tissues become well hydrated, the black crust may gradually separate from the ulcer bed. Some use antibiotic ointments in cases requiring an additional antibacterial effect. Hydrogel preparations may also be considered in view of their water-donating properties.

■ **Soaking/Hydration.** Soaking the affected limb (and ulcer) in a bath of water may soften the crust. However, for patients with leg ulcers, especially those with diabetes, this procedure is not desirable, since it may result in maceration and damage to healthy skin.

In order to limit water exposure to the ulcer area, hydration can be carried out as demonstrated in Fig. 20.5: Apply several layers of gauze or cloth (not one layer only, as in the case of a secreting ulcer) saturated with water, Ringer's lactate or saline solution, in the form of a compress. Wetting should be done several times per day, each time for 15–20 min. In this way, evaporation is not possible and the crust becomes hy-

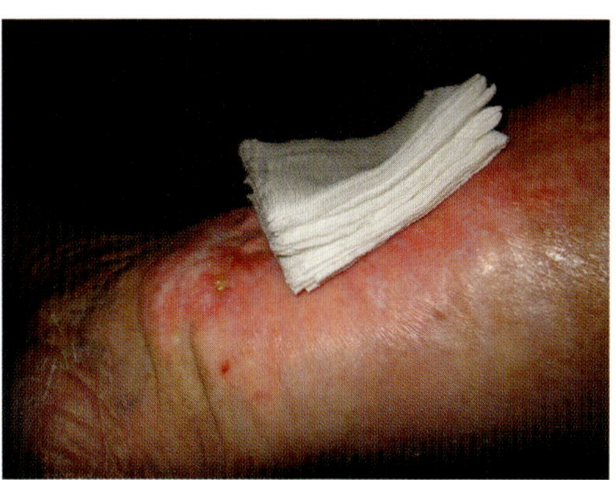

Fig. 20.5. Hydration, using several layers of gauze saturated with water

drated and soft. This can be combined with the use of ointments on the ulcer bed.

■ **Surgical Debridement.** In more severe cases, surgical debridement is the treatment of choice. Hydration with saturated gauzes, as described above, or application of fatty ointment prior to the surgical procedure may help soften the dry material and ease its removal. See Fig. 20.6 for a therapeutic approach to a dry black ulcer.

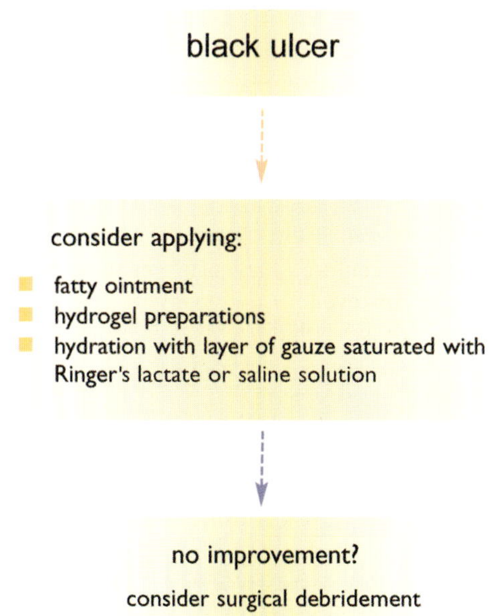

Fig. 20.6. Therapeutic approach to a black, dry ulcer

20.4 'Sloughy' Ulcers

In addition to the three classical types of ulcers, as previously mentioned, we feel that an additional type should be included to complete the classification. The term 'sloughy ulcer' has already been described by others [8]. We refer to these as 'sloughy' ulcers, whose surface is covered with material, which may be yellow, green or gray/white in appearance. It is usually soft in consistency, ranging from a liquefied mass to semi-solid or relatively solid material; it is composed of necrotic proteins, devitalized collagen and fibrin (Fig. 20.7 a, b). It is essential to remove or dissolve the necrotic layer to enable appropriate healing of the ulcer.

When there is clearly defined devitalized material, which can be cut away and removed

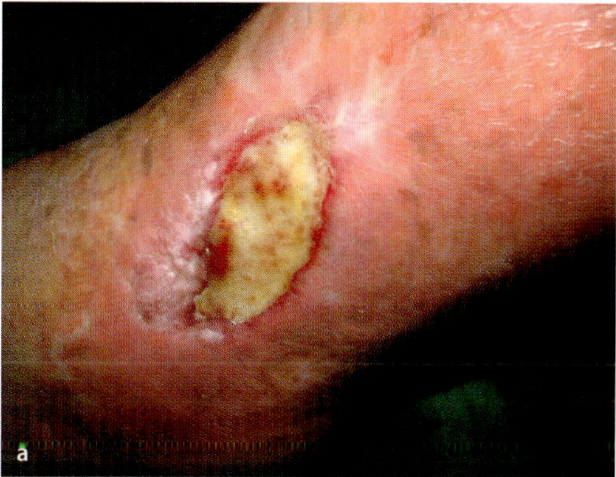

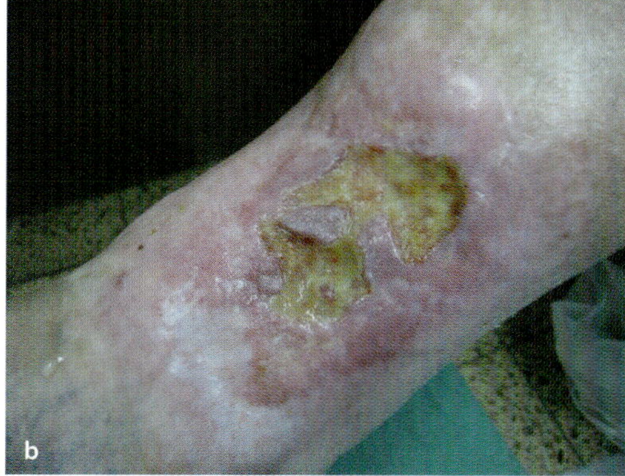

Fig. 20.7 a, b. Sloughy ulcers (Note: Sometimes it is difficult to differentiate between a picture of a sloughy ulcer and a picture of a yellow ulcer, as opposed to seeing them in real life)

without damaging healthy and vital tissue, surgical debridement may be carried out. When nearing vital tissue, the procedure should be discontinued and further debridement may be accomplished by using an alternative method.

However, in many cases, there is no clear border between the sloughy and healthy tissue. Surgical debridement, in that situation, may result in the unnecessary loss of healthy tissue.

Note that in cases where the amount of slough is minimal and the ulcer seems to appear relatively clean, one may consider shaving surgical debridement (which is immediately followed by the application of growth factors or composite grafting). This method is detailed below in the section on a clean red ulcer.

When surgical debridement cannot be used, other methods should be employed to dissolve the necrotic material. The therapeutic options presented below (and in Fig. 20.8) should be considered in accordance with the ulcer type, etiology, the patient's general health, and the availability of each method.

■ **Soaking/Hydration.** Soaking the ulcer in water (or hydration, as described above) may soften the necrotic material and ease its removal. A modification of this method is the use of a product which combines multi-layered polyacrylate dressing with Ringer's lactate solution (Tenderwet®, see Chap. 8). The Ringer's lactate solution creates a moist environment, and may

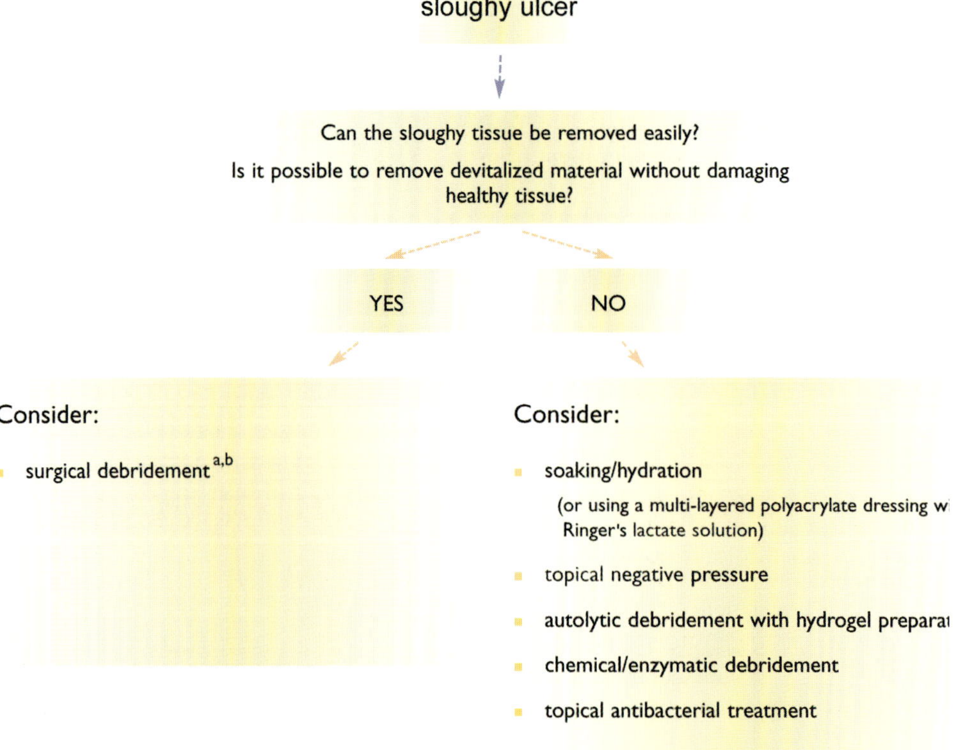

Fig. 20.8. Therapeutic approach to a sloughy ulcer

soften and loosen the slough, resulting in its detachment from the ulcer bed.

■ **Topical Negative Pressure.** Another reasonable method of treatment is to use a dressing applying topical negative pressure (vacuum-assisted closure®). This method helps to absorb necrotic material, secretions, and debris from the ulcer bed.

■ **Chemical or Autolytic Debridement.** Chemical or autolytic debridement may also be used (see Chap. 9).

■ **Antibacterial Preparations.** In most cases, this wound type is associated with bacterial colonization. Therefore, antibacterial preparations may be used, according to the general guidelines detailed in Chap. 10.

20.5 Clean 'Red' Ulcers

A clean red ulcer is the so-called 'ideal' ulcer a physician would like to achieve, with the best chances for complete healing. When dealing with the three other types of ulcers described above, the purpose is to convert them to this clean red form. The desired hue lies somewhere in the spectrum between dark-red and purple (Fig. 20.9 a, b). Red ulcers may manifest a scale of hydration states – from relatively dry red to moist red.

The surface area of a 'red' ulcer, i.e., the ulcer bed, is covered by granulation tissue, which is composed mainly of numerous blood vessels, leukocytes (mainly macrophages), and fibroblasts. It serves as a substrate on which the healing proceeds, until the whole ulcer bed is covered by epithelial cells. The various cells of the granulation tissue secrete growth factors that regulate and enhance the healing processes.

The term 'granulation' is derived from the general appearance of the tissue. On close inspection, the tissue seems to contain numerous tiny granules, which are actually young blood vessels.

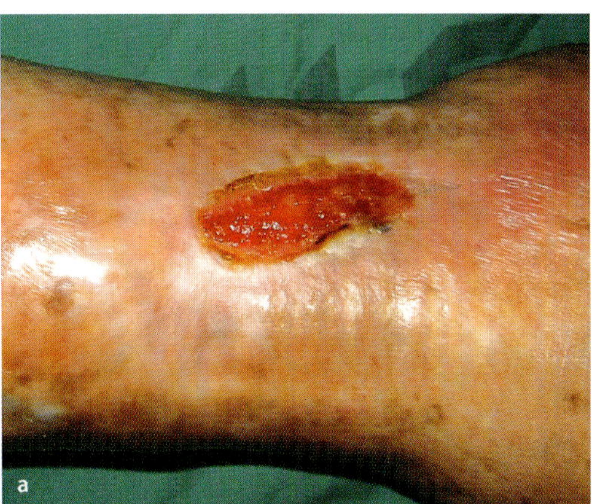

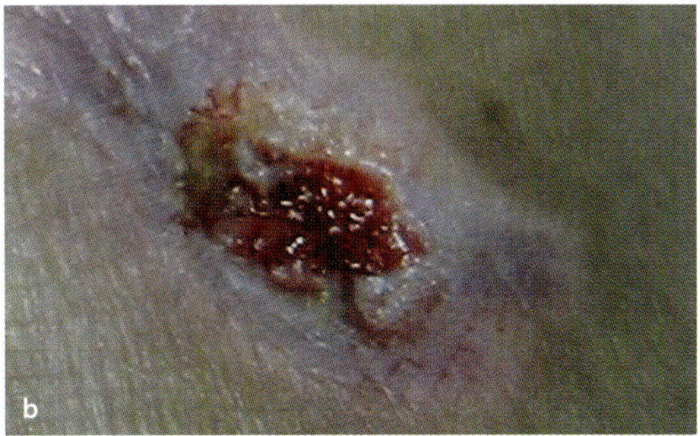

Fig. 20.9 a, b. Clean red ulcers

Normal granulation tissue is dark red to purple. This is in contrast to ischemic ulcers, which occur in elderly patients suffering from peripheral vascular disease, where the granulation tissue tends to be relatively bright red or even pink.

Note that certain infected ulcers may manifest an exuberant deep reddish-brown granulation tissue, which tends to bleed easily [9, 16]. This is not the desired red-to-purple color of clean red wounds.

The decision on how to treat a clean red wound should be determined by the speed (if at all) at which the ulcer heals. It is important to distinguish between an ulcer that gradually improves and advances towards healing and a 'stagnant' ulcer, which does not.

20.5.1 Ulcers Advancing Towards Healing

When positive parameters such as re-epithelialization and progressive wound contraction are observed, it may suffice to merely supply an ideal moist environment. The significance of the moist environment in the ulcer area for normal healing is detailed in Chap. 8

There are several methods for providing a moist environment:

■ **Saline or Ringer's Lactate Solution.** An ulcer can be kept moist by applying a moistened woven gauze to the surface. The following simple traditional method was presented by Pham et al. [17]: A layer of saline-moistened gauze is placed over the wound bed, followed by a layer of dry gauze. A layer of petrolatum gauze (or a plastic wrap) is then placed over that and the area is wrapped with a layer of conforming gauze bandage. The secondary dressing should be changed twice a day.

Since, under these circumstances, the ulcer is occluded, it is important to keep a close watch on the area to identify and prevent maceration or infection. Moreover, when using saline solution on an ulcer bed, a layer of a protective preparation (such as zinc paste) should be applied to the healthy skin around the ulcer to prevent maceration of intact surrounding skin.

A similar therapeutic approach uses a very slow, continuous drip of saline solution which provides a moist environment and also removes bacteria from the ulcer's surface [18]. The rate of the drip should be adjusted to the level of hydration of the ulcer – the dryer the ulcer the faster the drip rate should be. Frequent monitoring is mandatory. The continuous drip is a relatively old method. Similar techniques were developed at the beginning of the twentieth century, as shown in Fig. 20.10.

■ **Hydrocolloid or Hydrogel Dressings.** The more widely accepted approach to achieving a relatively moist environment is to use occlusives such as hydrocolloid dressings. Certain hydrogel dressings may also be used for this purpose, due to their water-donating properties (see Chap. 8).

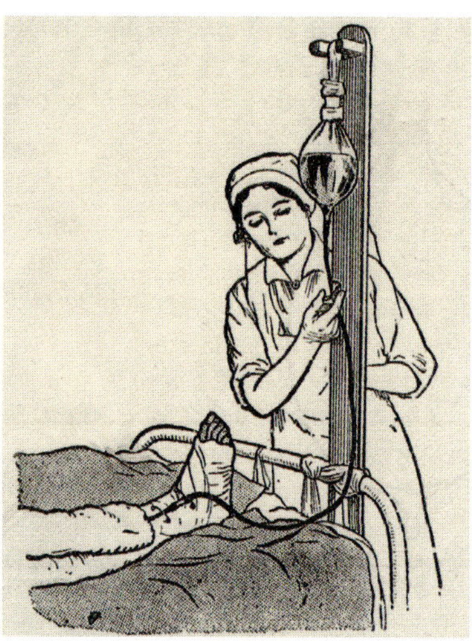

Fig. 20.10. A device for instilling antiseptic liquid under the dressing. The preparation used in this case is Dakin's solution. (From *The Treatment of Infected Wounds*, by Carrel & Dehelly, published by The Macmillan Company of Canada, 1917)

20.5.2 'Stagnant' Ulcers

When dealing with ulcers that do not show any sign of improvement, a more active approach is needed. Significant enhancement of healing may be achieved by the application of preparations containing growth factors. Alternatively, other advanced treatment modalities may be used, such as keratinocyte grafts, autologous skin grafts, or composite grafts.

Note: Advanced therapeutic modalities such as growth factors or composite grafting are intended for clean red ulcers. There is no justification for using them on a secreting ulcer or on an infected ulcer. Nevertheless, there is documented evidence that such treatments may have some antibacterial effect, or that they may enhance the patient's immune function [19–21]. Therefore, one may consider using these treatment modalities even for ulcers that are not 'perfectly clean', preferably combined with one of the treatments for 'yellow' or 'sloughy' ulcers, as discussed above. Figure 20.11 summarizes the therapeutic approach to a clean red ulcer.

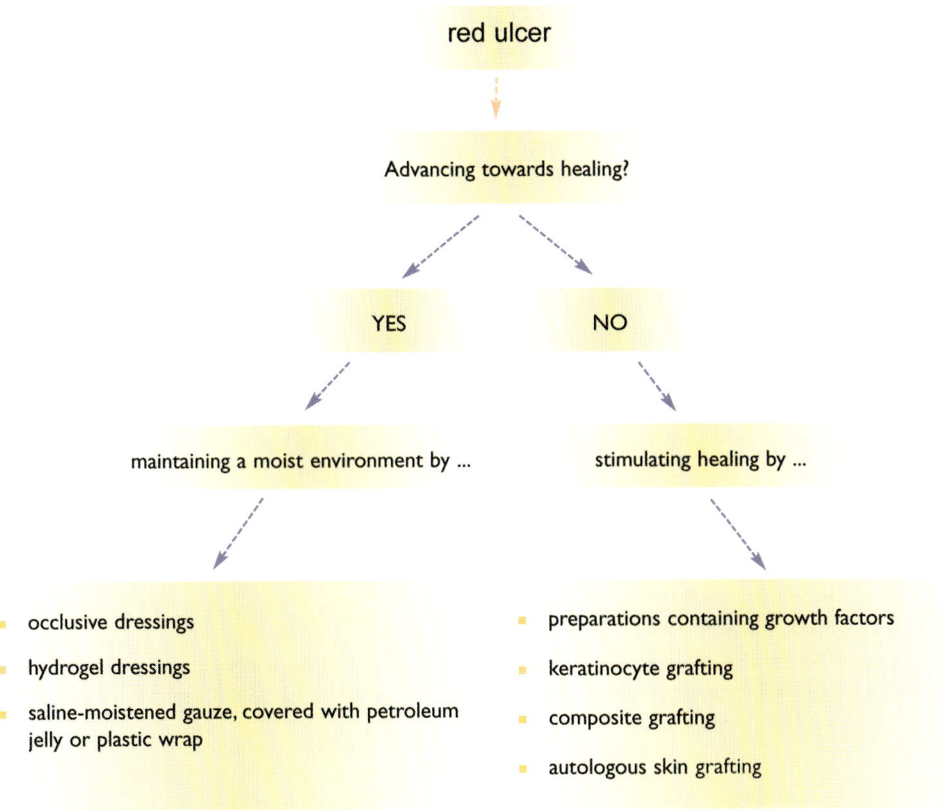

Fig. 20.11. Therapeutic approach to a red clean ulcer

20.6 'Unresponsive' Ulcers

We do not always have a clear and scientific explanation as to why, in some cases, certain modes of therapy do not improve healing, whereas in other cases they do. For the time being, there are several 'black holes' in the understanding of wound healing.

Certain sloughy ulcers benefit from autolytic debridement, while others benefit from enzymatic debridement. Certain clean wounds improve only when treated with saline-moistened gauze and do not heal when treated with hydrocolloid dressings. In many cases, there is an element of trial and error in the treatment of cutaneous ulcers. When a certain regimen aggravates the ulcer, treatment should be changed. If an ulcer does not improve within 10–14 days with one mode of therapy, another approach should be considered. However, the treatment should not be changed too often; a reasonable amount of time is required to let a certain treatment take effect.

For an unresponsive ulcer, consider one of the following options:
- Hospitalizing patients whose self-treatment seems to be inadequate. In many cases, cutaneous ulcers do not respond to accepted treatment because it is carried out inappropriately [22]. In cases where a patient is not capable of treating the ulcer as required, the ulcer may deepen and worsen.

— Hyperbaric oxygen therapy, when appropriate.
— An alternative/additional topical therapy (see Chaps. 17 and 18).

As stated above, for a stagnant red ulcer, one should consider the use of growth factors or composite grafting.

In any case the workup to determine the ulcer's etiology should be revised. Complications such as osteomyelitis should be ruled out (see Table 7.3).

20.7 'Mixed' Ulcers

Often, cutaneous ulcers are not uniform in color. Some ulcers may present slough together with black crusting on the surface. In others, one may discern clean red areas as well as yellow secreting or sloughy areas.

In these cases, the guiding principles are as follows:
— Avoid any damage to healthy granulation tissue; e.g., clean red areas of the ulcer bed should not be exposed to enzymatic preparations.
— Secreting or sloughy areas should be treated first, since these areas are more prone to the development of infection.

20.8 Additional Comments

— Healing of a cutaneous ulcer is a dynamic process, subject to changes. Treatment should be adjusted according to the ulcer's current clinical appearance. When a yellow secreting wound becomes clean and

red, the therapeutic approach should be modified accordingly.
— Consider combining some of the treatment modalities as presented above. For example, repeated wetting together with application of an antibacterial cream, or with special dressings.
— Several researchers have suggested that Ringer's lactate solution may be preferable to saline for rinsing and/or wetting wounds and cutaneous ulcers. It is considered to be more 'friendly' to the ulcer tissue in respect to pH and electrolyte content (e.g. calcium). Currently, there are insufficient data to confirm this approach.

20.9 Treating Hypergranulation Tissue

Hypergranulation tissue above a wound or ulcer's surface may impair normal healing (Fig. 20.12 a). This is superfluous tissue that impedes epithelialization and wound closure. Thus, the excess tissue should be removed. This may be done surgically (preferably followed by advanced therapeutic modalities such as growth factors, or keratinocyte grafting, or skin grafting).

Alternative methods are as follows [23–25]:
— Applying a preparation containing a low-potency corticosteroid for a short period, once or twice daily, which may decrease the amount of excessive granulation tissue (Fig. 20.12 b).
— Some suggest using semipermeable instead of impermeable dressings, since low oxygen tension may enhance the formation of granulation tissue. As described in Chap. 8, this may be so when dealing with acute wounds, but not necessarily for chronic ulcers.

- A polyurethane foam dressing has been shown to have a beneficial effect.

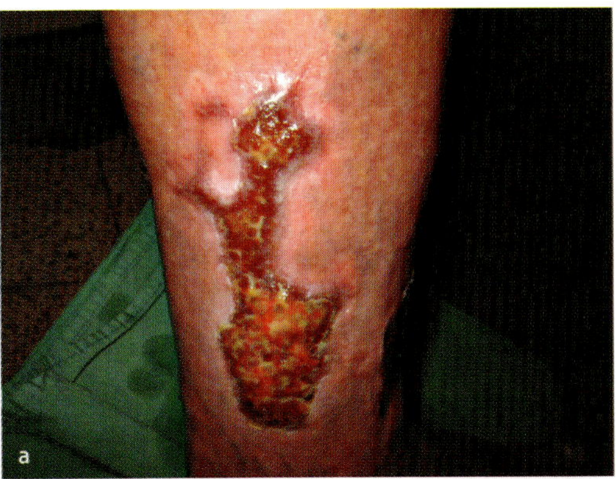

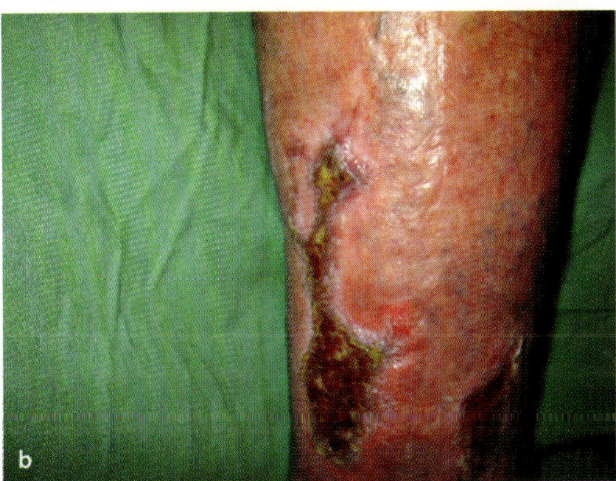

Fig. 20.12. a. Excessive granulation tissue. b. The same ulcer following two weeks' daily application of a preparation containing low-potency corticosteroids

20.10 Addendum: Dressings that Apply Topical Negative Pressure

Topical negative pressure (TNP) (vacuum-assisted closure®) is currently being used on acute traumatic wounds as well as on chronic cutaneous ulcers and has already been studied by many investigators [26–31].

At present, not all mechanisms by which TNP exerts its beneficial effects have been identified. The main mechanisms suggested are as follows [32, 33]:

- Absorption of fluid and debris from the ulcer bed, with subsequent reduction of wound edema
- Increasing blood flow and dermal perfusion, with enhancement of granulation tissue formation
- Mechanical effect, intended to draw the ulcer's edges towards its center, thereby accelerating wound contraction
- Reducing the amount of stagnant fluid and bacterial load

The TNP dressing is a porous foam material. Tubes are embedded in the dressing, while their proximal part is connected to an adjustable vacuum pump (Fig. 20.13). The dressing should be trimmed to conform to the shape of the ulcer into which it is inserted. While activated, the vacuum device creates a continuous and controlled negative pressure.

In our experience, the TNP dressing has shown a relatively high level of efficacy in 'cleaning' the chronic ulcer bed, leading to the development of healthy granulation tissue. This is especially evident in venous ulcers and ulcers related to lymphedema. However, TNP has also been documented as accelerating healing of ulcers of various other etiologies. In any case, more research studies are required to examine the most appropriate guidelines for TNP use.

During TNP therapy patients are immobilized and continuously attached to the TNP device. Therefore, during the treatment period, patients (especially elderly patients for whom immobilization carries a risk of deep venous thrombosis or pneumonia) should be encouraged to detach themselves from the device a few times each day, to walk and activate their legs.

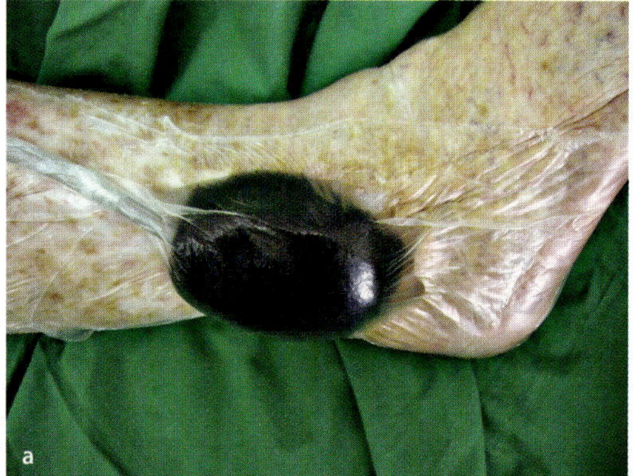

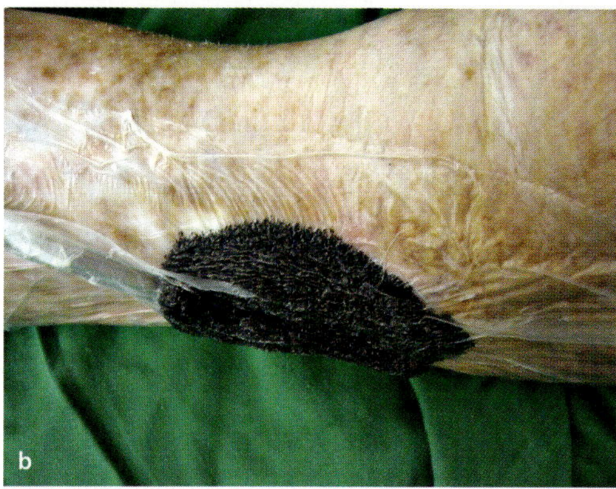

Fig. 20.13 a, b. A dressing applying negative pressure. Tubes connect the vacuum device to the porous dressing covering the ulcer. **a.** Before applying negative pressure. **b.** Flattening of the dressing following the application of negative pressure

References

1. Hellgren L, Vincent J: A classification of dressings and preparations for the treatment of wounds by second intention based on stages in the healing process. Care Sci Pract 1986; 4:13–17
2. Stotts NA: Seeing red and yellow and black. The three-color concept of wound care. Nursing 1990; 20:59–61
3. Hellgren L, Vincent J: Debridement: an essential step in wound healing. In: Westerhof W (ed) Leg Ulcers: Diagnosis and Treatment. Amsterdam: Elsevier. 1993; pp 305–312
4. Eriksson G: Local treatment of venous leg ulcers. Acta Chir Scand 1988; [Suppl] 544:47–52
5. Goldman RJ, Salcido R: More than one way to measure a wound: An overview of tools and techniques. Adv Skin Wound Care 2002; 15:236–245
6. Findlay D: Modern dressings: What to use. Aust Fam Physician 1994; 23: 824–839
7. Romanelli M, Gaggio G, Piaggesi A, et al: Technological advances in wound bed measurements. Wounds 2002; 14:58–66
8. Thomas S: Wound dressings. In: Rovee DT, Maibach HI (eds) The Epidermis in Wound Healing. Boca Raton: CRC Press. 2004; pp 215–241
9. Browne A, Dow G, Sibbald RG. Infected wounds; definitions and controversies. In: Falanga V (ed) Cutaneous Wound Healing, 1st edn. London: Martin Dunitz. 2001; pp 203–219
10. Parish LC, Witkowski JA: The infected decubitus ulcer. Int J Dermatol 1989; 28:643–647
11. Niedner R, Schopf E. Wound infections and antibacterial therapy. In: Westerhof W (ed) Leg Ulcers: Diagnosis and Treatment. Amsterdam: Elsevier. 1993; pp 293–303
12. Lipsky BA, Berendt AR: Principles and practice of antibiotic therapy of diabetic foot infections. Diabetes Metab Res Rev 2000; 16 [Suppl 1]:S42–S46
13. Robson MC: Wound Infection: a failure of wound healing caused by an imbalance of bacteria. Surg Clin North Am 1997; 77:637–650
14. Winter GD: Formation of the scab and the rate of epithelization of superficial wounds in the skin of the young domestic pig. Nature 1962; 193:293–294
15. Hinman CD, Maibach H: Effect of air exposure and occlusion on experimental human skin wounds. Nature 1963; 200:377–378
16. Cutting KF, Harding KG: Criteria to identify wound infection. J Wound Care 1994; 3:198-201
17. Pham HT, Rosenblum BI, Lyons TE, et al: Evaluation of a human skin equivalent for the treatment of diabetic foot ulcers in a prospective, randomized, clinical trial. Wounds 1999; 11:79–86
18. Marquez RR: Wound debridement and hydrotherapy. In: Gogia PP (ed) Clinical Wound Management, 1st edn. New Jersey: Slack Incorporated. 1995; pp 115–130
19. Schmid P: Apligraf – phenotypic characteristics and their potential implications for the treatment of diabetic foot ulcers. A satellite symposium at the 36th annual meeting of the European association for the study of diabetes (EASD). Jerusalem, Israel. September 2000
20. Gough A, Clapperton M, Rolando N, et al: Randomized placebo-controlled trial of granulocyte- colony stimulating factor in diabetic foot infection. Lancet 1997; 350:855–859
21. De Lalla F, Pellizzer G, Strazzabosco M, et al: Randomized prospective controlled trial of recombinant granulocyte colony- stimulating factor as adjunctive therapy for limb- threatening diabetic foot infection. Antimicrob Agents Chemother 2001; 45: 1094–1098
22. Haram RB, Dagfinn N: Errors and discrepancies: a patient perspective on leg ulcer treatment at home. J Wound Care 2003; 12:195–199
23. Feedar JA: Clinical management of chronic wounds. In: McCulloch JM, Kloth LC, Feedar JA (eds) Wound Healing – Alternatives in Management, 2nd edn. Philadelphia: FA Davis. 1995; pp 137–185

24. Harris A, Rolstad BS: Hypergranulation tissue: a nontraumatic method of management. Ostomy Wound Manage 1994; 40:20–22,24,26–30

25. Thomas S, Leigh IM: Wound dressing. In: Leaper DJ, Harding KG (eds) Wounds: Biology and Management. Oxford: Oxford University Press. 1998; pp 166–183

26. Evans D, Land L: Topical negative pressure for treating chronic wounds: a systematic review. Br J Plast Surg 2001; 54:238–242

27. Argenta LC, Morykwas MJ: Vacuum-assisted closure: A new method for wound control and treatment: Clinical experience. Ann Plast Surg 1997; 38:563–576

28. Banwell PE, Teot L: Topical negative pressure (TNP): the evolution of a novel wound therapy. J Wound Care 2003; 12:22–28

29. McCallon SK, Knight CA, Valiulus JP, et al: Vacuum-assisted closure versus saline-moistened gauze in the healing of postoperative diabetic foot wounds. Ostomy Wound Manage 2000; 46:28–32,34

30. Joseph E, Hamori CA, Bergman S, et al: A prospective, randomized trial of vacuum-assisted closure versus standard therapy of chronic non-healing wounds. Wounds 2000; 12:60–67

31. Evans D, Land L: Topical negative pressure for treating chronic wounds (Cochrane Review). In: The Cochrane library, Issue 4, 2001. Oxford: Update software

32. Morykwas MJ, Argenta LC, Shelton-Brown EI, et al: Vacuum assisted closure: a new method control and treatment: animal studies and basic foundation. Ann Plast Surg 1997; 38:553–562

33. Mendez-Eastman S: Guidelines for using negative pressure wound therapy. Adv Skin Wound Care 2001; 14:314–322

Appendix: Guidelines for Patients and Medical Staff

Contents

21.1 General Patient Guidelines for the Treatment of Ulcers or Wounds at Home

- Take care to wash your hands with soap and water before and after the treatment.
- When the dressing is changed, any materials removed from the wound should be placed directly into a plastic bag set aside earlier for that purpose. Make sure that the infected dressings do not come into contact with the floor, the furniture, or any other object, so as to avoid as far as possible any spread of infectious bacteria to the surroundings.
- The skin around the wound may be cleaned using a very dilute, mild soap. Ensure that all the residual soap is thoroughly rinsed off, using a gentle stream of lukewarm water. Avoid using soap directly on the wound.
- After being rinsed with water, the wound should be dried by gentle patting/dabbing only. Never scrub or rub the wound.
- Any medical substance that needs to be placed on the wound bed should be applied using an object such as a spatula, or tongue depressor. Never apply the substance directly from its container, and never use bare fingers to apply it.
- To remove dressings that have become stuck to the wound because of dried secretions on the wound surface, moisten them with saline or tap water and leave them wet for a few minutes. They can usually then be removed relatively easily without causing any damage to the bed of the wound.
- Ensure that the dressing is not too tight or pressing too hard on the wound, since a tightly applied dressing may interfere with the blood flow.
- Use an elastic net dressing (e.g., flexible elastic net bandages; stockinette) to hold the dressing on the wound. Avoid the use of adhesive plaster directly on the skin.
- Smoking is strictly forbidden!!!

21.2 Patient Guidelines for the Management of Skin Ulcers Caused by Venous Insufficiency

- Avoid standing as much as possible.
- While seated, make sure your legs are elevated, if possible slightly above the level of your buttocks.
- When lying down, it is advisable to elevate the legs slightly on a cushion or folded blanket.
- It is advisable to walk every day for at least 30–60 min; do not stand still during this time.
- When seated or lying down, move your legs (twisting, cycling motion, etc.) several times a day for 10–15 min each time.
- If your doctor advises you to use support stockings, you should put them on in the morning, after your legs have been elevated for a few hours, so that your legs will not be swollen when you put the stockings on.
- Smoking is strictly forbidden!!!

21.3 General Guidelines for Patients with Diabetes or Peripheral Arterial Disease

The following guidelines should be implemented by patients with diabetes or peripheral arterial disease, in order to prevent formation of cutaneous ulcers.

- Wash your feet at least once a day with a mild soap under running water. Make sure you rinse off all traces of the soap, particularly between the toes.
- Use only lukewarm, not hot water.
- After washing, dry your feet thoroughly, including between the toes, since moisture in that area can lead to infections. Usually a normal towel is not adequate; use absorbent paper in addition.
- It is recommended you walk at least 30–60 min every day. It is also advisable to move your legs while lying down or sitting (twisting or cycling movements, etc.) several times a day, for 10–15 min each time. In the case of a neuropathic ulcer consult your doctor as to the appropriate mode of physical activity and pressure off-loading.
- Cutting toenails: Avoid cutting the corners; trim the toenails straight across. If necessary, get someone to help you, so you don't injure yourself. Do not 'dig' with a sharp instrument in the angle between the nail and the flesh.
- Examine your legs and feet once a day, using a mirror, or get someone to help if necessary.
- Treatment of wounds, corns, blisters should be carried out only under medical supervision. Should areas of dry skin, rashes, scaling, or changes in the skin color appear, seek medical advice.
- Cold and heat injury: Avoid exposure to cold; keep the feet warm in winter. However, do not sit too close to a heater or fire. Don't use a hot water bottle. Do not use an electric blanket without a thermostat. Before washing your feet, test the water temperature with your hand.
- Wear comfortable, well-fitting shoes. A poorly fitted shoe may cause corns, because of uneven pressure distribution on the foot when walking. Before putting your shoes on, shake them out to remove any small stones. Don't wear shoes without socks. Cotton socks

are preferable. Change your socks at least once a day. Avoid sandals or thongs, since they do not protect the foot from injury.

— Smoking is strictly forbidden!!!

21.4 Treatment of Edema

Once the cause of edema has been identified, treatment should be done accordingly (see Chap. 7).

In addition, the following steps should be considered:

— Elevation of the extremities: The patient should be given clear instructions to raise the affected extremity. In the case of leg ulcers the patient should be instructed to avoid prolonged standing as much as possible and to raise the leg while sitting or lying down.

— Physical activity: The patient should be advised to engage in physical activity and to exercise the leg muscles. Physical activity can reduce the degree of leg edema [1, 2].

— Physical therapy: The patient should be referred for a special form of therapy known as *manual lymph drainage*. This is a massage technique designed to reduce edema. It is effective for edema of the lower extremities and can aid in the healing of cutaneous ulcers associated with edema [2–9]. Kurtz et al. [8] found that this procedure may lead to the mobilization of up to 1 l of urine from reabsorption and transport of interstitial fluid. Gentle pressure is applied to lymph nodes and lymph vessels with the finger tips to evacuate lymphatic content. The rhythm of applied pressure is different from that of traditional massage

techniques [3, 4]. The basic principle is that central regions of lymph drainage, such as the lower abdomen and proximal thigh, should be emptied initially to provide space for the drainage of peripheral fluid. After the proximal region of a limb has been cleared of its lymph, distal areas are massaged to mobilize the fluid proximally. The scheduling of therapeutic sessions depends on the size of the ulcer, the amount of edema, and the patient's general condition. It is usual to conduct two to three sessions per week [4], but daily sessions should be considered under certain circumstances.

— Compression therapy is done using stockings or elastic bandages. Compression therapy has a proven value as a means of treating venous insufficiency and its ensuing leg ulcers [10–13].

— Administration of diuretics should be considered, depending on the clinical data.

References

1. Ciocon JO, Galindo Ciocon D, Galindo DJ: Raised leg exercises for leg edema in the elderly. Angiology 1995; 46:19–25
2. Casley-Smith JR, Casley-Smith JR: The nature of complex physical therapy. In: Casley-Smith JR, Casley-Smith JR (eds) Modern Treatment for Lymphoedema, 5th revised edn. Adelaide: The Lymphoedema Association of Australia. 1997; p 131
3. Casley-Smith JR, Casley-Smith JR: Massage techniques for lymphoedema. In: Casley-Smith JR, Casley-Smith JR (eds) Modern Treatment for Lymphoedema, 5th revised edn. Adelaide: The Lymphoedema Association of Australia. 1997; pp 134–152
4. Stahel HU: Manual Lymph Drainage. Curr Probl Dermatol 1999; 27:148–152
5. Hoffmann A, Petzoldt D: Manual lymph drainage. Hautarzt 1978; 29:463–466
6. Evrard-Bras M, Coupe M, Laroche JP, et al: Manual lymphatic drainage. Rev Prat 2000; 50:1199–1203
7. Derdeyn A, Aslam M, Pflug JJ: Manual lymph drainage – mode of action. Lymphology 1994; 27 [Suppl]: 527–529

8. Kurz W, Kurz R, Litmanovitch YI, et al: Effect of manual lymph drainage massage on blood components and urinary neurohormones in chronic lymphedema. Angiology 1981; 32:119–127

9. Francois A, Richaud C, Bouchet JY, et al: Does medical treatment of lymphedema act by increasing lymph flow? Vasa 1989; 18:281–286

10. Partsch H: Compression therapy for venous ulcers. Curr Probl Dermatol 1999; 27:130–140

11. Cullum N, Nelson EA, Fletcher AW, et al: Compression for venous leg ulcers (Cochrane Review). In: The Cochrane Library. Issue 1, 2003; Oxford: Update Software

12. Phillips TJ, Dover JS: Leg ulcers. J Am Acad Dermatol 1991; 25:965–987

13. Yasuhara H, Shigematsu H, Muto T: A study of the advantages of elastic stockings for leg lymphedema. Int Angiol 1996; 15:272–277

21.5 Guidelines for Nurses: Outpatient Management of Cutaneous Ulcers

- Warn the patient not to touch any object, furniture, or any other item in the clinic unnecessarily, to reduce the spread of bacteria to the surroundings.
- Both the patient and the nurse should wash their hands before and after the treatment. Show the patient how to wash his/her hands correctly. Hands should be washed under running water, for about 15–20 sec, with 3–5 ml of a cleaning agent [1]. Another accepted disinfecting method is to use an alcohol-based hand-rub solution (containing about 70% alcohol). Recently, the latter has been documented as the best method for reducing transmission of infection [2, 3].
- The patient should avoid placing his/her treated foot directly on the floor. The treated foot should be placed on a stool covered by plastic and a clean cloth or sheet [4] (Fig. 21.1).
- Should the ulcer need to be rinsed extensively with saline, ensure that there are sheets of plastic on the floor or bench.
- Place a plastic bag near the patient, in which you can readily dispose of all the dressing materials removed from the ulcer (Fig. 21.2). Ensure that used dressing materials removed from the ulcer do not come into contact with the floor, the furniture, or any other object in the clinic.
- Throughout the treatment procedures the nurse must wear gloves. It is advisable to change the gloves after removing the old dressing. Use a new pair of gloves when applying the fresh dressing to the wound.
- Enter information into the patient's record after completing the dressing procedure, removing the gloves, and washing your hands.
- Between one patient and the next, clean the treatment area with antiseptic solution.
- After treating an ulcer that is likely to be heavily infected (such as a cutaneous ulcer known to contain methicillin-resistant *Staphylococcus aureus* or resistant *Pseudomonas* strains) or a heavily secreting ulcer, clean the treatment room thoroughly with soap and sodium-hypochlorite solution. Free available chlorine at 500 ppm is documented as being the most effective compound against most nosocomial pathogens [5].

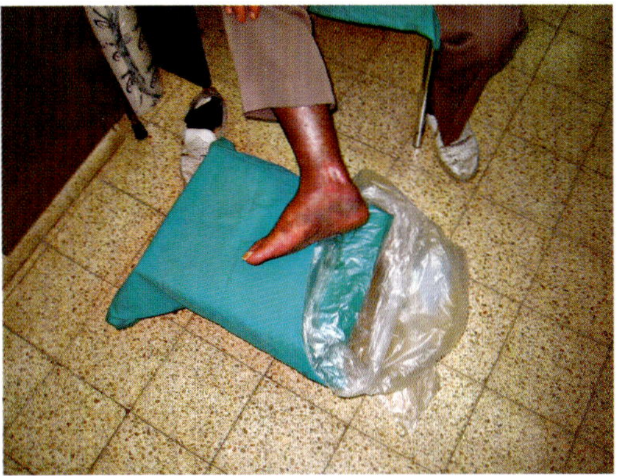

Fig. 21.1. The patient's leg is placed on a stool

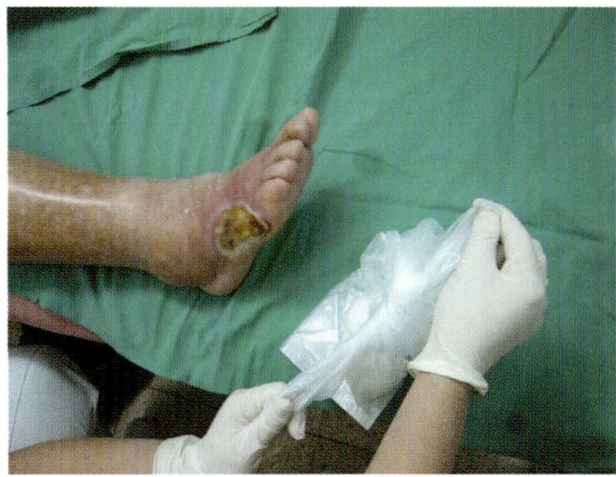

Fig. 21.2. A plastic bag is used for disposal of the dressing materials removed from the ulcer

References

1. Larson E: APIC guideline for hand washing and hand antisepsis in health-care settings. Am J Infect Control 1995; 23:251–269
2. Hugonnet S, Pittet D: Hand hygiene revisited: Lessons from the past and present. Curr Infect Dis Rep 2000; 2:484–489
3. Teare L, Cookson B, Stone S: Hand hygiene. Use alcohol hand rub between patients: they reduce transmission of infection. Br Med J 2001; 323:411–412
4. Shai A, Bilenko N, Ben-Zeev R, et al: Use of infection control procedures in an out-patient clinic for leg ulcers and the rate of contamination with methicillin-resistant Staphylococcus aureus. Wounds 2004; 16: 193–200
5. Zaidi M, Wenzel RP: Disinfection, sterilization, and control of hospital waste. In: Mandell GL, Bennett JE, Dolin R (eds) Mandell, Douglas and Bennett's Principles and Practice of Infective Diseases, 5th edn. Philadelphia: Churchill Livingstone. 2000; pp 2995–3005

Subject Index